D1608265

SPINAL CORD INJURY

Medical Management and Rehabilitation

THE REHABILITATION INSTITUTE OF CHICAGO
PUBLICATION SERIES

Don A. Olson, PhD, Series Coordinator

Spinal Cord Injury: A Guide to Functional
Outcomes in Physical Therapy Management

Lower Extremity Amputation: A Guide to Functional
Outcomes in Physical Therapy Management, Second Edition

Stroke/Head Injury: A Guide to Functional
Outcomes in Physical Therapy Management

Clinical Management of Right Hemisphere Dysfunction

Clinical Evaluation of Dysphasia

Spinal Cord Injury: A Guide to Functional
Outcomes in Occupational Therapy

Spinal Cord Injury: A Guide to Rehabilitation Nursing

Head Injury: A Guide to Functional Outcomes in
Occupational Therapy Management

Speech/Language Treatment of the Aphasias: Treatment Materials
for Auditory Comprehension and Reading Comprehension

Speech/Language Treatment of the Aphasias: Treatment Materials
for Oral Expression and Written Expression

Rehabilitation Nursing Procedures Manual

Psychological Management of Traumatic Brain Injuries
in Children and Adolescents

Medical Management of Long-Term Disability

Psychological Aspects of Geriatric Rehabilitation

Clinical Management of Dysphagia in Adults and Children,
Second Edition

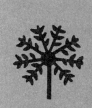

Rehabilitation
Institute of
Chicago
PROCEDURE
MANUAL

SPINAL
CORD
INJURY

Medical Management and Rehabilitation

Edited by

Gary M. Yarkony, MD
Spinal Cord Injury Rehabilitation Program
Rehabilitation Institute of Chicago
Associate Professor of Physical Medicine
and Rehabilitation
Northwestern University Medical School
Adjunct Associate Professor
Pritzker Institute of Medical Engineering
Illinois Institute of Technology
Chicago, Illinois

AN ASPEN PUBLICATION®
Aspen Publishers, Inc.
Gaithersburg, Maryland
1994

Library of Congress Cataloging-in-Publication Data

Spinal cord injury : medical management and rehabilitation / edited by
Gary M. Yarkony.
p.   cm. — (Rehabilitation Institute of Chicago procedure
manual) (Rehabilitation Institute of Chicago publication series)
"An Aspen publication."
Includes bibliographical references and index.
ISBN 0-8342-0553-X
1. Spinal cord—Wounds and injuries—Patients—Rehabilitation.
2. Spinal cord—Wounds and injuries—Treatment. I. Yarkony, Gary
M. II. Series. III. Series: Rehabilitation Institute of Chicago
publication series.
RD594.3.S6654   1994
617.4′82044—dc20
94-14208
CIP

Aspen Publishers, Inc., grants permission for photocopying for limited personal or internal use. This consent does not extend to other kinds of copying, such as copying for general distribution, for advertising or promotional purposes, for creating new collective works, or for resale. For information, address Aspen Publishers, Inc., Permissions Department, 200 Orchard Ridge Drive, Suite 200, Gaithersburg, Maryland 20878.

The authors have made every effort to ensure the accuracy of the information herein. However, appropriate information sources should be consulted, especially for new or unfamiliar procedures. It is the responsibility of every practitioner to evaluate the appropriateness of a particular opinion in the context of actual clinical situations and with due consideration to new developments. Authors, editors, and the publisher cannot be held responsible for any typographical or other errors found in this book.

Editorial Resources: Ruth Bloom

Library of Congress Catalog Card Number: 94-14208
ISBN: 0-8342-0553-X

Printed in the United States of America

1 2 3 4 5

Table of Contents

EDITOR

Gary M. Yarkony, MD
Spinal Cord Injury Rehabilitation Program
Rehabilitation Institute of Chicago
Associate Professor of Physical Medicine
    and Rehabilitation
Northwestern University Medical School
Adjunct Associate Professor
Pritzker Institute of Medical Engineering
Illinois Institute of Technology
Chicago, Illinois

CONTRIBUTORS

David Chen, MD
Associate Director, Spinal Cord Injury Program
Rehabilitation Institute of Chicago
Assistant Professor of Physical Medicine and
    Rehabilitation
Northwestern University Medical School
Chicago, Illinois

Frederick S. Frost, MD
Assistant Professor of Medicine (Rehabilitation)
Case Western Reserve University Medical School
Chief, Spinal Cord Injury Rehabilitation
MetroHealth Medical Center
Cleveland, Ohio

Judy Hill, OTR/L
Director of Occupational Therapy
Rehabilitation Institute of Chicago
Chicago, Illinois

Susan S. Holstein, MS, MEd, PhD
Psychologist in private practice
Geneva, Illinois

Robert Harold Jackson, BA, CIRS
President
Robert H. Jackson & Associates, Inc.
Oak Brook, Illinois

Robert Jaeger, PhD
Associate Professor of Medical Engineering
Illinois Institute of Technology
Adjunct Associate Professor of Physical
    Medicine and Rehabilitation
Northwestern University Medical School
Chicago, Illinois

Richard T. Katz, MD
Associate Professor
St. Louis University
Medical Director
SSM Rehabilitation Institute
St. Louis, Missouri

Mary Elizabeth Keen, MD, MRM
Clinical Assistant Professor
Departments of Pediatrics and Orthopedic
    Surgery
Loyola University Medical School
Maywood, Illinois
Director of Pediatric Programs
Marianjoy Rehabilitation Hospital and Clinics
Wheaton, Illinois

Kirsten M. Kohlmeyer, MS, OTR/L
Clinical Specialist
Rehabilitation Institute of Chicago
Chicago, Illinois

Alojz Kralj, Dipl Eng, MSc, DSc
Professor
Biomedical Engineering and Robotics
Head
Laboratory for Biomedical Engineering and
    Laboratory for Robotics
University of Ljubljana
Ljubljana, Slovenia

Richard B. Lazar, MD
Executive Vice President and Medical Director
Schwab Rehabilitation Hospital and Care
    Network
and
Northwestern University Medical School
Chicago, Illinois

Victor L. Lewis, Jr, MD
Associate Professor of Clinical Surgery
Northwestern University Medical School
Chicago, Illinois

Thomas H. McPike, MS
Supervisor
Therapeutic Recreation
Chicago Park District
Professor, Department of Health and Physical
    Education
Chicago State University
Certified Therapeutic Recreation Specialist
Chicago, Illinois

Jeri Morris, PhD
Assistant Professor
Department of Psychiatry and Behavioral Sciences
and
Department of Rehabilitation Medicine
Northwestern University Medical School
Chicago, Illinois

John B. Nanninga, MD
Associate Professor of Urology
Northwestern University Medical School
Consultant in Urology
Rehabilitation Institute of Chicago
Chicago, Illinois

Don A. Olson, PhD
Director, Education and Training Center
Rehabilitation Institute of Chicago
and
Associate Professor
Departments of Physical Medicine and
    Rehabilitation and Neurology
Northwestern University Medical School
Chicago, Illinois

Christi Rom, OTR/L
Clinical Specialist/Driving Program Manager
Rehabilitation Institute of Chicago
Chicago, Illinois

Elliot J. Roth, MD
Director
Center for Stroke Rehabilitation
Rehabilitation Institute of Chicago
Associate Professor
Department of Physical Medicine and
    Rehabilitation
Northwestern University Medical School
Chicago, Illinois

Sue Stevens, PT
Senior Physical Therapist
Rehabilitation Institute of Chicago
Chicago, Illinois

Jennifer Ueberfluss, PT
Senior Physical Therapist
Rehabilitation Institute of Chicago
Chicago, Illinois

Brian C. Walker, MS, JD
Attorney at Law
Hoey and Farina
Chicago, Illinois

Yeongchi Wu, MD
Associate Professor of Physical Medicine and
    Rehabilitation
Northwestern University Medical School
Chicago, Illinois

Linda Yasukawa, PT
Clinical Supervisor
Department of Physical Therapy
Rehabilitation Institute of Chicago
Chicago, Illinois

Series Foreword

The patient benefits most when the health care team understands the role, the abilities, and the shared knowledge of each member of the team involved with that patient. This book presents the information needed by the spinal cord injury team that works to maximize the outcome potential of the individual with spinal cord injury. Although the philosophy of care is primarily that of the Rehabilitation Institute of Chicago's (RIC's) programs, it also includes input ideas and approaches to care of individuals with spinal cord injury from other facilities, former patients, and other health care workers of RIC.

The book is written for use by physicians, nurses, allied health workers, the rehabilitation spinal cord team, the family, and the individual with spinal cord injury. Medical, psychological, allied health, social, vocational, and recreational aspects of the impact of spinal cord injury are presented for the reader to appreciate the range of information needed to maximize the quality of life and ensure community reintegration and the empowerment of the individual with spinal cord injury.

Although the number of spinal cord injury cases annually has been reduced from a once high of 12,000 to 14,000 in the 1970s to approximately 8,000 new spinal cord injuries currently, the severity of the problem makes it one of the most challenging rehabilitation problems facing the health care worker. This book attempts to stimulate the reader to use this material as a reference point and a basis for planning his or her unique and innovative approach to the management of the individual with spinal cord injury.

—Don A. Olson, PhD
Series Editor
and
Director, Education and Training Center
Rehabilitation Institute of Chicago
and
Associate Professor
Departments of Physical Medicine and
Rehabilitation and Neurology
Northwestern University Medical School
Chicago, Illinois

Foreword

Dr. Yarkony and his colleagues have brought us a valuable reference book for the management of the spinal cord injured person. This book is useful for educating health care professionals and, by extension, patients who have experienced a spinal cord injury. Physicians, resident physicians, nurses, and allied health professionals and other professionals associated with this unique and challenging population will enjoy having this text in their library.

Although it is popularly felt that the number of spinal cord injury each year has recently been reduced, the impact of this devastating injury to the individual remains one of the most interesting and challenging in the rehabilitation field. The experience of Dr. Yarkony and his colleagues, with the federally funded spinal cord injury centers and the program of the Rehabilitation Institute of Chicago, are revealed in the comprehensive approach to this problem as presented in this text. The need for a holistic approach including shared knowledge with professionals in prevention, acute care, rehabilitation care, vocational rehabilitation, and community issues is the overriding format of the book.

In this text, the early chapters deal primarily with the medical complications associated with spinal cord injury. The clarification of terminologies assists the health care professionals in using common words and explanations so that as a team, they can better serve the individual with spinal cord injury. Specific medical complications of spinal cord injury are presented as well as detailed descriptions on unique problems such as gastrointestinal dysfunction, neurogenic bladder, and management of the ventilator-dependent quadriplegic person. Also, the psychosocial aspects are handled in this section, and a helpful psychotherapy treatment philosophy is presented.

The last half of the book deals with functional aspects of rehabilitation for the spinal cord injured person. These chapters include the current status on functional electrical stimulation, driver assessment, vocational rehabilitation implications, and a detailed chapter on home modification of the physically challenged spinal cord injured person.

The text aims to be as complete as possible and is written with clarity. Although it strongly sets forth the management of the spinal cord injured person as carried out at the Rehabilitation Institute of Chicago, it succeeds in giving a complete state-of-the-art review of the management of the spinal cord injured individual. The text could readily become the standard medical, allied health, rehabilitation, and nursing reference text for spinal cord injury rehabilitation.

D.A.O.

Chapter 1

Overview of Spinal Cord Injury Rehabilitation in the Acute Phase, the Rehabilitation Team, and Classification of Spinal Cord Lesion

Gary M. Yarkony

Spinal cord injury can be one of the most devastating calamities in human life both for the patient and his or her family and friends (Guttmann 1976). Rehabilitation after a spinal cord injury seeks the fullest physical and psychological adjustment of individuals to their disability with a goal of reintegration into society.

History shows that this view of spinal cord injuries was not held until this century. The Edwin Smith Surgical Papyrus indicates that the ancient Egyptians did not consider it possible to treat a spinal cord injury. Until the 20th century, those sustaining a spinal cord injury died shortly afterward. President Garfield died shortly after a gunshot wound to the conus medullaris. In spite of Garfield's being treated by the U.S. Surgeon General, the nature of the injury to his spinal cord was unrecognized; he succumbed to the gunshot wound 79 days later. World War I saw no improvement in spinal cord care. The majority of patients with spinal cord injury died within a few weeks, and the small percentage who made it back to the United States died within a year. After surviving the rigors of World War II, General George S. Patton, Jr. died in 1945 within 2 weeks of sustaining a spinal cord injury in an automobile accident.

With the advent of comprehensive treatment centers, the chances for survival for patients with spinal cord injury improved, and rehabilitation methods advanced. The first centers were developed in the United States in the 1930s by Munro and in England in the 1940s by Guttmann. These centers strove to provide a coordinated system of care to enhance survival, decrease secondary complications, and provide life-long follow-up treatment. A comprehensive rehabilitation program that provides a full range of services and maximum patient participation improves the chances for favorable outcomes, promotes the resumption of a meaningful life, and facilitates opportunities for community reintegration (Yarkony et al. 1987).

The foundation of a comprehensive rehabilitation program is an interdisciplinary team functioning in an appropriate facility (Fordyce 1981). It is essential that an appropriate skill level be maintained by all staff members to provide the varied and comprehensive services required by individuals with spinal cord injury. The staff must be willing to work together while breaking down the boundaries of individual disciplines for the betterment of those they serve. Collaboration, not isolation, is the key to enhanced rehabilitation success.

Spinal cord injury remains relatively uncommon: There are approximately 10,000 injuries each year in the United States (Anderson & McLaurin 1980) and an estimated 250,000 persons with spinal cord injuries living in the United States (Stover & Fine 1986). The average age of those injured is 19.7 years (median, 25.0 years), with most injuries occurring in the 16- to 30-year range. Motor vehicle accidents are the most common cause (47.7%), followed by falls (20.8%), acts of violence (14.6%), and sporting injuries (14.2%). The majority of sporting injuries are diving accidents. The typical individual with spinal cord injury is a white (73.9%) male (82.0%), although there is a greater proportion of nonwhites sustaining spinal cord injuries than in the general population. The leading cause of spinal cord injury in the white population is motor vehicle accidents; among nonwhites, acts of violence are the leading cause. Etiology varies by age as well. Motor vehicle accidents are the leading cause below age 45, and falls are the leading cause above age 45. Spinal cord injuries most commonly occur in July, and Saturday is the most common day. Alcohol or substance abuse plays a major role in these accidents.

Approximately half of all spinal cord injuries are cervical and one third are thoracic. The most frequently occurring neurologic level of injury is the fifth cervical segment, with the fourth and sixth cervical and twelfth thoracic levels following in frequency. Half of all spinal cord injuries are complete.

Neural recovery can generally be predicted by the initial extent of injury and the time course of functional recovery (Maynard et al. 1979). The majority of complete injuries remain complete upon discharge. Those admitted with sparing of motor function below the level of the injury have a better chance of being discharged with useful motor function compared with those admitted with only sensory sparing. Another guideline to recovery is the clinical course of the patient: The speed of return of motor function and its clinical course are good guidelines. As time progresses with little change, further major recovery outside the zone of injury is unlikely.

REHABILITATION IN THE ACUTE CARE PHASE

The primary objective in the immediate postinjury period is to save the life of the injured person, stabilize the spine to prevent further damage, and decompress the spinal cord if indicated. During this process, it is important to begin certain aspects of the rehabilitation process while realizing that basic life support may prevent attainment of these goals.

Heinemann and associates (1989) have documented the benefits of spinal cord center acute short-term care. In their study, patients treated initially in a spinal cord acute care unit as opposed to a general hospital had shorter acute care lengths of stay (27.5 as opposed to 60.8 days) because general hospitals tend not to be aware of skin issues, which are an important factor. Noncenter patients had a greater incidence of spine instability. Center patients made functional gains with greater efficiency. These results provide and lend support for the concept of spinal cord centers.

Prevention of joint contractures generally is accomplished through range of motion and orthotic management. The flaccid patient may require daily ranging. Because joints may be affected by local trauma or edema, daily range of motion exercises may not be satisfactory. The development of spasticity generally requires additional passive range of motion exercises. These exercises may be necessary two or three times daily, and availability of the therapist may be limited, so that other team members such as nurses may assist in contracture prevention. Involved family members may be of some assis-

tance. Orthotic management is often necessary for the wrists and hands. Resting hand splints or long opponens orthoses may be fabricated. Care should be taken not to overstretch the finger flexors in quadriplegics at the sixth cervical level who will be using tenodesis as part of their daily activities. Equinovarus deformities may be prevented by splinting the ankle in neutral. When orthotic management of the ankle is required, particular attention must be paid to prevention of pressure ulceration of the heels. The shoulder requires particular attention. Keeping the shoulders abducted in some external rotation has been suggested as a means of preventing adhesive capsulitis. Loss of range of motion or a painful shoulder can severely limit progress and prevent goal attainment in rehabilitation. A painful shoulder often is due to impingement and the deltoid being under more strain than the rotator cuff. Studies of contractures in individuals with spinal cord injury have shown a decreased incidence when care is given initially in a specialized spinal cord injury acute care unit (Yarkony et al. 1985). Contractures develop most commonly in the hips, knees, and ankles.

Pressure ulceration of the skin is prevented by skin inspection, positioning, and frequent turning. Initially the patient is turned every 2 hours. Skin is to be clean and dry. Transfers should be performed carefully to avoid shearing forces, which can significantly decrease the amount of pressure needed to cause skin ulceration. Although designed to prevent skin ulceration, the Rotorest bed may actually be a contributing factor if the bed is stopped frequently when care is provided or if the pelvis is allowed to slide to and fro during turning. Sacral and heel sores are the areas most commonly affected by pressure ulceration during the acute care phase. The head can be protected by orthotic devices that elevate it off the bed completely to prevent pressure ulcers.

There are numerous options in urological management during the acute care phase. Fluid and electrolyte balance and careful monitoring of intake and outputs often require use of an indwelling catheter. Intermittent catheterization should be considered if catheterization can be performed regularly and volumes can be maintained at less than 450 mL. Generally this requires catheterization every 4 hours. An indwelling catheter is more appropriate than a poorly managed intermittent catheterization program. Early intermittent catheterization (Lloyd et al. 1986) does not produce any long-term advantages to patients with spinal cord injury in terms of urinary infection rates, upper tract pathological abnormalities, or ultimate bladder drainage method. Use of an indwelling catheter for more than 3 months increases the risks of urethral complications; these can be decreased by suprapubic cystotomy.

Concurrent brain and spinal cord injury may require early medical intervention and behavioral therapy. This may affect the patient's ability to cooperate with the program initially and may require alternative teaching methods and the involvement of the neuropsychologist and/or speech pathologist and occupational therapist to teach strategies for structuring the patient's environment.

THE REHABILITATION TEAM

Collaboration by an interdisciplinary team is the key to successful spinal injury rehabilitation (Fordyce 1981). Each team member must be aware of the others' skills and areas of knowledge so that joint solutions can be reached. Wheelchair seating and community reentry are examples of two areas where collaboration is essential. A physician coordinates the rehabilitation team, attempting to prevent and, if necessary, treating medical complications that may occur as a result of the spinal cord injury. Care is provided on a lifelong basis. The physician should have specialized training in spinal cord injury and dedicate the majority of his or her practice to the care of individuals with spinal cord injury. This physician, who is generally a physiatrist, may work with consultants in orthopedic surgery, neurosurgery, plastic surgery, psychiatry, urology, and internal medicine. The spinal cord injury specialist coordinates all care with the patient's input and consent.

The rehabilitation nurse or nurse therapist (Matthews & Carlson 1987) provides numerous services in addition to basic nursing care. Nurses collaborate with the physician in the management of both skin lesions and the neurogenic bladder and bowel. Teaching the patient and family both practical and preventive aspects of the secondary complications of spinal cord injury is a major role of the nurse therapist. This includes techniques of bowel and bladder management, skin care, and the actions and side effects of medications. Complications such as autonomic dysreflexia, deep venous thrombosis, pulmonary embolism, and urinary tract complications must be recognized by the patient and caregiver and prevented. The nurse works closely with the therapists to ensure that skills learned in therapy are carried over to the nursing unit.

The physical therapist's primary role (Bromley 1981; Nixon 1985) is enhancement of mobility skills, which often entails the provision of assistive devices. Basic skills such as balance, sitting, and turning in bed are taught initially. With time more complex tasks are learned, such as wheelchair use, transfers, and, for some patients, gait training. The physical therapist is involved in the prescription of equipment such as wheelchairs and shower equipment. Physical therapists also are involved in respiratory function, especially in the quadriplegic, as well as in wheelchair prescription, seating, and cardiopulmonary endurance.

Occupational therapy (Hill 1986) stresses activities of daily living such as grooming, bathing, dressing, feeding, writing, homemaking, driving, and sexual functioning. Orthotic management is an important component of these activities. Splints may be fabricated to maintain range of motion, or they may be dynamic devices for grasping objects. Training in the use of environmental controls allows for increased independence,

particularly at high levels of injury. Nursing and occupational therapy often collaborate in adaptive techniques for the individual, such as catheterization or bowel management. Occupational therapists also are involved in vocational rehabilitation, work-site evaluations, and vocational activities.

The rehabilitation engineer provides varied services for individuals with spinal cord injuries. The design and modification of wheelchair seating systems may help improve posture, prevent pressure ulcers, and increase function. Systems for communication, environmental controls, and electric wheelchairs may be modified by engineers to enable persons with various levels of injury to benefit from their use. They may assist in the design of modifications for the home to overcome architectural barriers.

Vocational rehabilitation seeks to assist the patient's return to work or school. This may involve former employers or representatives of various state agencies. The goal may be to return the individual to school, a former job, or a new career.

The social worker assists the patient and team throughout the rehabilitation stay, coordinates discharge planning, and plays a big role in assisting the patient in setting up finances. When psychosocial problems arise, close coordination with the psychologist may be required. The social worker coordinates the team and family members and may do some counseling.

The clinical psychologist provides counseling services to the patient and family members (Trieschmann 1976). Because adaptation to a spinal cord injury is rarely without difficulty, these services are provided to all patients. Neuropsychological testing may be needed to assess concurrent brain injury or for vocational purposes and driving. The psychologist works with team members to improve interactions with patients who are having difficulties adapting to their injuries or the rehabilitation unit and those with behavioral problems.

Speech pathology and audiology services are provided to patients with feeding problems and speech and language problems secondary to brain injury. Swallowing problems may result from the position of the head and neck in a halo vest, from local trauma as a result of postoperative complications, or from traumatic brain injury. Nonverbal communication of the patient on a ventilator may require augmentation.

Therapeutic recreation encourages socialization and provides for new or adapted recreational activities after injury while supplementing the skills taught by other team members. Recreation activities may occur in the patients' rooms, on the nursing unit, in special recreation areas, or in the community as their medical condition allows. The recreation therapist collaborates with the planning and implementation of community reentry programs with the other disciplines. Wheelchair sports are often a major component of the therapeutic recreation programs for those with spinal cord injury.

Driver education requires close collaboration with the occupational therapist to determine upper extremity functional abilities for driving and transfer skills to obtain an adequate seating system.

Other team members include the chaplain, the dietitian, state agencies such as the department of rehabilitation services, the third party payer, and the patient and family. Case managers and insurers should be informed of progress in therapy, the team goals, and equipment needs. Collaboration with these representatives leads to better communication and improved patient outcomes.

NEUROLOGICAL CLASSIFICATION

The American Spinal Injury Association (ASIA, 1992) has developed guidelines to classify the level and extent of a spinal cord injury. Guidelines such as these allow for improved communication in clinical care and research. The discussion that follows is based on ASIA guidelines.

Spinal cord injury refers to injury within the neural canal from the foramen magnum to and including the cauda equina. Injuries to the brachial plexus or lumbar plexus are excluded. Damage to neural elements within the cervical area of the spinal cord results in quadriplegia and various degrees of motor and sensory impairment in the arms, trunk, legs, bowel, and

bladder. Damage to the thoracic, lumbar, or sacral segments, including the conus medullaris or cauda equina, results in paraplegia. There is a variable degree of loss of motor and sensory function in the trunk, legs, bowel, and bladder. The arms are spared in paraplegia.

The neurological level of injury is determined by the motor and sensory examination to determine the most caudal normal segments. There are key muscle groups to determine the level of most segments. As a result of overlap of innervation of these muscles from more than one segment, fair (antigravity) strength is considered sufficient to classify the muscle as normal if the segments above have good to normal strength. The key muscles for C-5 lesions are the elbow flexors (biceps and brachialis); for C-6, the wrist extensors (extensor carpi radialis longus and brevis); for C-7, the elbow extensors (triceps); for C-8, the finger flexors (flexor digitorum profundus) to the middle finger; and for T-1, the small finger abductors (abductor digiti minimi). The diaphragm is used for C-4. The key muscle groups in the lower extremity for L-2 are the hip flexors (iliopsoas); for L-3, the knee extensors (quadriceps); for L-4, the ankle dorsiflexors (tibialis anterior); for L-5, the long toe extensors (extensor hallucis longus); and for S-1, the ankle plantar flexors (gastrocnemius and soleus).

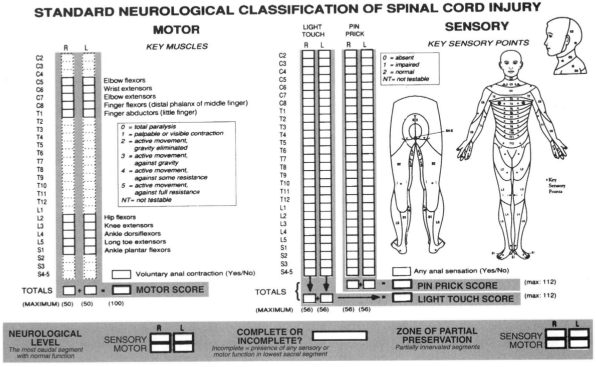

Figure 1–1 Standard neurological classification of spinal cord injury.

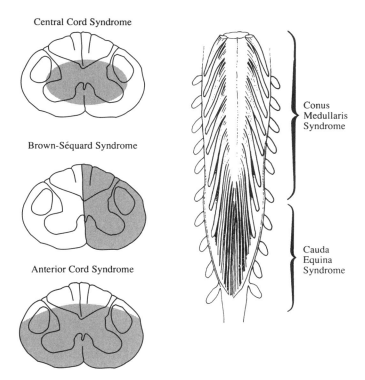

Central Cord Syndrome

Brown-Séquard Syndrome

Anterior Cord Syndrome

Conus Medullaris Syndrome

Cauda Equina Syndrome

Figure 1–2 Spinal cord injury syndromes.

The sensory examination determines the level above C-4, from T-2 through L-1 and from S-2 through S-5. Because the sensory level may not correspond to the motor level, the sensory level is determined by using the dermatome chart (Figure 1–1). A motor and sensory level is recorded for each side. The dermatome chart indicates by a black dot the key areas to test for each dermatome. Examples are the xiphoid for T-6, the umbilicus for T-10 and the occipital protuberance for C-2.

An injury may be classified as complete or incomplete. A complete injury is defined as the absence of sensory and motor function in the lowest sacral segment. An incomplete injury is defined as the presence of sensory and/or motor functions be-

low the neurological level of injury and must include the lowest sacral segments. Sensation can be present at the anal mucocutaneous junction or deep in the anus. Motor function is considered incomplete if sensation is absent but there is voluntary contraction of the external anal sphincter upon digital examination.

The Frankel classification (ASIA 1992; Frankel et al. 1969) has been replaced by the ASIA Impairment Scale and is similar to it. An ASIA Impairment Scale classification A indicates a complete lesion: There is no motor or sensory function preserved in the sacral segments S4–5. ASIA scale B is an incomplete lesion in which only sensation is present below the neurological level, including the sacral segments S4–5. ASIA scale C indicates an incomplete lesion with motor function below the neurological level and the majority of muscles having a grade less than 3. ASIA scale D is an incomplete lesion with motor function preserved below the neurological level and the majority of key muscles below the level having a muscle grade of 3 or greater. ASIA scale E indicates that motor and sensory function is normal.

The Functional Independent Measure is now recommended as a means of assessing activities of daily living. The reader is referred to the 1992 edition of *Standards for Neurological and Functional Classification of Spinal Cord Injury* (ASIA 1992).

Injuries to the spinal cord may result in commonly recognized syndromes if the damage is confined to limited areas of the cord (Figure 1–2). Brown-Séquard syndrome results in paralysis with loss of posterior column sensory function on the same side as the lesion and a contralateral loss of pain and temperature sensation. The central cord syndrome (Roth et al. 1990) is caused by damage to the central area of the cervical spinal cord and results in greater weakness in the arms than the legs. These individuals may ambulate but have partial or complete upper extremity paralysis. The anterior cord syndrome spares the posterior columns but results in paralysis and loss of pain and temperature sensation. Injuries to the conus medullaris generally result in lower limb paralysis with an areflexic bowel and bladder; injuries to the cauda equina may be more asymmetric.

REFERENCES

American Spinal Injury Association (ASIA). 1992. *Standards for neurological and functional classification of spinal cord injury.* Chicago, Ill.: ASIA.

Anderson, D.W., and R.L. McLaurin. 1980. The national head and spinal cord injury survey. *J. Neurosurg.* 53:S1–S43.

Bromley, I. 1981. *Tetraplegia and paraplegia: A guide for physiotherapists.* 2d ed. New York, N.Y.: Churchill Livingstone.

Fordyce, W.E. 1981. On interdisciplinary peers. *Arch. Phys. Med. Rehabil.* 62:51–53.

Frankel, H., et al. 1969. The value of postural reduction in the initial management of closed injuries to the spine with paraplegia and tetraplegia. *Paraplegia* 7:179–192.

Guttmann, L. 1976. *Spinal cord injuries comprehensive and management research.* 2d ed. Boston, Mass.: Blackwell Scientific.

Heinemann, A.W., et al. 1989. Functional outcome following spinal cord injury: A comparison of specialized spinal cord injury center vs. general hospital short-term care. *Arch. Neurol.* 46:1098–1102.

Hill, J.P. 1986. *Spinal cord injury: A guide to functional outcomes in occupational therapy.* Gaithersburg, Md.: Aspen.

Lloyd, L.K., et al. 1986. Initial bladder management in spinal cord injury: Does it make a difference? *J. Urol.* 135:523–527.

Matthews, P.J., and C.E. Carlson. 1987. *Spinal cord injury: A guide to rehabilitation nursing.* Gaithersburg, Md.: Aspen.

Maynard, F.M., et al. 1979. Neurological prognosis after traumatic quadriplegia. *J. Neurosurg.* 50:611–616.

Nixon, V. 1985. *Spinal cord injury: A guide to functional outcomes in physical therapy management.* Gaithersburg, Md.: Aspen.

Roth, E.J., et al. 1990. Traumatic central cord syndrome: Clinical features and functional outcomes. *Arch. Phys. Med. Rehabil.* 71:18–23.

Stover, S.L., and P.R. Fine. 1986. *Spinal cord injury: The facts and figures.* Birmingham, Ala.: University of Alabama.

Trieschmann, R.B., ed. 1976. *Spinal cord injuries: Psychological, social and vocational adjustment.* Elmsford, N.Y.: Pergamon.

Yarkony, G.M., et al. 1985. Contractures complicating spinal cord injury: Incidence and comparison between spinal cord center and general hospital acute care. *Paraplegia* 23:265–271.

Yarkony, G.M., et al. 1987. Benefits of rehabilitation for traumatic spinal cord injury: Multivariate analysis in 711 patients. *Arch. Neurol.* 44:93–96.

Chapter 2

Functional Outcome after Spinal Cord Injury Rehabilitation

Kirsten M. Kohlmeyer and Gary M. Yarkony

Patients with spinal cord injury generally are admitted to the rehabilitation facility when they are medically stable. The spinal column must be stabilized so that the individual can participate fully in the rehabilitation program. Any precautions or restrictions due to spinal orthoses or associated injuries should be communicated to all team members.

The majority of persons with spinal cord injury benefit from admission to a spinal cord injury rehabilitation unit, particularly those individuals who functioned independently before their injury. The clinical course of older individuals before admission to the rehabilitation center is often subject to more medical complications, such as pneumonia, deep venous thrombosis, and urinary tract infection; once stabilized, however, older persons generally will do as well functionally as their younger counterparts. Complex transfers and activities of daily living such as dressing may pose a problem for older individuals, particularly complete paraplegics (Yarkony et al. 1988a). For quadriplegics and incomplete paraplegics, the major limiting factor appears to be motor function, not age.

Concurrent brain injury (Davidoff et al. 1985), often seen with spinal cord injury, necessitates expertise in dealing with both these impairment issues. Special nursing needs of individuals with spinal cord injury often prohibit their admission to a brain trauma unit.

The unit should foster an environment that encourages peer interaction. Individuals with spinal cord injury gain from the experience of other current patients at various points in their rehabilitation stay as well as from peer visitors. Individuals readmitted for training in more advanced skills or for compli-

cations such as pressure ulcers help newly injured individuals better grasp potential future needs. This may occur informally through interactions on the unit or via scheduled group sessions.

Prediction of functional abilities after a spinal cord injury generally follows the degree of motor function (Bergstrom et al. 1985; Douglas et al. 1983; Woolsey 1985; Yarkony et al. 1987). Individuals will benefit from rehabilitation at all levels of injury. If a particular skill cannot be performed by the individual, he or she should be taught to direct others in its performance. An educational program for individuals with spinal cord injury and their family, friends, and caregivers is an essential component of the rehabilitation program. Everyone involved in the care of the individual must be trained to prevent and recognize the physical and medical complications that can occur. Skills learned in the rehabilitation setting must be generalized to the home environment and community before discharge to optimize the chances for successful postdischarge reintegration into society. Therapeutic weekend passes and community activities conducted during the rehabilitation stay are two means of accomplishing this. Skills learned in the protected environment of the spinal cord unit often require modification after discharge because of environmental barriers. Both paraplegics and quadriplegics maintain the skills learned in rehabilitation for at least 3 years after their discharge (Yarkony et al. 1988b).

A description of functional outcomes and equipment considerations by motor level follows. Although there is an interplay of numerous psychological and physical factors, motor function is the primary determinant of functional outcomes (Long & Lawton 1955; Yarkony et al. 1987).

These are general guidelines, not an exhaustive description of all possible functional outcomes and equipment needs. It is essential that the rehabilitation program address the needs and goals of the individual. Patients who are motivated may achieve goals expected for individuals with greater motor function if given the opportunity. The injured individual should be given the opportunity to attempt any task with proper guidance for safety to facilitate understanding of physical abilities and limitations. The actual attempts, as opposed to staff explanations, usually reduce conflict.

C1–4 QUADRIPLEGIA

Rehabilitation of high quadriplegics requires sophisticated electronic equipment and a staff trained in dealing with the potential pulmonary complications. Patients with lesions at C-1 and C-2 may have sparing of the phrenic nerve and be managed with implanted phrenic nerve pacemakers (Lee et al. 1989). Pacing of the diaphragms may be simultaneous or alternating. These patients benefit from a lesser need for equipment than ventilator-dependent patients and are often easier to manage and discharge from the rehabilitation environment. They may also have their tracheostomies plugged or discontinued if secretions are not a problem. Patients with lesions above C-4 who are ventilator dependent participate in similar rehabilitation programs as those with phrenic nerve pacemakers, although the equipment, respiratory circuitry, and tracheostomy often interfere with communication and lead to greater discharge challenges. Patients at the C-4 level will often be free of respiratory equipment beyond the initial acute care stage but still have the same functional equipment needs as ventilator-dependent injuries.

A major component of rehabilitation with these individuals is the use of technical aids, such as environmental controls (Hill 1986). Cooperation between an occupational therapist and a rehabilitation engineer often is necessary to modify commercially available equipment for the individual patient. Equipment that may be necessary includes an emergency call system, a computer, a speaker telephone, an electric page turner, an automatic door opener, and environmental control units (ECUs). ECUs may access these devices, or these devices may be prescribed individually.

ECUs may be simple or complex. Access options include breath control (sip and puff, from bed or wheelchair), mouthstick, or tread switch. Simple systems that are commercially available often require hand function. Voice-activated systems have become available as their price has diminished, but they still are prescribed less frequently. Furthermore, development of cost-efficient and commercially available robotics may facilitate return to work for a greater number of high quadriplegics and increased independence at home. Robotic

systems are now beginning to enter the marketplace. Many typewriters and computers now can be controlled with eye blink.

Power wheelchairs are essential at these levels of injury (Nixon 1985). They may be operated by breath control, chin control, head control, voice-activation, or hand control in patients with spared function. These chairs may be reclined by head-, chin-, or eyebrow-activated switches to perform pressure reliefs. A manual wheelchair will be necessary in addition to the power wheelchair, which may not be accessible to all environments, is not easily transportable, and may be in need of charging and repair. Lifts such as the Hoyer or Transaid may be necessary for transfers because patients are dependent at this level (see Chapter 17).

C-5 QUADRIPLEGIA

Individuals at the C-5 level have functional deltoid and/or biceps musculature. The presence of functional biceps and appropriate splinting often allow for significant improvements in activities of daily living (Yarkony et al. 1988c). These individuals may initially require use of a balanced forearm orthosis for enhanced arm placement during activities such as feeding and typing (Figure 2–1). This device is particularly useful for patients with partial C-4 lesions with inadequate elbow flexors. A long opponens orthosis with utensil slots and pen holders provides wrist stability to allow these individuals to perform activities such as feeding, writing, and typing. Other less commonly used devices include cable-driven, electrically powered, or ratchet orthosis that provide tenodesis,

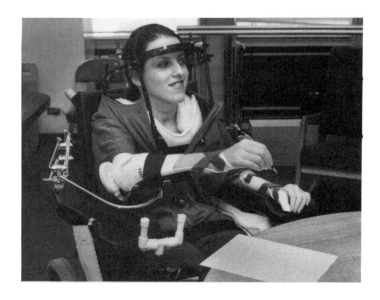

Figure 2–1 Quadriplegic using a balanced forearm orthosis.

similar to those used by C-6 quadriplegics. With assistive devices and set-up, most C-5 quadriplegics should be able to feed themselves, perform oral facial hygiene, participate in tabletop communication and leisure activities, and assist with upper extremity dressing.

Power wheelchair propulsion may be performed with a hand control. A manual wheelchair with oblique hand-rim projections may be propelled indoors on smooth surfaces and occasionally on uneven surfaces for short distances.

C-6 QUADRIPLEGIA

Active wrist extension and the presence of the C-6 component in the proximal musculature enhance functional independence (Yarkony et al. 1988d). Wrist extensor recovery is common in C-6 quadriplegics, although its return can be delayed. Tenodesis, opposition of the thumb to the index finger, and finger flexion with wrist extension, are used for functional activities. The Rehabilitation Institute of Chicago tenodesis orthosis (Figure 2–2) is fabricated easily for tenodesis training during the early phases of recovery. Some patients are provided with a wrist-driven flexor hinge orthosis (Figure 2–3) to perform tasks requiring increased pinch strength, such as catheterization and work skills. Because of poor follow-through and high cost and maintenance issues, these devices are not often used after discharge. Patients at this level often use short opponens orthosis with utensil slots, writing splints with simple D-ring Velcro handles, and cuffs to assist in performing feeding, writing, and oral facial hygiene. C-6 quadriplegics usually feed themselves when food is served and cut, perform their oral and facial hygiene and upper extremity dressing independently, and assist with or are independent

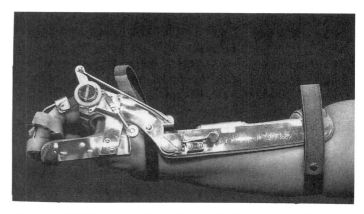

Figure 2–3 Wrist-driven flexor hinge splint (Rancho design).

with lower extremity dressing. They may catheterize themselves and perform their bowel program with assistive devices.

Manual wheelchair propulsion is generally independent on level surfaces but will be limited on rough terrain. Vertical wheelchair projections and coated hand rims may be required in conjunction with wheelchair gloves. Some patients may require power wheelchairs for work and school, where distance and need for speed may be factors. Transfers may be independent or assisted on level surfaces with a sliding board. Driving may be possible with an appropriately equipped van.

C7–8 QUADRIPLEGIA

The addition of functional triceps at C-7 greatly improves transfer and mobility skills. C-7 quadriplegics may also exhibit and benefit from enhanced finger extension and wrist flexion, which enhance grasp strength. Short opponens or tenodesis splints may be used to assist in activities of daily living. Most activities of daily living are independent at this level. Active elbow extension facilitates wheelchair and transfer skills, and wheelchair propulsion is improved on rough terrain and slopes. The Rehabilitation Institute of Chicago has reported a case of a C-7 quadriplegic who was able to walk a short distance with a specially modified walker (Yarkony et al. 1986). Although this is far from the norm, it is an example of the importance of allowing a patient to attempt functional skills far beyond that predicted at a given level of injury.

C-8 quadriplegics have flexor digitorum profundus function. Although hand function is not normal, there is the opportunity for total independence from a wheelchair level. C-8 quadriplegics may be able to balance their wheelchairs on the rear wheels (do "wheelies") and independently transfer their wheelchairs into cars. A van may no longer be necessary for independent transportation. Homemaking tasks are performed more easily or at a greater level of independence.

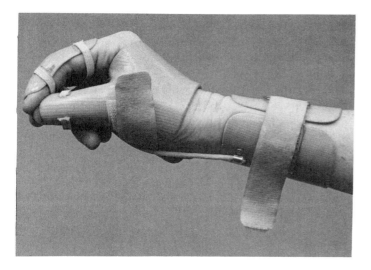

Figure 2–2 The Rehabilitation Institute of Chicago tenodesis orthosis.

THORACIC PARAPLEGIA

The T-1 level is the first level with normal hand function. As thoracic levels proceed caudally, intercostal and abdominal musculature recovery is present, providing for improved respiratory function and trunk balance. Patients at all thoracic levels should be independent from a wheelchair level and should be able to manage their bowel and bladder functions. Variable outcomes at the thoracic level are often described based on various levels of injury within the thoracic spinal cord. Our studies in a large series of thoracic patients show that this is not generally true. Patients at all levels should attempt complex transfers, standing, and ambulation because most descriptions based on thoracic level are artificial (Yarkony et al. 1990).

There are numerous orthotic devices that have been developed for paraplegic ambulation. Figure 2–4 depicts three of these devices. Standard metal upright knee-ankle-foot orthoses (KAFOs) generally have upper and lower thigh bands, drop locks, a calf band, and a single-action (Klenzak) or double-action type ankle joint. A pelvic band and hip joint rarely are added, except for children, because they add increased weight and energy requirements and are not necessary as patients can extend at the hips using the ligaments of the hip

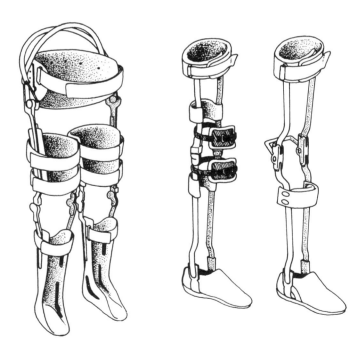

Figure 2–4 Three orthoses commonly used for ambulation in paraplegic persons: left, Louisiana State University reciprocal gait orthosis (RGO); center, knee-ankle-foot orthosis (KAFO); right, Scott Craig orthosis.

to stabilize (American Academy of Orthopaedic Surgeons 1975). The Scott Craig (O'Daniel & Hahn 1981) design, with a bale lock at the knee, a patellar tendon strap, and a rigid ankle support, provides a lighter-weight orthosis. The knee is eccentrically placed, and lower thigh and calf band closures are eliminated. Improved donning and doffing, better standing, and more efficient ambulation result.

There are two recent designs of orthosis that attempt to restore a reciprocating gait pattern. These are the reciprocating gait orthosis (RGO) or Louisiana State University orthosis (Douglas et al. 1983) and the adult hip guidance orthosis (Parawalker or HGO; Patrick & McClelland 1985). The RGO uses the Bowden cable system commonly used in prosthetic devices, which allows alternative hip flexion because the hip is lifted and forces are transferred from the weight-bearing side via extension. Although this system yields a more esthetic gait pattern, RGOs are less efficient than the Scott Craig orthosis and more cumbersome and expensive (Jaeger et al. 1989). The Parawalker combines a pair of rigid leg braces and a rigid pelvic brace articulating with ball-bearing hinges. Hybrid systems with this brace or the RGO and functional neuromuscular stimulation have demonstrated the possibility of ambulation combining these two techniques. The Orlau swivel walker (Seymour et al. 1982) and the pneumatic orthosis (Lehmann et al. 1977; Ragnarsson et al. 1975) are not in common use today. The recently developed Vannini boot sets the ankle in plantarflexion to keep the knee extended. Its utility appears limited.

In spite of the development of several orthotic systems, it is uncommon for paraplegics to ambulate at the community level (Coughlin et al. 1980; Heinemann et al. 1987; Mikelberg & Reid 1981; Natvig & McAdam 1978–79; O'Daniel & Hahn 1981; Rosman & Spira 1974). Rejection rates in these series are as high as 75%. In one series, only 4% of the individuals used their braces more than their wheelchairs. Numerous studies have shown that with the six determinants of gait loss the energy requirement per unit distance is at least six times normal levels (Merkel et al. 1984; Miller et al. 1984). As in other disabilities, gait slows to a more tolerable level. The rejection of KAFOs for functional ambulation is therefore common (Heinemann et al. 1987; Jaeger et al. 1989). Ambulation is not the only reason to prescribe leg braces. Standing for short periods to reach objects at home or work or for short exercise periods during the day is found to be of value. Many paraplegics exercise with their KAFOs in home parallel bars or with a walker or crutches. Brief periods of ambulation may be necessary in environments that are not wheelchair accessible. Many patients report that bowel function improves from periodic standing or walking. Osteoporosis is not improved by passive standing.

There are numerous recommended approaches in dealing with the paraplegic individual who would like to ambulate (Waters & Miller 1987). Although we advise our patients of the difficulties associated with ambulation, the high energy requirements, and the dangers of falling, the decision to attempt ambulation is the patient's. Temporary KAFOs are available, so that custom fitting is not necessary. Patients should not feel they were denied their chance to walk and must discover on their own whether ambulation is feasible. Conjoint goal setting often enhances cooperation and mastery of functional skills at the wheelchair level, especially for those individuals whose only stated goal is to "walk out of here." After learning prerequisite wheelchair skills, gait training is attempted so that individuals can determine independently the feasibility of walking and can focus on realistic rehabilitation goals (Yarkony et al. 1990).

LUMBAR PARAPLEGIA

Most lumbar patients are independent of the wheelchair level, and ambulation is common. Hussey and Stauffer (1973) concluded that community ambulators generally have proprioception at the hips and ankles, good pelvic control, hip flexors, and a functional quadriceps muscle on one side. Lack of hip extension and abduction could be compensated for by canes or crutches and loss of ankle control with ankle foot orthoses. The ambulatory motor index (AMI; Waters et al. 1989), which grades muscles on a 4-point scale (0, absent; 1, trace or poor; 2, fair; 3, good; and 4, normal), may be helpful in determining the potential for community ambulation. The muscle groups graded are hip flexion, hip abduction, hip extension, knee extension, and knee flexion. The percentage of the maximum possible score of 30 is the AMI. Community ambulators that meet Hussey and Stauffer's guidelines have an AMI of 60% or greater. With an AMI of less than 40%, two KAFOs and two crutches are required to ambulate.

Hip flexion is present at the L-2 level, knee extension at L-3, and ankle dorsiflexion at L-4. The L-5 level adds the ex-

tensor hallucis longus, and the S-1 level adds the gastrocnemius and the soleus muscles.

SEATING AND POSITIONING

Proper seating in a wheelchair and in bath equipment is of the utmost importance. Positioning can prevent deformity, decrease pain, prevent tissue damage, upgrade sitting tolerance and balance, enhance respiratory function, enhance functional abilities, and enhance mobility. A team approach among the patient, occupational therapy, physical therapy, rehabilitation engineering, and vendor is essential. Evaluation of the patient's range of motion, tone, sensation, motor function, trunk and pelvic mobility, and activities done in the wheelchair precedes positioning. The pelvis is key, followed by the trunk, head, and upper extremities. Fixed deformities must be accommodated; flexible deformity may be corrected.

The wheelchair cushion distributes pressure, minimizes shear, and provides a stable base of support. No one cushion is ideal for all patients. Ultimately independent, timely, and effective pressure relief must be performed. Our spinal cord injury center commonly prescribes the ROHO or JAY cushion. Considerations in choosing cushions include effect on transfer skills, direct pressure loading on the buttocks, shear forces created with tissue movement, and moisture evaporation.

Determination of the best option(s) for wheelchair mobility depends on positioning needs, safety, and energy-efficient operation. Integration of posture, pressure management, and mobility maximizes function. Interfacing with technology, patient/family education, and periodic reevaluation are also necessary components of seating and positioning. Final considerations include funding, patient preference, and discharge environment (i.e., accessibility, transportation, and maintenance issues).

REFERENCES

American Academy of Orthopaedic Surgeons. 1975. *Atlas of Orthotics.* St. Louis, Mo.: Mosby.

Bergstrom, E.M.K., et al. 1985. Physical ability in relation to anthropometric measurements in persons with complete spinal cord lesion below the sixth cervical segment. *Int. Rehabil. Med.* 7:51–55.

Coughlin, J.K., et al. 1980. Lower extremity bracing in paraplegia—A follow-up study. *Paraplegia* 18:25–32.

Davidoff, G., et al. 1985. Closed head injury in spinal cord injured patients: Retrospective study of the loss of consciousness and post-traumatic amnesia. *Arch. Phys. Med. Rehabil.* 66:41–46.

Douglas, R., et al. 1983. The LSU reciprocation gait orthosis. *Orthopedics* 6:834–839.

Heinemann, A.W., et al. 1987. Mobility for persons with spinal cord injury: An evaluation of two systems. *Arch. Phys. Med. Rehabil.* 68:90–93.

Hill, J.P. 1986. *Spinal cord injury: A guide to functional outcomes in occupational therapy.* Gaithersburg, Md.: Aspen.

Hussey, R.W., and E.S. Stauffer. 1973. Spinal cord injury: Requirements for ambulation. *Arch. Phys. Med. Rehabil.* 50:544–547.

Jaeger, R.J., et al. 1989. Rehabilitation technology for standing and walking after spinal cord injury. *Am. J. Med. Rehabil.* 68:128–133.

Lee, M.Y., et al. 1989. Rehabilitation of quadriplegic patients with phrenic nerve pacers. *Arch. Phys. Med. Rehabil.* 70:549–552.

Lehmann, J.F., et al. 1977. Pneumatic and standard double upright orthoses: Comparison of their biomechanical function in three patients with spinal cord injuries. *Arch. Phys. Med. Rehabil.* 58:72–80.

Long, C., and E.B. Lawton. 1955. Functional significance of spinal cord lesion level. *Arch. Phys. Med. Rehabil.* 36:249–255.

Merkel, K.D., et al. 1984. Energy expenditure of paraplegic patients standing and walking with two knee-ankle-foot orthoses. *Arch. Phys. Med. Rehabil.* 65:121–124.

Mikelberg, R., and S. Reid. 1981. Spinal cord lesions and lower extremity bracing: An overview and follow-up study. *Paraplegia* 19:379–385.

Miller, N.E., et al. 1984. Paraplegic energy expenditure during negotiation of architectural barriers. *Arch. Phys. Med. Rehabil.* 65:778–779.

Natvig, H., and R. McAdam. 1978–79. Ambulation without wheelchairs for paraplegics with complete lesions. *Paraplegia* 16:142–146.

Nixon, V. 1985. *Spinal cord injury: A guide to functional outcomes in physical therapy management.* Gaithersburg, Md.: Aspen.

O'Daniel, W.E., and H.R. Hahn. 1981. Follow-up usage of the Scott-Craig orthosis in paraplegia. *Paraplegia* 19:373–378.

Patrick, J.H., and M.R. McClelland. 1985. Low energy reciprocal walking for the adult paraplegic. *Paraplegia* 23:113–117.

Ragnarsson, K.T., et al. 1975. Pneumatic orthosis for paraplegic patients: Functional evaluation and prescription considerations. *Arch. Phys. Med. Rehabil.* 56:479–483.

Rosman, N., and E. Spira. 1974. Paraplegic use of walking braces: A survey. *Arch. Phys. Med. Rehabil.* 55:310–314.

Seymour, R.J., et al. 1982. Paraplegics use of the ORLAU swivel walker: Case report. *Arch. Phys. Med. Rehabil.* 63:490–494.

Waters, R.E., and L. Miller. 1987. A physiologic rationale for orthotic prescription in paraplegia. *Clin. Prosthet. Orthot.* 11:66–73.

Waters, R.L., et al. 1989. Determinants of gait performance following spinal cord injury. *Arch. Phys. Med. Rehabil.* 70:811–818.

Woolsey, R.M. 1985. Rehabilitation outcome following spinal cord injury. *Arch. Neurol.* 42:116–119.

Yarkony, G.M., et al. 1986. Jones-Hedman walker modifications for C7 quadriplegic patient: Case study in team cooperation. *Arch. Phys. Med. Rehabil.* 67:54–55.

Yarkony, G.M., et al. 1987. Benefits of rehabilitation for traumatic spinal cord injury: Multivariate analysis of 711 patients. *Arch. Neurol.* 44:93–96.

Yarkony, G.M., et al. 1988a. Spinal cord injury rehabilitation outcome: The impact of age. *J. Clin. Epidemiol.* 41:173–177.

Yarkony, G.M., et al. 1988b. Functional skills after spinal cord injury rehabilitation: Three-year longitudinal follow-up. *Arch. Phys. Med. Rehabil.* 69:111–114.

Yarkony, G.M., et al. 1988c. Rehabilitation outcomes in C5 quadriplegia. *Am. J. Phys. Med. Rehabil.* 67:73–76.

Yarkony, G.M., et al. 1988d. Rehabilitation outcomes in C6 tetraplegia. *Paraplegia* 26:177–185.

Yarkony, G.M., et al. 1990. Rehabilitation outcomes in patients with complete thoracic spinal cord injury. *Am. J. Phys. Med. Rehabil.* 69:23–27.

Part II

Medical and Surgical Management

Chapter 3

Medical and Physical Complications of Spinal Cord Injury

Gary M. Yarkony

AUTONOMIC DYSREFLEXIA

Autonomic dysreflexia, also known as autonomic hyperreflexia, is a potentially fatal complication of spinal cord injury characterized by exaggerated autonomic responses to stimuli that are innocuous in normal individuals (Erickson 1980; Head & Riddoch 1917; Kewalramani 1980; Thompson & Witham 1948). Individuals with spinal cord injury with lesions at or above T-6 generally are considered at risk for dysreflexia because the lesion is above the sympathic outflow from the spinal cord. Reports of this syndrome occurring in a man with a lesion at T-8 and in a T-10 paraplegic woman during the postpartum period indicate that level alone should not be the sole factor in the diagnosis of autonomic dysreflexia (Gimousky et al. 1981; Moeller & Scheinberg 1973). Those persons who develop this condition often state that they are "going hyper."

Autonomic dysreflexia may be considered a disorder of autonomic homeostasis (Erickson 1980; Kurnick 1956). Sensory input from bladder distension or other noxious stimuli induce generalized sympathetic activity, resulting in vasoconstriction and hypertension. Norepinephrine is released from sympathetic postganglionic fibers. There is an exaggerated response to the norepinephrine as a result of the lack of supraspinal vasomotor reflexes.

The incidence of dysreflexia has been reported to range from 48% to 85% of those susceptible (Bors 1956; Kumar & Mallican 1986; Kursh et al. 1977). The primary differential diagnosis is pheochromocytoma (Manger et al. 1979) or other catecholamine-secreting tumors (Thorn-Alquist 1975) and toxemia during pregnancy. The initial onset usually is after the first 2 months after injury, and 92% of cases occur within the first year. It may occur for the first time as late as 15 years after injury (Ciliberti et al. 1953; Guttmann et al. 1965–66). The syndrome develops in both complete and incomplete lesions.

Autonomic dysreflexia results from a noxious stimulus below the level of the lesion. Distension of pelvic viscera, such as the bladder, colon, or rectum, or uterine contractions during labor generally represent the inciting stimulus for autonomic dysreflexia (Erickson 1980; Kewalramani 1980). When associated with uterine contractions, the hypertension begins within a few seconds of the onset of a contraction and may diminish or dissipate completely between contractions (Robertson & Guttmann 1963). Other possible stimuli include menses, catheterization, urinary tract infection, ingrown toenails, hemorrhagic cystitis, testicular torsion, sexual intercourse, intraabdominal catastrophes, surgical manipulation of the pelvis or abdomen, pressure ulcers, and tight clothing, shoes, or leg-bag strapping. Bladder distension is the most common stimulus, followed by rectal distension (fecal impaction). In women, ovarian cysts (Kumar & Mallican 1986) and breast feeding (Devenport & Swenson 1983) have been reported to be the inciting stimuli. Men undergoing vibratory ejaculation or electroejaculation may develop the syndrome.

Symptoms include headache (generally described as pounding), hyperhydrosis, cutaneous vasodilation, nasal obstruction, piloerection (goose flesh), and paresthesias. Anxiety and the desire to void may be experienced (Lindan et al. 1980).

Examination reveals hypertension, hyperhydrosis, splotches on the face or neck, and, in general, bladder distension, fecal impaction, or uterine contractions. If the patient is evaluated early in the course of the episode, bradycardia may be present. It is most common to have a normal pulse rate or tachycardia. Other findings include a prominent Horner syndrome. If an ECG is obtained, a rhythm disturbance may be present (Guttmann et al. 1965–66).

Hypertension is the primary cause of the morbidity and mortality associated with autonomic dysreflexia (Kursh et al. 1977) and may result in loss of consciousness, seizures, intracerebral bleeding (Wackwitz et al. 1982), and death (Yarkony et al. 1986). The syndrome may present with seizures and may be treated as a primary seizure disorder, with the autonomic dysreflexia going unrecognized.

Proper medical management of skin, bowel, and bladder should prevent the syndrome from occurring. Annual genitourinary follow-up is essential to detect bladder or kidney stones, which may cause dysreflexia. When an episode does occur, the patient should have the head of the bed elevated or sit up, tight clothing should be removed, and the inciting stimulus should be sought. A distended bladder is generally found and is relieved by performing a straight catheterization, unkinking an indwelling catheter, emptying a leg bag, or changing a clogged indwelling catheter. If irrigation of a Foley leads to cessation of the syndrome, the catheter still should be changed. Episodes due to rectal distension may resolve spontaneously, but if rectal examination is required, an anesthetic ointment should be used.

If mechanical means do not resolve the syndrome, medical management is then directed to a reduction in blood pressure. Agents that generally have been successful include diazoxide (Hyperstat), nitroprusside (Nipride), hydralazine (Apresoline), chlorpromazine (Thorazine), nifedipine, and amyl nitrate. Nifedipine can be given orally and is preferred by many for this reason. The nitrates are administered easily as well. Recurrent episodes not responsive to successful bladder or bowel management generally are treated with α-blockers or ganglionic blockers such as phenoxybenzamine (Dibenzyline; McGuire et al. 1976; Scott & Morrow 1978; Sizemore & Winternitz 1970), mecamylamine (Inversine; Braddom & Johnson 1969), and guanethidine (Ismelin; Young 1963). Many patients have dysreflexia at predictable times, such as with their bowel program. They may premedicate themselves with nitro paste, for example, and then remove the paste when the program is completed.

Autonomic dysreflexia is a well-recognized complication of urologic and other surgeries in individuals with spinal cord injury. Numerous anesthetic approaches have been attempted. These techniques either prevent the syndrome from occurring, which is preferred, or treat the resultant hypertension. Ganglionic blocking agents such as hexamethonium or tetraethylammonium chloride were among the first successful agents to be reported (Ciliberti et al. 1953). More recently, trimethaphan (Arfonad) has been shown in several case reports to be useful (Thorn-Alquist 1975). This approach allows the dysreflexia to develop as opposed to preventing its onset. Bilateral paravertebral sympathetic blocks are insufficient to prevent dysreflexia. Spinal anesthesia has been shown to prevent the reflex and to eliminate the associated hypertension and headache. One series of 97 patients confirmed this (Schonwald et al. 1981). Bradycardia is unpredictable and may occur suddenly with spinal anesthesia. Technical difficulties in individuals with spinal cord injury who have lumbar injuries are also a problem. Epidural anesthesia may be effective (Ciliberti et al. 1953; Guttmann et al. 1965–66), but there is a danger of inadvertent subarachnoid injection, and acute apneic episodes may occur (Schonwald et al. 1981). The height of the block with these techniques may be difficult to determine, and hypotension may occur (Thorn-Alquist 1975).

General anesthesia may pose a problem because of decreased vital capacity, bronchial secretions, and diminished cough. Nitrous oxide plus narcotics is less effective than halothane or enflurane anesthesia with assisted ventilation. Dysrhythmias have been reported in patients receiving general anesthesia without assisted ventilation. Hypotension is also a risk but may be diminished with preoperative hydration. Nondepolarizing muscle relaxants should be used because succinylcholine has been shown to induce hyperkalemia and subsequent cardiac arrest in lower motor neuron lesions (Brooke et al. 1978).

DEEP VENOUS THROMBOSIS

Deep venous thrombosis (DVT) is a major complication after spinal cord injury, but recent advances should provide for a decrease in its incidence (Green et al. 1988; Merli et al. 1988). In one series from our center (Rehabilitation Institute of Chicago) the incidence was 72%, but others have reported the incidence to be 100%. Fatal pulmonary embolism has been reported to range from 2% to 16% of patients within 2 to 3 months of spinal cord injury.

Virchow's triad of stasis, hypercoagulability, and vascular injury was the initial mechanism proposed to lead to DVT. Stasis clearly is a major factor after spinal cord injury. Blood viscosity may increase as a result of dehydration and edema. Protein catabolism may lead to decreased antithrombin III, and decreased fibrinolytic activity results from diminished release of plasminogen activator, which is dependent on muscular contraction. Pulmonary emboli generally arise from the proximal veins of the legs.

Diagnosis of DVT

Physical Examination

DVT may cause venous obstruction and/or inflammatory signs about the thrombus (Browse 1978). Venous obstruction may lead to leg swelling, dilatation of the superficial veins, increased skin temperatures, or, rarely, a bluish discoloration in the distal lower extremities. The individual may complain of pain and tenderness. Pain and tenderness are unreliable because they may result from numerous other causes; edema is especially common after a spinal cord injury (Green et al. 1982). Two thirds of persons with thrombosis have no clinical signs (Turpie 1989). Fever may be present in these patients as the only sign (Green 1990). The section of this chapter on heterotopic bone below discusses this important differential diagnosis. Laboratory diagnosis is essential for this condition.

Doppler Ultrasound

This noninvasive technique uses low-frequency ultrasound (5 to 10 Hz) to detect venous flow signals (Browse 1978; Flanigan et al. 1978; Green 1990). These signals may be audible or reproduced via a recordable analog wave form. The venous flow characteristics permit the detection of thrombosis in both superficial and deep veins. This is accomplished by compressing the upstream tissues of the vein to increase the rate of blood flow. It is most accurate in detecting thrombi in the proximal veins large enough to cause an obstruction, but it may miss smaller, more fragile, nonobstructing thrombi and calf thrombi. False positives may result from external compression such as a Baker cyst. Not all veins (internal iliac) are accessible with this technique.

Impedance Plethysmography

Impedance plethysmography (Browse 1978; Flanigan et al. 1978; Green 1990) uses electrical impedance to measure calf volume and to examine the changes produced by venous congestion and the rate of emptying of the calf after release of the congestion. Thrombi that produce a significant obstruction to flow are detected. Accuracy is low for calf vein thrombosis but high for major femoral and iliac thrombosis.

Fibrinogen Leg Scanning

Fibrinogen leg scanning (Browse 1978; Flanigan et al. 1978; Green 1990) depends on the incorporation of circulating radioactive fibrinogen into a forming or recently formed thrombus to a degree sufficient to make the thrombus detectable by external scintillation counting. There is a danger of viral hepatitis dissemination from the fibrinogen that significantly reduces this technique's utility. It is highly accurate below the middle of the thigh. False positives occur with local trauma, arthritis, or edema, and false negatives occur if the thrombus is more than 5 days old. Disadvantages include its cost, the 24-hour delay from injection to reading, failure to detect established thrombi, and the danger of viral transmission.

B-Mode Imaging (Duplex Ultrasonography)

This recent, noninvasive technique (Aitken & Godden 1987; Longsfeld et al. 1987) uses real-time imaging to diagnose DVT. It provides longitudinal and transverse real-time images and can reveal clots in the ileal femoral, popliteal, and calf veins. These clots need not be large enough to cause audible hemodynamic changes. Limitations include the need for skilled and experienced technicians, the inability to image the iliac veins, and difficulties with calf veins.

Venography

The gold standard (Aitken & Godden 1987; Browse 1978; Green 1990; Ramchandau et al. 1981; Satiani 1981) for diagnosis of DVT is still venography. Radiopaque contrast media are injected into a dorsal vein of the foot; clots are diagnosed by the presence of a persistent filling defect or complete occlusion of a vein with presence of dye above and below and collateral filling, allowing the examination of all lower extremity veins except the deep femoral and internal iliac. This is an invasive technique, and side effects include pain, superficial thrombophlebitis at the injection site, and dye allergies. It probably detects 95% of thrombi (Browse 1978). False positives may occur with inadequate mixing of the blood and contrast from blood entering an opacified vein.

Diagnosis of Pulmonary Embolism

There are no characteristic signs or symptoms of pulmonary embolism (Rosenow et al. 1981). Pulmonary embolisms may be silent. Common symptoms include dyspnea, tachypnea, tachycardia, fever, and chest pain. These findings are nonspecific. ECG changes are transient and nonspecific, and, except for sinus tachycardia, dysrhythmias are uncommon and usually atrial in origin. An elevated hemidiaphragm may be seen, but chest radiography is generally normal or nonspecific. A pleural effusion may be present, but this is often transient as well. Arterial oxygen tension may be normal. A pulmonary infarction may be present with cough, hemoptysis, and pleuritic chest pain.

Ventilation-perfusion lung scanning is useful in the diagnosis of pulmonary embolism. A normal scan essentially rules out an embolus. An abnormal scan does not necessarily indicate a pulmonary embolus. A ventilation-perfusion mismatch is an area of abnormal perfusion with normal ventilation. A high-probability scan with two or more segmental or larger perfusion defects with normal ventilation is diagnostic, but results other than normal are not as helpful. Impedance plethysmography may be helpful if the scan is nondiagnostic (Green et al. 1990). If a DVT is present, anticoagulation is indicated anyway. A pulmonary angiogram is the definitive test. It should be performed within 24 to 72 hours to avoid a false negative due to clot resolution.

Prevention of Thromboembolism

Numerous techniques have been proposed to prevent DVT after a spinal cord injury. Early remobilization would be of obvious benefit, but generally this is not possible. Lower extremity passive range of motion may be of some benefit. Compression stockings (TED hose) are not a preventive measure (Guttmann 1976).

External pneumatic calf compression (Green et al. 1982; Rossi et al. 1980) has been demonstrated at our center to result in a significant reduction in DVT, but the incidence with its use is still unacceptably high (40%). In that study, aspirin and dipyridamole led to further reductions in the incidence of DVT, but bleeding complications prohibit their usage. Functional electrical stimulation (FES) (Katz et al. 1987) may change plasma fibrinolytic activity and promote venous return in the lower extremities. Merli et al. (1988) combined FES with low-dose heparin and obtained a significant reduction of thrombosis. This study included patients as late as 2 weeks after injury and excluded 34 of 87 patients, so that many at greater risk may have been excluded. The other difficulty with FES is that it may not be practical once the patient is in the rehabilitation phase.

Heparin is more practical to administer as a prophylactic agent. It can be used in both acute care and rehabilitation. Studies from our center (Green et al. 1988) demonstrated that, if the activated partial thromboplastin time (APTT) is kept at 1.5 times control after a spinal cord injury, thromboembolism can be reduced. Unfortunately there were several episodes of bleeding on this regimen. This technique should be used in individuals at low risk for bleeding.

Low–molecular weight heparin (Turpie et al. 1986), which can be given once daily and has greater bioavailability than standard heparin, led to a significant reduction of thromboembolic complications in our center. Logiporin was used in our study, which at the time of this writing is not commercially available (Green et al. 1990). It was found to be far superior to heparin, 5,000 U subcutaneously every 8 hours. Pending its availability, heparin, 5,000 U subcutaneously every 8 hours, or adjusted-dose heparin should be given if the bleeding risk is low. FES or intermittent compression may be beneficial in combination with lose-dose heparin.

Treatment

Heparin given intravenously to prolong the APTT 1.5 times control will prevent new thrombus or extension of existing thrombus but not embolization from existing thrombus. Warfarin should be initiated at day 3 to 5 and overlap for 5 days with heparin. Patients with calf DVT may receive intravenous heparin followed by subcutaneous heparin, but they should be monitored carefully with serial impedance plethysmography for thrombus extension. In that situation, warfarin or increased subcutaneous heparin may be needed.

HETEROTOPIC OSSIFICATION

Heterotopic ossification (HO) is known by several names (Kewalramani 1977; Lal 1990; Stover 1989): ectopic bone os-

sification, paraosteoarthropathy, neurogenic HO, and myositis ossificans. It is bone that develops in abnormal anatomic locations, generally in the soft tissue. Myositis ossificans progressiva begins soon after birth and eventually leads to death. Myositis ossificans traumatica (Samuelson & Coleman 1976) or circumscripta is the most common form, occurring as a result of local trauma. The bone developing after a spinal cord injury is a nonprogressive idiopathic form that many consider best called neurogenic HO (Jensen et al. 1988). It may also occur after cerebrovascular accidents, traumatic closed head injury, brain injury, polio, and multiple sclerosis.

The incidence of HO after spinal cord injury has been reported to range from 5% to 50% (Hernandez et al. 1978-79) and varies from center to center and from year to year at any location. It occurs most commonly in the hips (Tibone et al. 1978), followed by the knees; it may also occur in the shoulders, elbows, or paravertebral area or along the femur. Occurrence in the hands and feet is uncommon (Lynch et al. 1981). It is more common in complete lesions (Nicholas 1973). It is not related to human leukocyte antigens or racial groups (Minaire et al. 1980; Scher 1976).

HO (Jensen et al. 1988) develops along tendons, aponeuroses, ligaments, and fasciae and is associated with soft tissue atrophy. It generally does not involve the periosteum. The joint space and joint capsule generally are preserved. Mature HO is cancellous bone with haversian canals, blood vessels, and cortex. Bone marrow is present, but hematopoiesis is minimal. The initial immature inflammatory mass is hypervascular with numerous immature cells. As the mass develops, immature amorphous calcium phosphate is replaced by hydroxyapatite crystals. Mature bone begins to appear at 6 months.

The initial clinical presentation is variable (Jensen et al. 1988). Decreased range of motion may be noted in a joint, or HO may be an incidental finding on radiography. Typically, localized swelling develops with associated warmth, redness, and loss of range of motion. An associated joint effusion may be present, and the patient may be febrile. The differential diagnosis includes local trauma or fracture, thrombophlebitis, cellulitis, periostitis, hematoma, and joint infection. HO can mimic DVT (Venier & Ditunno 1971; Yarkony et al. 1989) by compressing the vasculature and resulting in distal edema, as is sometimes seen with DVT. HO may lead to false-positive Doppler studies, impedance plethysmography, and B-mode ultrasonography. A venogram may be necessary to confirm the presence of a DVT because long-term anticoagulation outweighs the risks of a venogram. Figure 3–1 presents our suggestions for evaluating DVT and HO in spinal cord injury.

The onset of HO generally is 1 to 4 months after injury. It is unusual to begin after 1 year, but this may occur with systemic illness, local trauma, or pressure ulcers. Laboratory diagnosis has centered on serum alkaline phosphatase, plain film, and bone scanning. Serum alkaline phosphatase may be elevated, but this is common in patients with spinal cord injury as a re-

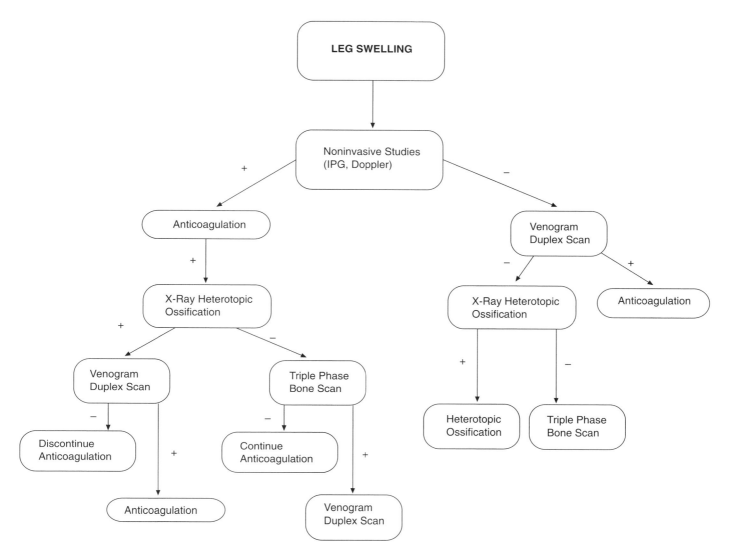

Figure 3–1 Evaluation of deep venous thrombosis in the presence of heterotopic ossification. *Source:* Reprinted from Yarkony, G.M., Lee, M.Y., Green, D., and Roth, E.J. Heterotopic Ossification Pseudophlebitis, *The American Journal of Medicine*, Vol. 87, p. 343, with permission of Yorke Medical Publishers, Copyright © 1989.

sult of associated fractures. Plain radiographic findings may lag as long as 2 weeks behind clinical findings. Triple-phase bone scan generally will be positive when there are clinical findings. In the early stages of HO, the first phase may be the only positive finding because of the increased vascularity (Orzel & Rudd 1985; Rossier et al. 1973).

Post–spinal cord injury prevention of HO has remained elusive. Radiation therapy is effective for prevention in total hip replacement but has not been studied in spinal cord injury (Ayers et al. 1986) because that population is younger and there may be a danger of malignancy. Indomethacin (McLaren 1990) is beneficial after total hip surgery and acetabular fractures but has not been studied in spinal cord injury. Range of motion exercises do not appear to predispose to HO (Stover et

al. 1975). If the exercises are not performed once HO is present, ankylosis will occur.

Etidronate disodium (Didronel) is the major treatment measure in spinal cord injury (Finerman & Stover 1981; Garland et al. 1983; Rassel & Smith 1973). It inhibits (Fleisch et al. 1970; Francis et al. 1969) the crystalline growth of hydroxyapatite crystals by blocking the transformation of amorphous calcium phosphate into hydroxyapatite crystals. When given prophylactically (Stover et al. 1976a), the final incidence is about the same, but the amount of bone deposited is considerably less (Stover et al. 1976b). Prophylaxis should begin about 3 weeks after injury and be given for 12 weeks. Side effects are mainly gastrointestinal. The initial dose is 20 mg/kg for 2 weeks followed by 10 mg/kg for 10 weeks (Stover 1989).

Surgical intervention requires careful evaluation (Garland & Orwin 1984). Complications include bleeding, infection, and recurrence. Resection is indicated for functional difficulties or pressure areas caused by the HO (Hassard 1975). HO tends to recur if surgery is performed while the bone is immature. Plain films are not reliable because mature and immature areas may be superimposed. Alkaline phosphatase is not a reliable indicator either. Bone scans (Tanaka et al. 1977) are the most accurate, but they should be performed serially to demonstrate decreasing uptake.

Etidronate disodium should be given preoperatively and postoperatively for 1 year (Stover et al. 1976b). The dosage is 20 mg/kg for 2 weeks preoperatively followed by 10 mg/kg for 12 months. Range of motion exercises should slowly increase the range of motion soon after surgical drains are removed. A wedge resection of bone may lead to a better surgical result than complete resection of the bony mass because surgical trauma and bleeding are limited.

CONTRACTURES

Joint contractures are a complication of immobilization; they are defined as a fixed high resistance to passive stretch of a muscle resulting from fibrosis of the muscles (Yarkony et al. 1985) and joints or from disorders of muscle fibers.

Frequent motion is required to maintain the normal relationships of the connective tissues about a joint (Frank et al. 1984). With immobilization, the meshwork of collagen in the connective tissue shortens to the length to which it is maximally stretched (Kottke 1966). In addition, with immobilization there is decreased proteoglycan synthesis, resulting in decreased fluids and shortening of the connective tissue (Woo et al. 1971).

An immobilized joint will develop fibrofatty proliferation, resulting in a decreased size or obliteration of the joint space (Enneking & Horowitz 1972). With continued immobilization, it may blend with the articular cartilage. Bony ankyloses may occur if the process continues. This process is hastened by local trauma, edema, or impaired circulation.

In spinal cord injury, contractures occur most commonly about the hips, knees, ankles, and shoulders. As with other secondary complications, the goal is prevention based primarily on positioning and range of motion.

Proper positioning is critical during the acute care phase. The arm should be abducted and externally rotated. Foot drop can be prevented by positioning the ankles in dorsiflexion. Passive splinting of the wrists and ankles may be helpful. Range of motion exercises should be performed daily at a minimum. As spasticity increases, the program should be upgraded as needed. The best guide to the need for range of motion exercises is continued monitoring of range of motion. If range of motion decreases, then passive range of motion must be increased in frequency. Pillows beneath the knees should

be avoided. Prevention of contractures allows for better positioning to prevent pressure ulcers.

If contractures develop, prolonged stretch is the basic treatment technique (Kottke et al. 1966). Splinting and casting may be necessary with more severe contractures (Cherry 1981). Heat (Lehmann et al. 1970) or ultrasound before stretch assists in the treatment of contractures. Simple cutaneous surgical methods of contracture release may be necessary if conservative management fails (Bedbrook 1981).

PULMONARY COMPLICATIONS

Pneumonia and other pulmonary complications are a leading cause of morbidity and mortality after spinal cord injury (Devivo et al. 1989). Therefore, it is essential that rehabilitation efforts be directed to optimizing the musculature for breathing and cough to diminish future complications.

The diaphragm is the major muscle of inspiration. If the intercostal muscles and abdominal muscles are paralyzed, it may be the only muscle contributing to inspiration. When the diaphragm contracts the thoracic cavities, vertical diameter increases, and the negative intrathoracic pressure for inspiration results. In spinal cord injury, the actions of the external intercostals to increase the anteroposterior diameter at the chest may be partially or completely lost, depending on the level of injury.

Expiration is a passive process. The abdominal contents, with the help of the tone of the abdominal musculature, return the diaphragm to the resting position. Particularly important and often lacking after a spinal cord injury is the force for cough, which is provided by the abdominal musculature (DeTroyer & Estenne 1991).

In quadriplegics with lesions below C-4, the capacity fills to approximately 58% (Morgan et al. 1986), although there is much individual variation. Initially after injury the reduction may be more, but this generally improves during the first 6 months (McMichan et al. 1980). The total lung capacity is reduced, and the residual volume rises. The decreased vital capacity is due largely to the decrease in expiratory volume. This results from the paralysis at the expiratory musculature. Pulmonary function tests will show a restrictive pattern with a decrease in all lung volumes (Fugel-Meyer 1971; McMichan et al. 1980). A paradoxical breathing pattern results when the abdomen rises and the anteroposterior diameter of the chest decreases.

Rehabilitation efforts are directed to improving vital capacity, maintaining mobility, preventing chest deformity, and improving cough. These efforts assume greater importance the more proximal in the spinal cord that the lesion occurs.

An abdominal binder is helpful for two reasons: It improves venous return, and it improves lung volumes. When the quadriplegic patient sits up, the diaphragm descends. This reduces the excursion at the diaphragm and increases the work of breathing. The abdominal binder (or corset) provides additional abdominal support, and the diaphragm is elevated to a higher, more functional resting position (Maloney 1979). It should be positioned over the lower ribs to the iliac crests bilaterally. If a corset is used, the lower straps should be higher than the upper ones.

Strengthening of the inspiratory musculature is an important component of any rehabilitation program for persons with spinal cord injury who have diminished vital capacity. Incentive spirometry is useful because it helps set a goal that can be visualized by the patient. The feedback is more useful than simple deep-breathing exercises. These exercises help prevent atelectasis, expand the chest wall to improve ventilation and exercise the inspiratory muscles. Inspiration exercises using a graded resistance also can improve strength and endurance (Gross et al. 1980).

Other techniques include resistance using weights in the epigastric area to provide resistance to diaphragmatic excursion. Exercises to increase thoracic expansion and to strengthen the intercostal musculature (if functioning) are helpful in maintaining the mobility of the chest wall (Haas et al. 1979). Proper wheelchair positioning, described elsewhere in this text, helps prevent chest deformity.

Glossopharyngeal breathing takes air into the mouth, traps it in the pharynx, and then forces it into the lungs (Nixon 1985; Zumwalt et al. 1956). This technique is known as frog breathing and can improve vital capacity and assist with cough. It can also decrease atelectasis and improve chest expansion (Metcalf 1966; Montero et al. 1967).

Atelectasis and pneumonia often develop from ineffective cough resulting in retained secretions. The most common method to decrease the complications is cough assist. This technique can increase the force of the cough and improve clearance of secretions (Kirby et al. 1966).

This technique is performed in two ways. The hands are placed in the epigastric area and pressure is applied in an upward fashion, or the hands are placed laterally over the ribs and pressure is applied (Bromley 1985). Assistive cough may result in deformation and caudal migration of Greenwald filters used to treat DVT (Balshi et al. 1989).

Currently under investigation is the application of neuromuscular stimulation to augment cough after spinal cord injury in quadriplegics. Although still under investigation, electrical stimulation at the abdominal musculature appears to be more effective than volitional cough and as effective as assistive cough (Turba et al. 1992). Further research is needed to determine the practicality of this technique.

The clavicular portion at the pectoralis major muscle has been shown to be an expiratory muscle in quadriplegia (DeTroyer et al. 1986). This muscle is strengthened, cough is improved, and expiratory volume is increased (Estenne et al. 1989); it is unclear, however, how effective this training is in the overall management of persons with spinal cord injury in decreasing long-term complications.

REFERENCES

Aitken, A.G.F., and D.J. Godden. 1987. Real-time ultrasound diagnosis of deep vein thrombosis: A comparison with venography. *Clin. Radiol.* 38:309–313.

Ayers, D.C., et al. 1986. The prevention of heterotopic ossification in high-risk patients by low dose radiation therapy after total hip arthroplasty. *J. Bone Joint Surg. Am.* 68:1423–1430.

Balshi, J.D., et al. 1989. Complications of caval interruption by Greenwald filter in quadriplegics. *J. Vasc. Surg.* 9:552–558.

Bedbrook, G. 1981. *The care and management of spinal cord injuries.* New York, N.Y.: Springer-Verlag.

Bors, E. 1956. Challenge of quadriplegia: Some personal observations in series of 233 cases. *Bull. Los Ang. Neurol. Soc.* 21:105–123.

Braddom, R.L., and E.W.L. Johnson. 1969. Mecamylamine in control of hyperreflexia. *Arch. Phys. Med. Rehabil.* 50:488–453, 456.

Bromley, I. 1985. *Tetraplegia and paraplegia: A guide for physiotherapists.* 2d ed. New York, N.Y.: Churchill Livingstone.

Brooke, M.M., et al. 1978. Paraplegia: Succinylcholine induced hyperkalemia and cardiac arrest. *Arch. Phys. Med. Rehabil.* 59:306–308.

Browse, N. 1978. Diagnosis of deep-vein thrombosis. *Br. Med. Bull.* 34:163–167.

Cherry, D.B. 1981. Review of physical therapy alternatives for producing muscle contracture. *Phys. Ther.* 61:1601–1603.

Ciliberti, B.J., et al. 1953. Hypertension during anesthesia in spinal cord injuries. *Anesthesiology* 15:273–279.

DeTroyer, A., and M. Estenne. 1991. The expiratory muscles in tetraplegia. *Paraplegia* 29:359–363.

DeTroyer, A., et al. 1986. Mechanism of active expiration in tetraplegia subjects. *N. Engl. J. Med.* 413:740–744.

Devenport, J.K., and J.R. Swenson. 1983. An unusual case of autonomic dysreflexia. *Arch. Phys. Med. Rehabil.* 64:485 (abstract).

Devivo, M.J., et al. 1989. Cause of death in patients with spinal cord injuries. *Arch. Intern. Med.* 149:1761–1766.

Enneking, W.F., and M. Horowitz. 1972. The intra-articular effects of immobilization on the human knee. *J. Bone Joint Surg. Am.* 54A:973–985.

Erickson, R.P. 1980. Autonomic hyperreflexia: Pathophysiology and medical management. *Arch. Phys. Med. Rehabil.* 61:431–440.

Estenne, M., et al. 1989. The effect of pectoralis muscle training in tetraplegic subjects. *Am. Rev. Respir. Dis.* 1218–1222.

Finerman, G.A.M., and S.L. Stover. 1981. Heterotopic ossification following hip replacement or spinal cord injury: Two clinical studies with EHDP. *Metab. Bone Dis. Relat. Res.* 4/5:337–342.

Flanigan, D., et al. 1978. Vascular-laboratory diagnosis of clinically suspected acute deep vein thrombosis. *Lancet* 2:331–334.

Fleisch, H.A., et al. 1970. The inhibitory effect of phosphonates on the formation of calcium phosphate crystals in vitro and on aortic and kidney calcification in vivo. *Eur. J. Clin. Invest.* 1:12–18.

Francis, M.D., et al. 1969. Diphosphonates inhibit formation of calcium phosphate crystals in vitro and pathological calcification in vivo. *Science* 165:1264–1266.

Frank, C., et al. 1984. Physiology and therapeutic value of passive joint motion. *Clin. Orthop.* 185:113–125.

Fugel-Meyer, A.R. 1971. Effects of respiratory muscles paralysis in tetraplegic and paraplegic patients. *Scand. J. Rehabil. Med.* 3:141–150.

Garland, D.E., et al. 1983. Diphosphonate treatment for heterotopic ossification in spinal cord injury patients. *Clin. Orthop.* 176:198–200.

Garland, D.E., and J.F. Orwin. 1984. Resection of heterotopic ossification in patients with spinal cord injuries. *Clin. Orthop.* 242:169–176.

Gimousky, M.L., et al. 1981. Management of autonomic hyperreflexia associated with a low thoracic spinal cord lesion. *Obstet. Gynecol.* 153:223–224.

Green, D. 1990. *Medical management of long term disability.* Gaithersburg, Md.: Aspen.

Green, D., et al. 1982. Deep vein thrombosis in spinal cord injury: Effect of prophylaxis with calf compression, aspirin and dipyridamole. *Paraplegia.* 20:227–234.

Green, D., et al. 1988. Fixed vs. adjusted dose heparin in the prophylaxis of thromboembolism in spinal cord injury. *J.A.M.A.* 260:1255–1258.

Green, D., et al. 1990. Prevention of thromboembolism after spinal cord injury using low molecular weight heparin. *Ann. Intern. Med.* 113:571–574.

Gross, D., et al. 1980. The effects of training on strength and endurance of the diaphragm in quadriplegia. *Am. J. Med.* 68:27–35.

Guttmann, L. 1976. *Spinal cord injuries comprehensive management of research.* 2d ed. Boston, Mass.: Blackwell Scientific.

Guttmann, L., et al. 1965–66. Cardiac irregularities during labour in paraplegic women. *Paraplegia* 3:141–151.

Haas, A., et al. 1979. *Pulmonary therapy and rehabilitation: Principles and practice.* Baltimore, Md.: Williams & Wilkins.

Hassard, G.H. 1975. Heterotopic bone formation about the hip and unilateral decubitus ulcers in spinal cord injury. *Arch. Phys. Med. Rehabil.* 56:355–358.

Head, H., and G. Riddoch. 1917. Autonomic bladder, excessive sweating and some other reflex conditions in gross injuries of spinal cord. *Brain* 40:188–263.

Hernandez, A.M., et al. 1978–79. The para articular ossification in our paraplegics and tetraplegics: A survey of 704 patients. *Paraplegia.* 16:272–275.

Jensen, L.L., et al. 1988. Neurogenic heterotopic ossification. *Am. J. Phys. Med.* 66:351–363.

Katz, R.T., et al. 1987. Functional electric stimulation to enhance systemic fibrinolytic activity in spinal cord injured patients. *Arch. Phys. Med. Rehabil.* 68:423–426.

Kewalramani, L.S. 1977. Ectopic ossification. *Am. J. Phys. Med.* 56:99–121.

Kewalramani, L.S. 1980. Autonomic dysreflexia in traumatic myelopathy. *Am. J. Phys. Med.* 59:1–21.

Kirby, N.A., et al. 1966. An evaluation of assisted cough in quadriplegic patients. *Arch. Phys. Med. Rehabil.* 47:705–710.

Kottke, F.J. 1966. The effects of limitation of activity upon the human body. *J.A.M.A.* 196:117–122.

Kottke, F.J., et al. 1966. The rationale for prolonged stretching for correction of shortening of connective tissue. *Arch. Phys. Med. Rehabil.* 47:345–352.

Kumar, U.N., and C.N. Mallican. 1986. Ovarian cyst and autonomic dysreflexia. *Arch. Phys. Med. Rehabil.* 70:547–548.

Kurnick, N.B. 1956. Autonomic hyperreflexia and its control in patients with spinal cord lesions. *Ann. Intern. Med.* 44:678–686.

Kursh, E.D., et al. 1977. Complications of autonomic dysreflexia. *J. Urol.* 118:70–72.

Lal, S. 1990. "Heterotopic ossification." In *Medical management of long-term disability,* ed. D. Green, 133–152. Gaithersburg, Md.: Aspen.

Lehmann, J.F., et al. 1970. Effect of therapeutic temperatures on tendon extensibility. *Arch. Phys. Med. Rehabil.* 51:481–487.

Lindan, R., et al. 1980. Incidence and clinical features of autonomic dysreflexia in patients with spinal cord injury. *Paraplegia* 18:285–292.

Longsfeld, M., et al. 1987. Duplex B-mode imaging for the diagnosis of deep venous thrombosis. *Arch. Surg.* 122:587–591.

Lynch, C., et al. 1981. Heterotopic ossification in the hand of a patient with spinal cord injury. *Arch. Phys. Med. Rehabil.* 62:291–293.

Maloney, F.P. 1979. Pulmonary function in quadriplegia: Effects of a corset. *Arch. Phys. Med. Rehabil.* 60:261–265.

Manger, W.M., et al. 1979. Autonomic hyperreflexia and its differentiation from pheochromocytoma. *Arch. Phys. Med. Rehabil.* 60:159–161.

McGuire, E.J., et al. 1976. Treatment of autonomic dysreflexia with phenoxybenzamine. *J. Urol.* 115:53–55.

McLaren, A.C. 1990. Prophylaxis with indomethacin for heterotopic bone. *J. Bone Joint Surg. Am.* 72:245–247.

McMichan, J.C., et al. 1980. Pulmonary dysfunction following traumatic quadriplegia. *J.A.M.A.* 243:528–531.

Merli, G.T., et al. 1988. Deep vein thrombosis: Prophylaxis in acute spinal cord injured patients. *Arch. Phys. Med. Rehabil.* 69:661–664.

Metcalf, V.A. 1966. Vital capacity and glossopharyngeal breathing in traumatic quadriplegia. *J. Am. Phys. Ther. Assoc.* 46:835–838.

Minaire, P., et al. 1980. Neurologic injuries, paraosteoarthropathies, and human leukocyte antigens. *Arch. Phys. Med. Rehabil.* 61:214–215.

Moeller, B.A., and D. Scheinberg. 1973. Autonomic dysreflexia in injuries below the sixth thoracic segment. *J.A.M.A.* 224:1295.

Montero, J.C., et al. 1967. Effects of glossopharyngeal breathing on respiratory function after cervical cord transection. *Arch. Phys. Med. Rehabil.* 48:650–653.

Morgan, M.D.L., et al. 1986. "The respiration system of the spinal cord injured patient in block." In *Management of spinal cord injuries,* ed. R.F. Block and M. Bausbaum, 78–116. Baltimore, Md.: Williams & Williams.

Nicholas, J.J. 1973. Ectopic bone formation in patients with spinal cord injury. *Arch. Phys. Med. Rehabil.* 54:354–359.

Nixon, V. 1985. *Spinal cord injury: A guide to functional outcomes in physical therapy management.* Gaithersburg, Md.: Aspen.

Orzel, J.A., and T.G. Rudd. 1985. Heterotopic bone formation: Clinical laboratory and imaging correlation. *J. Nucl. Med.* 26:125–132.

Ramchandau, P., et al. 1981. Deep vein thrombosis: Significant limitations of noninvasive tests. *Radiology* 156:47–49.

Rassel, R.G.G., and Smith, R. 1973. Diphosphonates: Experimental and clinical aspects. *J. Bone Joint Surg. Br.* 55:66–86.

Robertson, D.N.S., and L. Guttmann. 1963. The paraplegic patient in pregnancy and labour. *Proc. R. Soc. Med.* 56:381–387.

Rosenow, E.C., et al. 1981. Pulmonary embolism. *Mayo Clin. Proc.* 56:161–178.

Rossi, E.C., et al. 1980. Sequential changes in factor VIII and platelets preceding deep vein thrombosis in patients with spinal cord injury. *Br. J. Haematol.* 45:143–151.

Rossier, A.B., et al. 1973. Current facts on para-osteo-arthropathy (POA). *Paraplegia* 11:36–78.

Samuelson, K.M., and S.S. Coleman. 1976. Nontraumatic myositis ossificans in healthy individuals. *J.A.M.A.* 23S:1132–1133.

Satiani, B. 1981. Diagnostic methods in acute deep venous thrombosis. *Cardiovasc. Rev. Rep.* 2:61–70.

Scher, A.T. 1976. The incidence of ectopic bone formation in post traumatic paraplegic patients of different racial groups. *Paraplegia* 14:202–206.

Schonwald, G., et al. 1981. Cardiovascular complications during anesthesia in chronic spinal cord injured patients. *Anesthesiology* 55:550–558.

Scott, M.B., and J.W. Morrow. 1978. Phenoxybenzamine in neurogenic bladder dysfunction after spinal cord injury. I autonomic dysreflexia. *J. Urol.* 119:483–484.

Sizemore, G.W., and W.W. Winternitz. 1970. Autonomic hyperreflexia—Suppression with α-adrenergic blocking agents. *N. Engl. J. Med.* 282:795.

Stover, S.L. 1989. "Heterotopic ossification after spinal cord injury." In *Management of spinal cord injuries,* ed. R.F. Block and M. Bausbaum, 284–301. Baltimore, Md.: Williams & Wilkins.

Stover, S.L., et al. 1975. Heterotopic ossification in spinal cord injured patients. *Arch. Phys. Med. Rehabil.* 56:199–204.

Stover, S.L., et al. 1976a. Disodium etidronate in the prevention of heterotopic ossification following spinal cord injury (preliminary report). *Paraplegia* 14:146–156.

Stover, S.L., et al. 1976b. Disodium etidronate in the prevention of postoperative recurrence of heterotopic ossification in spinal cord injury patients. *J. Bone Joint Surg. Am.* 58:683–688.

Tanaka, T., et al. 1977. Quantitative assessment of para-osteo-arthropathy and its maturation on serial radionuclide bone images. *Radiology* 123:217–221.

Thompson, C.E., and A.C. Witham. 1948. Paroxysmal hypertension in spinal cord injuries. *N. Engl. J. Med.* 23:291–294.

Thorn-Alquist, A. 1975. Prevention of hypersensitive crises in patients with high spinal lesions during cystoscopy and lithotripsy. *Acta Anaesth. Scand.* 57(suppl.):79–82.

Tibone, J., et al. 1978. Heterotopic ossification around the hip in spinal cord injured patients. *J. Bone Joint Surg. Am.* 60:769–775.

Turba, R.M., et al. 1992. Cough in spinal cord injury: Augmentation by electrical stimulation. *Arch. Phys. Med. Rehabil.* 73:1972 (abstract).

Turpie, A.G.G. 1989. "Thrombosis prevention and treatment in spinal cord injured patients." In *Management of spinal cord injuries,* ed. R.F. Block and M. Bausbaum, 212–240. Baltimore, Md.: Williams & Wilkins.

Turpie, A.G.G., et al. 1986. A randomized controlled trial of a low–molecular-weight heparin (enoxaparin) to prevent deep venous thrombosis in patients undergoing elective hip surgery. *N. Engl. J. Med.* 315:925–929.

Venier, L.H., and J.F. Ditunno. 1971. Heterotopic ossification in the paraplegic patient. *Arch. Phys. Med. Rehabil.* 52:475–479.

Wackwitz, D.L., et al. 1982. Autonomic dysreflexia: Cause of postoperative hemorrhage. *J. Bone Joint Surg. Am.* 64:297–299.

Woo, S.L., et al. 1971. Connective tissue response to immobility. *Arthritis Rheum.* 18:257–269.

Yarkony, G.M., et al. 1985. Contractures complicating spinal cord injury: Incidence and comparison between spinal cord center and general hospital acute care. *Paraplegia* 23:265–271.

Yarkony, G.M., et al. 1986. Seizures secondary to autonomic dysreflexia. *Arch. Phys. Med. Rehabil.* 67:834–835.

Yarkony, G.M., et al. 1989. Heterotopic ossification pseudophlebitis. *Am. J. Med.* 87:342–344.

Young, J.S. 1963. Use of guanethidine in control of sympathetic hyperreflexia in persons with cervical and thoracic cord lesions. *Arch. Phys. Med. Rehabil.* 44:204–207.

Zumwalt, J., et al. 1956. Glossopharyngeal breathing. *Phys. Ther. Rev.* 36:455–460.

Chapter 4

Gastrointestinal Dysfunction in Spinal Cord Injury

Frederick S. Frost

SCOPE OF THE PROBLEM

As survival rates for persons with spinal cord injury (SCI) have improved, more attention has been directed toward quality of life issues. Despite the fact that gastrointestinal (GI) disorders rank seventh as the cause of death in this population (Apple & Hudson 1990), dysfunction of this system has a profound impact on medical morbidity, maintenance of body image, and the need for caregiver support. More than one third of surveyed paraplegics ranked the loss of bowel and bladder control as the most significant functional losses associated with their respective injury, more important than the loss of the use of their legs (Hanson & Franklin 1976). Dependence in the area of bowel emptying can have an impact on virtually every aspect of life, presenting a potential handicap in terms of fulfillment of interpersonal, sexual, and employment roles.

Each year, diseases of the GI tract account for a large percentage of outpatient clinic visits, hospital admissions, and major surgical procedures in the United States, placing a huge economic burden upon the health care system. Studies of GI complications in patients with SCI have traditionally focused upon the acute, postinjury period. Gore et al. (1981) reviewed 567 admissions to an SCI center and identified ileus and gastric ulcer as the most common disorders of the digestive system during the first 4 weeks after injury. As might be expected, during the next 3 months the investigators found that morbidity was more likely to be attributable to lower tract dysfunction, noting the most common problem to be fecal impaction (*n* = 46).

More recent investigations have taken a broader view and have attempted to assess the importance of GI problems over the long term using large outpatient clinic populations that allow for the assessment of chronic GI morbidity. Stone et al. (1990), in a study of 90 SCI outpatients, found that 29% reported GI dysfunction that required therapy or altered their life styles, with an increase in bowel-related problems associated with complete neurologic lesions and a postinjury period of greater than 5 years. In a similar study in 1990, Albert et al. (1990) found that 6% of 1,100 patients with SCI with an average follow-up of 3.8 years exhibited GI complications. Approximately half these complications were due to GI bleeding. Among patients with chronic injuries, the deleterious effects of 20 or more years of suppository use, digital evacuation, and chronic constipation are only now being elucidated as more individuals appear regularly in clinics complaining about their bowel function.

NUTRITION

Although most medical personnel agree about the importance of nutrition in the maintenance of good health, few appreciate the myriad factors that serve as a deterrent to adequate dietary intake in the population with SCI. It is particularly unfortunate to note that in most cases only cursory attention is paid to these matters in the rehabilitation setting, particularly because poor nutrition is the most remediable of factors in the development of disease. In addition, nutrition often takes on a larger meaning than simple food intake: Feeding may be seen as an important issue in independence and socialization or simply as a pleasurable sensory experience for an individual who is otherwise deprived of sensory input.

The physiological, psychological, and environmental causes for malnutrition in this population are not difficult to delineate. During the acute period, persons with SCI invariably will fall behind on protein intake relative to the huge protein losses associated with recovery from major trauma (Peiffer et al. 1981). In fact, the careful resumption of oral intake may be a major goal during the critical care period because concomitant trauma to the GI tract or disorders associated with acute neurologic injury may preclude feeding. Although careful attention may be given to these issues in the critical care setting with the utilization of hyperalimentation and nutritional supplements, carryover of nutritional issues into the postacute period often falls short of the mark. After discharge from intensive care, nutritional status may decline for a number of reasons.

Many of those discharged from intensive care simply may not feel well enough to eat. Often patients are constipated upon admission to the rehabilitation setting, a remediable cause of nausea and poor appetite. Resumption of a higher level of activity and involvement in a more stimulating environment usually will result in an increased appetite. For patients with quadriplegia at the C-5 level and below, mealtime occupational therapy for training in feeding skills takes on extreme medical and psychological importance. Moreover, a patient's appetite may be further discouraged by unpalatable hospital food. Although most facilities encourage the patient's family and friends to bring food from home, this practice is not inherently laudable. Particularly in the pediatric and teenage populations, increased vigilance is necessary to ensure that some semblance of a balanced diet is maintained. Particular emphasis must be placed upon dietary fiber and protein intake. Despite protein supplementation, most patients with SCI show evidence of poor assimilation of ingested protein during the acute injury period (Cooper et al. 1950).

Sophisticated and complicated nutritional assessment of this patient population rarely is necessary. Whether due to issues of inconvenience or lack of proper equipment and personnel, the most important measures in nutritional assessment—the patient's weight and calorie count—often are not performed. Weekly weights for newly injured persons with quadriplegia constitute an important standard of medical care. Blood tests for serum creatinine, albumin, and hemoglobin by themselves are of questionable use in their application to this patient population (Ring et al. 1974) and are not a viable alternative to the performance of a calorie count for the patient who is failing to maintain body weight.

The maintenance of appropriate body weight is of obvious importance for the person with a chronic disability. Small changes in body weight can restrict physical mobility in per-

sons with borderline function and can have devastating implications for those individuals prone to pressure sores (Greenway et al. 1969). In a study of persons with chronic SCI, Peiffer et al. (1981) found that 44% of persons in both quadriplegic and paraplegic groups were more than 10% below their ideal body weight even after allowance had been made for their neurologic injury. For persons with paraplegia, the recommended guideline was 10 to 15 lb below the standard calculated nondisabled body weight for sex and height, adjusting for body frame and build. For persons with quadriplegia, a decrement of 15 to 20 lb was allowed by standard calculated values for the nondisabled person. Persons falling 10% or more below these standards, with caloric and protein intake less than calculated maintenance levels, must be considered at nutritional risk.

SWALLOWING

In the acute assessment of a person with cervical spine trauma, the evaluation of the patency of the esophagus and the ability to swallow is of critical importance. Because the posterior wall of the pharynx lies adjacent to the anterior aspect of the cervical vertebrae, severe cervical trauma may cause bony elements to impinge upon or even perforate the pharynx or esophagus. Elderly patients with cervical osteoarthritis may develop esophageal dysphagia, even in the absence of trauma, because large anterior cervical osteophytes encroach upon passage of a food bolus. Although the incidence of esophageal rupture in these patients is low, the index of suspicion on the part of the clinician must be high. The leakage of saliva and food into adjacent cervical tissue planes may result in the formation of a mediastinal abscess, a condition with disastrous consequences. Initial evaluation by endoscopy or water-soluble radiographic contrast studies is recommended if the clinical suspicion of perforation is present. Examination of a lacerated GI tract with barium sulfate is not recommended if mediastinal extension is a consideration (Gelfand 1980).

Although the neurologic mechanisms of swallowing should be unaffected even in high-level quadriplegic injuries, a variety of mechanical and medical causes of swallowing disorders may predispose the patient to aspiration of saliva or food material. Chief among these are the use of skeletal traction (usually holding the neck in forced extension) and the necessity of patient sedation, which may circumvent the basic components of airway protection. Because anterior cervical decompression and fusion procedures are gaining increased popularity in the acute setting, the swelling and local pain associated with these interventions along with the soreness related to oropharyngeal airway use may result in significant dysphagia.

Elderly patients and patients with premorbid psychiatric illness are at special risk for developing swallowing difficulties.

A lack of somatic sensory input, increased pulmonary secretions, and forced supine positioning in the intensive care setting, combined with claustrophobia and disorientation, may result in panic episodes and the sensation of drowning. For these reasons, patients who have been switched from tong traction to Halo vest immobilization must be observed carefully for the first few hours after application, and great caution must be exercised in making the decision to move the patient from the intensive care unit to the general nursing floor.

In the intensive care setting, interventions such as early tracheotomy and the use of a cuffed tracheostomy tube allow for better pulmonary hygiene and provide some airway protection against impaired swallowing; inflation of the tracheostomy tube cuff is not a foolproof protection against aspiration of swallowed substances, however, because liquids may pass around the cuff. In patients who are receiving mechanical ventilation, cuffless tubes, combined with appropriate ventilator adjustment to compensate for inflation volume loss, are often superior to cuffed tubes; particulate matter that collects around the cuffless tube may actually be blown into the oropharynx and swallowed during the ventilator inflation phase.

Tracheostomy tubes (especially those attached to heavy ventilator tubing) may further affect swallowing in these patients. By applying traction to the neck, these devices may inhibit the normal upward translation of the pharynx necessary to complete the swallowing action. Stable ventilator tubing brackets are an important component of the bedside equipment set-up and an essential part of a wheelchair prescription for a ventilator-dependent quadriplegic patient.

Little scientific analysis of the swallowing disorders in patients with high quadriplegia has been performed to date. In the evaluation of those with swallowing difficulty, there is preliminary evidence that the cricopharyngeal phase of swallowing is disrupted and that this may be remediable by instruction of the patient in the use of the Mendelsson maneuver (Logeman 1990). The pathophysiologic explanation for this deficiency is as yet undetermined.

ESOPHAGUS, STOMACH, AND SMALL BOWEL

Although CNS input closely controls both ends of the digestive tract (the upper esophagus and the external anal sphincter), the balance of the system can function fairly well in the absence of CNS input. Such autonomous activity is attributed to intrinsic reflexes mediated by nerve ganglia found within the walls of the visceral structures. For this reason, in persons with SCI the basic propulsive, secretory, and absorptive functions of the digestive system usually are maintained; the fine-tuning of these actions, however, depends upon the modulating influences of the autonomic nervous system and a variety of neurotransmitters and peptides (Wattchow et al.

1988). An injury to the spinal cord can result in derangement of these secondary regulating factors and have a significant effect upon digestive function.

GI REFLUX DISEASE

Symptoms of heartburn, dysphagia, retrosternal pain, hiccoughs, excessive salivation, or regurgitation may indicate excessive reflux of gastric contents into the esophagus. Several factors may be present in the patient with SCI that promote reflux disease (Exhibit 4–1). Symptoms of reflux disease are usually nonspecific, and actual esophagitis may not necessarily be present. In many instances, symptomatic therapy is instituted without endoscopic or histologic confirmation of esophagitis; radiologic or endoscopic study is critical when abdominal pain (rather than burning) or blood loss is present, however, or when pulmonary aspiration is suspected. In addition, perfusion of acid into the esophagus through a catheter (the Bernstein test) can be carried out to determine whether such a challenge reproduces the patient's symptoms. The conventional assumption that sensory fibers supplying the esophagus are vagal in origin (and therefore unaffected by SCI) has been reached through indirect evidence and animal studies. Thus it is likely that acid challenge testing would be reliable even in patients with high cervical cord lesions.

The treatment of reflux disease is directed at ameliorating the basic elements of this condition: poor esophageal acid clearance, impaired function of the lower esophageal sphincter, and increased acidity of stomach contents. Elevation of the head of the bed to 30° is nearly always helpful, but use of skeletal traction and orthopedic stability may preclude this maneuver during the acute phase after SCI. Dietary measures center on the restriction of fatty foods and reinstitution of a regular mealtime schedule with moderation in size of meals. In some instances, the cessation of cigarette smoking and restriction of caffeine and alcohol ingestion will result in resolution of symptoms without further therapy. If such simple measures

Exhibit 4–1 Factors Promoting GI Reflux in Persons with SCI

Medical:	recumbency and immobilization, delayed gastric emptying, increased gastrin and acid release, irregular mealtime patterns
Drugs (lower pressure in esophageal sphincter):	diazepam, theophylline, meperidine, anticholinergics, antispasmodics, tricyclic antidepressants, calcium channel blockers, nitrates
Miscellaneous:	cigarettes, fatty foods, chocolate, citrus juices, coffee

are not of benefit, antacids of the alginic acid type can be given four times a day. H$_2$ antagonists may be used to reduce the acidity of refluxed stomach contents. In those patients with documented esophagitis and refractory symptoms, bethanechol (25 mg four times daily) and metoclopramide (10 mg three times daily) may augment esophageal clearance while elevating lower esophageal sphincter pressures (Humphries & Castell 1981; McCallum et al. 1977). Newer pharmacologic agents that affect gut motility through noncholinergic mechanisms (cisapride and domperidone) have been used in this population and may be of benefit (Binnie et al. 1988; Smout et al. 1985). In refractory cases, surgery can be performed in hopes of restoring esophageal sphincter competence.

IMPAIRMENT OF GASTRIC EMPTYING

The clinical observation that gastric distension and ileus commonly occur after acute SCI is not surprising in that impairment of GI motility may be associated with major trauma, immobilization, or recumbency. The relative importance of the neurologic injury, with potential alteration in autonomic control of the GI tract, has been assessed by direct and indirect means.

When studied in the chronic stage of SCI, persons with spinal cord transection above the T-1 level have demonstrated prolonged gastric emptying and abnormal propagation of propulsive motor complexes in the stomach and duodenum compared with control subjects with lower spinal cord lesions (Fealey et al. 1984; Shuster 1981). This observation is interesting from both a clinical and a pathophysiologic standpoint because it implicates the thoracic sympathetic outflow (T5–10) as an important contributor to the digestive processes of the stomach and duodenum. Further confirmation of the relative importance of neurologic injury was provided by Peschiera and Beerman (1990), who found an extremely low incidence of intestinal dysfunction in patients who had sustained spinal fractures without neurologic injury.

In pointing out evidence that supports the concept of a neurologic component in the development of motility problems, it is important to avoid overstating the relative clinical importance of such phenomena. The underlying mechanisms behind the development of GI motility disorders are not well understood but are most certainly multifactorial. Gut motility is no doubt influenced by general health status, diet, physical activity, electrolyte disturbances, and a number of drugs commonly used in this population. The metabolic and endocrine changes associated with SCI (Claus-Walker & Halstead 1981) may also play a role.

Impairment of gastric emptying can manifest itself through a wide range of signs and symptoms. Not infrequently, a stomach distended with swallowed air will be noted on a plain chest radiograph during the acute phase of SCI; this finding must not be considered insignificant, however, even in patients with no active GI symptomatology. If it persists, such distension can restrict pulmonary ventilation and promote the development of atelectasis. In addition, these abnormalities in gastric emptying have been shown to decrease the bioavailability of orally administered drugs (Segal et al. 1985), a finding of considerable clinical importance. Incomplete GI drug absorption should be acknowledged as a possible cause of therapeutic failure. Most important, the presence of gastric distension may herald more serious GI pathology and the development of intestinal ileus. It is important to determine that actual gastric obstruction is not present before embarking upon a therapeutic plan. This condition is uncommon, but a delay in diagnosis can have disastrous implications.

Gastric outlet obstruction occurs most commonly as a result of peptic ulcer disease and may occasionally occur as the initial presentation of an ulcer. Less commonly, mechanical blockade may be caused by local tumor, pancreatitis, or inflammatory bowel disease.

The symptoms of nausea, epigastric distension, or anorexia are too nonspecific to be diagnostic in most situations when the patient appears acutely ill. The presence of vomiting, especially when it occurs 1 hour or more after meals, is particularly worrisome and usually warrants further investigation and intervention. A plain radiograph of the abdomen is helpful, primarily in determining whether free air is present in the peritoneal cavity, a sign of gastric perforation. The placement of a nasogastric tube will often provide objective evidence of obstruction. A saline load test can be performed by instilling 750 mL of isotonic saline into the stomach. The removal of more than 400 mL of fluid 30 minutes thereafter supports the diagnosis of obstruction. An upper GI series or radionuclide scintigraphy will further outline the problem.

A large percentage of patients with noncancerous obstruction will respond to medical management of this condition with an emphasis on gastric decompression (by nasogastric suction), correction of fluid and electrolyte disorders, and nutritional support. Persistent output of large gastric volumes after 72 hours is a poor prognostic sign, indicating that surgical correction may be necessary.

The nonobstructed delay in gastric emptying seen in many patients with SCI will prove less life threatening but no less bothersome to the patient. These patients may benefit from approaches utilized in persons with emptying disorders secondary to other conditions (diabetic gastroparesis, vagotomy, and viral illnesses), although no careful evaluation of the efficacy of these methods has been carried out in patients with SCI. Gastric motility will improve during the acute phase of SCI as electrolyte abnormalities are corrected and general health improves. From a pharmacologic standpoint, metoclopramide (10 mg 30 minutes before meals) is the best agent available at this time, but it is of little benefit when used over the long term. Cholinergic agents (e.g., 25 mg of bethanechol 30 minutes before meals) also are helpful in some instances. In the chronic setting, dietary management constitutes the most effective therapy. A change to small portions of soft cooked foods, chewed well, will almost always result in improvement of symptoms. For quadriplegic patients with severe and chronic gastric distension, placement of a gastrostomy tube for gaseous decompression has been shown to be effective (Cosman et al. 1991).

ILEUS AND INTESTINAL OBSTRUCTION

Although there is no evidence that CNS injury by itself causes impairment of transit through the small intestine, medical conditions associated with SCI no doubt have a significant impact on such processes. Intestinal obstruction is a frequent complicating factor after the acute injury and is a common cause of rehospitalization of patients in the chronic stage of disability (Gore et al. 1981).

Just as in the case of impaired gastric emptying, intestinal obstruction may be secondary to mechanical blockage or to disorders of bowel motility. Because persons with SCI may have impairment of pain appreciation, obstruction may initially be manifested only by nausea, obstipation and abdominal distension. If the blockage is distal in the colon, vomiting may not be seen until late in the clinical course. On examination, bowel sounds that are frequent and high pitched (suggestive of an early mechanical obstruction) or completely absent indicate a need to take action. Liberal use of diagnostic testing is necessary; plain abdominal radiographs, complete blood counts, and serum electrolyte determinations are critical in establishing a diagnosis.

Mechanical obstruction of the small bowel has been reported in the postacute stages of SCI (Greenfield 1948). A clear demarcation between proximal dilated bowel and distal collapsed bowel may be seen on plain radiographs. The treatment for such lesions is almost invariably surgical, and the cause for the obstruction (e.g., tumors, adhesions, or hernias) is rarely determined before surgical exploration.

As an exception, the superior mesenteric artery syndrome has been reported to occur with frequency in persons with quadriplegia (Roth et al. 1991). This condition has a characteristic prodrome: Such patients will exhibit epigastric pain (especially in the supine position) and may have frequent episodes of vomiting large volumes of material. A characteristic appearance is seen on fluoroscopy: A cut-off between the third and fourth portions of the duodenum is demonstrated in the supine posture, which disappears with the subject in the upright posture. This condition is usually found in immobilized patients who recently have undergone significant weight loss and is probably caused by a loss of the mesenteric fat that serves to shield the duodenum as it passes behind the superior mesenteric artery and in front of the lumbar spine and aorta.

This type of mechanical obstruction is also exceptional in that it may respond to medical management (upright body positioning and dietary support).

Intestinal obstructions of a nonmechanical nature often are termed adynamic (or paralytic) ileus or pseudo-obstruction. Adynamic ileus occurs as a response to a major trauma, anesthesia, surgery, or severe medical illness; because SCI often involves all these, signs and symptoms of adynamic ileus are seen commonly regardless of the level of injury. Although symptoms may mirror those seen in mechanical obstruction, they typically are less striking; adynamic ileus tends to follow an indolent course, developing gradually over 3 to 4 days. In the acutely injured patient, auscultation for bowel sounds must be carried out carefully and frequently, as the disappearance of bowel sounds may occur before symptomatology becomes evident. On plain films of the abdomen, dilatation is commonly present throughout the small intestine and colon. Every effort should be made, despite orthopedic restrictions, to obtain upright or lateral decubitus films to determine whether air–fluid levels are present.

Abnormalities in serum electrolytes and fluid status may occur as either a cause or an effect of adynamic ileus. Once ileus occurs, several liters of plasma volume may be sequestered into the edematous intestinal wall, making restoration of fluid balance difficult. Most often this picture is associated with hyponatremia and hypochloremia.

The treatment of adynamic ileus follows the same rationale as the treatment for gastric obstruction. In most cases the cause of the condition is multifactorial, with resolution being brought about by careful restoration of electrolyte balance and general supportive measures. Intestinal decompression through nasogastric suction is indicated and should be maintained until symptoms improve (with passage of stool or gas) and plain abdominal radiographs begin to show resolution of the abnormal gas patterns. Surface electrical stimulation has been shown to increase upper and lower GI motility and may aid in resolution of ileus during the acute period (Richardson & Cerullo 1979).

Chronic neglect of proper bowel emptying and poor general health, combined with baseline motility disorders of SCI, may predispose the patient to the development of intermittent episodes of ileus, more appropriately termed secondary intestinal pseudoobstruction. Although primary pseudoobstruction, a devastating and rare global disorder of bowel motility, is probably an inherited disorder, secondary pseudoobstruction involves recurrent episodes of ileus that occur as a response to a chronic condition (e.g., collagen vascular disease, drug effects, and neurologic motility disorders). Most commonly, this is seen in persons with chronic SCI who may be under hospitalization for conditions such as urosepsis or pneumonia and who exhibit symptoms of abdominal distension and signs of ileus on plain films of the abdomen. Treatment of the underlying medical condition is the key, although the management may be made more difficult because of the coincident presence of large amounts of stool in the colon.

In most cases, this clinical picture involves an acute decline in health status combined with the effects of hospitalization of a patient with poor baseline fitness. Admission to the hospital, by itself, will take the patient away from standard activity and from dietary and bowel-emptying routines. Health care providers often do not anticipate the need for artificial bowel emptying in these patients early in their admission. With the appearance of GI symptoms, abdominal radiographs are obtained, and the discovery of large amounts of stool in the colon, a normal finding in chronic SCI, often leads to the incorrect conclusion that fecal impaction is the primary problem. This in turn will lead to therapeutic maneuvers that may make the situation worse rather than better. Strong oral cathartics may be given to relieve the impaction, an action that serves only to fill a poorly motile gastrointestinal tract with more gas and fluid, worsening symptoms and producing further dilatation of the small bowel on radiographic study. In some instances, GI perforation can occur (Moses 1988). Fortunately, in most cases treatment of the primary medical illness is successful; general supportive measures result in a return of intestinal motility, and the pseudoobstruction resolves spontaneously. Of course, there will be instances where fecal impaction is indeed the cause of intestinal obstruction. Management of this condition is described below.

ABDOMINAL PAIN AND THE ACUTE ABDOMEN

The evaluation of abdominal pain and acute abdominal processes in persons with SCI is among the most frustrating problems of medical practice. In this population, many patients will exhibit impairment of visceral sensation, thereby eliminating many of the clues to diagnosis often gained by history and physical examination. In the case of an obstruction, perforated ulcer, or ruptured viscus, abdominal discomfort may not be present until the inflammatory process has reached the peritoneum of the upper abdominal quadrants, which carry the nerve supply from the upper cervical segments. In the acute SCI trauma setting, laparoscopy often is necessary to rule out the possibility of concomitant injury to the viscera.

In the rehabilitation and chronic care setting, acute abdominal complaints are too often incorrectly ascribed early in their course to pyelonephritis or constipation. In the emergency department, mild leukocytosis and pyuria are nonspecific findings in all SCI patients; it is the presence of constipation that puts these persons at even greater risk for acute abdominal disorders because it results in a higher incidence of diverticuli and rectal fistulas, increasing the likelihood of bowel perforation (Charney et al. 1975). Immobilization and atherosclerosis in older patients with SCI may predispose these patients to the development of mesenteric vascular thrombosis or infarct. Gallbladder disease is especially common in these patients,

probably as a result of dysmotility (Chassin et al. 1988). The predisposition for the development of biliary tract disease, combined with a high incidence of previous abdominal trauma and alcoholism in these patients, presents a clinical picture that is favorable for the development of acute pancreatitis. As a diagnosis of exclusion, neurogenic abdominal pain must be considered, particularly in paraplegic patients. A burning or lancinating pain, sometimes localized to the border between sensate and insensate skin, may represent a neurologic, dysesthetic pain syndrome.

Obviously, these points necessitate a particular vigilance on the part of the evaluating physician when confronted with vague abdominal symptomatology. Subtle clues, such as an increase in abdominal muscle spasticity, may be present early in the course of an abdominal perforation. As noted above, plain abdominal radiographs are essential to determine whether free air is present in the abdominal cavity. On examination, close attention is given to the presence and nature of bowel sounds. A serum amylase level and daily leukocyte counts are recommended. Noninvasive duplex ultrasound scanning can be used to determine whether vascular thrombosis is present. Computed tomography of the abdomen and pelvis should be performed when one is confronted with an SCI patient with malaise, leukocytosis, and an absence of localizing signs.

ULCER DISEASE AND BLEEDING

Bleeding from the upper GI tract is an infrequent but dangerous complication of SCI in both acute and chronic phases of injury. The reported incidence of GI bleeding and ulceration in patients with SCI varies from 0.5% to 22.0% (Kewalramani 1979). Kiwerski (1986) found that 52 of 2,000 (2.6%) patients with SCI had documentation of significant postinjury upper GI bleeding and noted that bleeding most often occurred in patients with a complete injury of the cervical spinal cord during the acute postinjury period. Most patients had no history of peptic ulcer disease. In the chronic stage of SCI, more than half those patients with nonspecific abdominal symptoms will be shown to have abnormalities on endoscopy (Tanaka et al. 1979).

Shortly after injury, multiple factors may predispose the patient to gastritis and ulceration, including stress, malnutrition, hypovolemic shock, and the use of steroids, antithrombotic agents, and nonsteroidal antiinflammatory drugs (NSAIDs). It has been postulated that the maintenance of vagal tone in the absence of effective thoracic sympathetic input to the stomach results in gastric hypersecretion and hyperacidity in these patients (Pollack & Finkelman 1954). In comparison with other types of severe injuries, those to the CNS have been shown to result in higher levels of serum gastrin (Bowen et al. 1974). This phenomenon could be explained, in part, by the possible association of peptic ulcer and corticosteroid therapy commonly implemented in patients with CNS trauma (Messer et al. 1983). Steroid treatment may also be associated with nonhemorrhagic perforation of the lower GI tract, especially if colonic diverticuli are present (Fadul et al. 1988). It remains to be seen whether recent trends involving the short-term use of large doses of glucocorticoids after acute trauma will result in a higher incidence of GI bleeding (Bracken et al. 1990).

Prevention of stress gastritis and ulcer disease during the acute injury period centers on the alteration of acid secretion. Both antacids and H_2 receptor blockers (cimetidine and ranitidine) have been shown to be superior to placebo treatment for the prevention of mucosa erosion in patients who are critically ill. Newer H_2 blockers (nizatidine and famotidine) as well as omeprazole, a powerful suppressant of gastric acid secretion, are still under evaluation for use in the acute setting. Sucralfate, through enhancing mucosal defenses, also has been shown to be effective in preventing acute GI bleeding in critically ill patients (Cannon et al. 1987). Misoprostol, an analog of prostaglandin E_1, inhibits gastric acid secretion and may prevent gastric ulceration caused by the effect of NSAIDs on the prostaglandin pathways. This drug, although expensive, may have greater use in the rehabilitation and chronic care setting, where NSAIDs have an important role in the treatment of pain and inflammation.

The suspicion of active upper GI bleeding invariably calls for endoscopic evaluation. This may be difficult if the patient is immobilized in a halo orthosis or if neck motion is limited by bony fusion. Barium studies should be avoided because the presence of contrast media may impair endoscopic therapeutic maneuvers should the patient have an acute decline in hemodynamic status. Contrast studies are also limited by the patient's ability to participate in the required position changes as a result of mobility restrictions. Treatment in this setting may involve coagulation or embolization via endoscope or infusion of intra-arterial vasopressin via arteriography.

THE COLON AND ANORECTUM

The term *neurogenic bowel* has been used to describe a number of disorders of bowel emptying in the population with SCI. This is unfortunate in that the term overemphasizes the importance of extrinsic innervation and central control of the lower GI tract and ignores the significant amount of reflex activity and local control that remains even in patients with profound neurologic deficits. A working knowledge of these local control mechanisms and how they can be manipulated provides a key to successful bowel management.

NEUROLOGIC AND HORMONAL CONTROL OF THE COLON

In contrast to the urinary bladder, the colon serves much more than a simple storage and expulsion function. Through-out its length, the mucosa of the large bowel plays a key role in the dynamic processing of the waste material before elimination. Control of its complicated functions is carried out through the input of the autonomic nervous system with significant contribution from GI peptide hormones that act either through the systemic circulation or as neurotransmitters released in the periphery.

A number of peptides have been identified that stimulate colonic motility through these mechanisms. Substance P, gastrin, enkephalin, and cholecystokinin have been implicated as colonic stimulants. The specific location of their action is still unclear because these substances have been identified in the circulation, within the wall of the colon, and within the axons of the myenteric nerve plexi (Wattchow et al. 1988). Secretin and glucagon have long been known to inhibit colonic function. Vasoactive intestinal peptide (VIP), a strong inhibitor of smooth muscle contractility, plays an important role in the forward propulsive activities of the gut (Koch et al. 1988). The discovery of VIP is especially interesting because this substance has been identified as a neurotransmitter in both the somatic and the autonomic nervous systems, perhaps serving as a neurochemical link that can help explain the obvious influence of the higher functions of the CNS over the baseline autonomic control of the bowel.

The extrinsic neural control of the colon has been studied extensively in animals, but significant anatomical differences found between species serve to cast doubt upon the relevance of these studies in outlining the nerve supply to the human colon. Recently, human studies involving direct electrical stimulation in quadriplegic patients have helped map human neural control of the bowel directly (Brindley et al. 1982).

Confusion arises over the terminology used to describe neurologic control over the propulsion of feces through the bowel. The maintenance of normal bowel activity involves a complex coordination of relaxation and contraction of the bowel wall. In this regard, a hypertonic bowel may impede waste flow if not accompanied by patterned relaxation. As a result, use of the terms *facilitation* and *inhibition* is confusing because the facilitation of smooth muscle tone may actually inhibit the flow of digested material. For this discussion, such terms will be applied solely to their effect on propulsion of intraluminal contents.

The parasympathetic output to the colon is almost exclusively stimulatory to the movement of feces. The vagus nerve supplies the GI tract to the level of the transverse colon, with the lower bowel being under the parasympathetic control of the sacral pelvic nerves. Sympathetic nervous system influences are inhibitory to the colonic propulsion. Sympathetic innervation is carried from the thoracolumbar segments of the spinal cord through the superior mesenteric ganglion and splanchnic nerves to the proximal colon. Distal colonic segments receive efferent sympathetic fibers from the lumbar colonic nerves through the inferior mesenteric ganglion. Sensory impulses arise primarily from mechanoreceptors in the wall of the colon, travel through peripheral parasympathetic nuclei, and send collateral fibers along preganglionic pathways to corresponding sacral dorsal root ganglia. The role of these sensory fibers is gaining increasing attention because local reflex loops are known to affect colonic motility in animals (Longhurst 1988).

Near the mucocutaneous junction in the rectum, GI smooth muscle merges with the striated fibers of the external anal sphincter, which is under somatic, voluntary control. Although the rectum derives its sensory supply from parasympathetic fibers, the anus sends cutaneous sensory impulses through the inferior hemorrhoidal nerves. Motor supply to the perianal striated musculature comes by way of the internal

pudendal nerve and the perineal branch of the fourth sacral nerve (Goligher et al. 1955).

Numerous areas of the brain, brain stem, and spinal cord have been shown to exert a direct influence over bowel function. Recent advances in brain stem imaging have allowed investigators to correlate specific CNS lesions with abnormalities in colonic motility studies in humans (Weber et al. 1985). It is likely that the higher levels of the CNS serve to inhibit spinal cord control centers for colonic function. This is clearly shown in patients with high spinal cord transection, who exhibit a generalized increase in colonic tone (Connell et al. 1963).

The spinal cord itself historically has been downplayed as a simple wiring system and relay center from the brain and brain

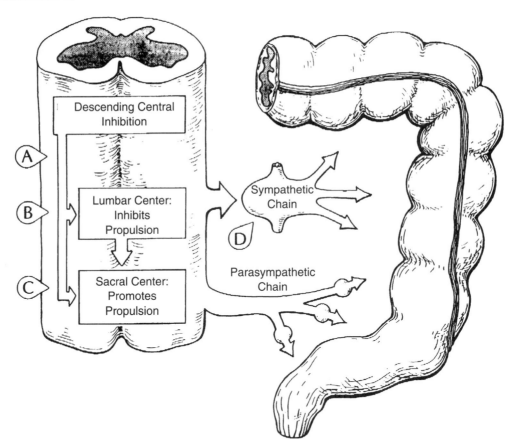

Figure 4–1 Schematic representation of extrinsic neurologic control of the descending colon and rectum. Fecal propulsion, involving regulation of relaxation and contraction of the bowel wall muscle, results from the interaction of extrinsic control with the enteric nervous system. A CNS lesion above the lumbar segments of the spinal cord (A) leaves the lumbar and sacral reflex centers intact, although a slight predominance of inhibitory influences from lumbar centers may develop. A lesion of the lumbar cord (B) decreases sympathetic inhibition and removes descending inhibition of the bowel from the sacral cord center, resulting in increased bowel propulsion. Lesions involving the sacral cord (C) or peripheral preganglionic parasympathetic fibers result in intractable loss of lower colonic tone and motility. Chemical or surgical sympathetic ablation (D) may have little effect on propulsion because the lumbar spinal cord remains intact, capable of modulating and inhibiting sacral promotion of bowel activity. *Source:* From Kahrilas, P.J., and Frost, F.S., "Disorders of Alimentation and Bowel Motility," in *Medical Management of Long-Term Disability*, D. Green, ed., p. 32. Copyright © 1990, Aspen Publishers, Inc.

stem; it is now clear, however, that the spinal cord plays an important role in processing information at segmental levels and that specific areas of the cord itself are important in the control of bowel and bladder function. Studies of patients with SCI at various levels have provided evidence of the importance of specific areas of the cord in relation to bowel activity (Figure 4–1). Individuals with spinal cord lesions of the lumbar cord may exhibit a marked increase in colonic motility, whereas patients with surgical or chemical lesions of the lumbar sympathetic chain show no significant changes in bowel function (Connell et al. 1963). These studies implicate the lumbar spinal cord as an inhibitory center for propulsion in the distal colon. In contrast, sacral lower motor neuron transections have been carried out in humans to facilitate bladder function, resulting in total elimination of colonic motility (Devroede & LaMarche 1974). These observations, along with several animal studies, point to a facilitory function present in the sacral nerves, as might be expected by the predominance of parasympathetic fibers in this region.

Despite being prevented from communicating with higher centers, the spinal cord below the level of a traumatic lesion usually is very much alive and active with considerable residual segmental reflex activity. Thus the patient with a high spinal cord lesion is usually left with functioning lumbar and sacral control centers removed from weak descending inhibitory influences. Although these individuals exhibit a generalized increase in bowel tone, the clinical function of the bowel is easier to manage than in those individuals with lumbar or sacral lesions.

At the peripheral level, basic propulsive properties of colonic smooth muscle are mediated by the myenteric nerve plexus. The neurologic influence promotes local relaxation, as shown by the increase in activity after the administration of neural antagonists and by the hypertonic bowel noted in humans with congenital absence of the myenteric plexus (Kaufman et al. 1988).

The study of colonic neurologic activity is fraught with problems. Disorders of colonic function usually are studied by colonic pressure recordings, or colonometrograms. Such motility investigations are limited by the large number of variables affecting bowel motility that are nearly impossible to control in experimental settings (e.g., diet, medications, and level of activity). It is therefore difficult to determine whether a change in motility has taken place as a result of a single experimental intervention. In light of this, strategies aimed at improvement of bowel function are best evaluated by assessing patient satisfaction. Studied in the electrophysiology laboratory, normal neural control at the local level of the bowel wall can be recorded by surface or needle electrodes as spike potentials and as slow waves, which are responsible for the mixing activity of the bowel. Abnormalities in the patterns of slow waves and spike potentials have been shown in SCI as well as in a wide variety of other neurologic conditions; the

utility of these findings is minimal in everyday practice, however. The range of normal physiologic activity measured in spike potentials and slow waves is quite wide, even when one is studying healthy control subjects.

The Bowel-Emptying Program

Sensing that the rectum is full, the nondisabled individual can get to the toilet and assume a body position appropriate for emptying. A low toilet is optimal because flexion of the knees and forward bending of the trunk increase abdominal pressure and put the rectum at the optimal angle for emptying. Next, the glottis is closed and intraabdominal pressure is raised, pushing the waste material downward toward the anorectal verge. With stretching of this area, the anorectal reflex is activated, relaxing the proximal anal region. Voluntary relaxation of the external sphincter completes the emptying process.

At each point of the defecation process, the patient with SCI may be at a disadvantage. Recumbency and impaired motility may prevent the mass movement of waste through the bowel. The gastrocolic reflex may be absent after spinal cord transection (Glick et al. 1984). The sensation of a full rectum may be impaired. Mobility deficits may make toileting impossible. In many instances, raised toilet seats are used to make transfers easier, placing the patient in an unfavorable posture for defecation. The lack of chest and abdominal wall muscle tone or the presence of a tracheostomy will result in the inability to raise intraabdominal pressures. If cauda equina or conus lesions are present, the patient may be devoid of reflex defecation mechanisms.

Simple interventions in these instances will benefit the patient. An abdominal binder will raise Valsalva pressures to the rectum. The patient can be situated in an upright position and flexed at the hip, or the program can be carried out in the right lateral sidelying position to take advantage of gravity and the natural rectal curvature. Most important, progressive physical mobilization will promote general health and normal mass movement of fecal material.

Upon admission to the rehabilitation unit, most patients will exhibit fecal impaction. Once this is treated (see below), the efficient bowel program calls for oral management of stool consistency through diet and rectal management of defecation through a combination of evacuants and/or manual removal. Ideally, oral cathartics will play a minimal role in this scenario. In practice, many of the oral medications used in the hospital for bowel management are discarded when the patient returns home to previous dietary habits. Particular attention must be given to all medications that the patient receives. Those that impair bowel function (e.g., clonidine, ferrous sulfate, codeine preparations, anticholinergics, and tricyclic antidepressants) will interfere with the establishment of a regular emptying pattern.

The role of dietary fiber in these instances is clear. Because the presence of liquid stool in the rectum is synonymous with incontinence in this group, maintenance of proper stool consistency is dependent upon regulation of fiber intake. Patients must achieve therapeutic constipation to maintain continence. Education about the fiber content of foods is essential; a change of only 25% in the amount of fiber in the diet can result in a significant change in stool consistency (Rousseau 1988). Experimentation with fiber intake must be supervised, however, especially in the case of bran fiber. Patients with erratic fluid intake or dehydration may develop intestinal obstruction because bran fiber increases stool bulk beyond the capacity of the body to saturate the waste material. If the patient is unable or unwilling to adhere to a healthy diet, the use of fiber supplementation in the form of commercial fiber preparations will be necessary.

Stool softeners, chiefly docusate preparations (Colace), are commonly used in the rehabilitation setting. The benefit of their use in this population is questionable (Chapman et al. 1985). They may act to soften by adding gas to fecal material, not by adding water (even the hardest stool is fully saturated). There is also the potential for hepatotoxicity because these products enhance the absorption of drugs that are metabolized by the liver.

In most instances, patients with spinal cord dysfunction should be encouraged to avoid the use of oral cathartic medications in their regular bowel routine. The time to onset of action is totally unpredictable in this population. Because sphincter control is not present, bowel accidents will be the rule rather than the exception. In addition, many of the commonly used cathartics have been shown to present significant risks when used over the long term. The regular use of cathartics in persons with refractory motility disorders and recurrent impaction is discussed below.

The final component of the bowel program, emptying of the rectum, is usually accomplished by artificial means. Occasionally, persons with incomplete injuries, good rectal sensation, and cooperative GI tracts are able to empty the rectum by abdominal massage and Valsalva maneuver; in most cases, however, external stimulation of rectal reflexes must be employed. The routine is best performed every other day or every third day. Insistence on daily emptying is unrealistic. It must be remembered that artificial means of emptying are being employed, and these means, if used every day, usually result in overstimulation of the rectal mucosa and increased production of mucus and gas. This increase in the net amount of fluid in the rectum will promote incontinence in those patients who have no control over the anal sphincter.

In this setting, manual removal of stool, suppositories, enemas, and digital stimulation of rectal reflexes are among the modalities used. In many instances, reliance on these measures means a loss of independence for the patient. Many physically disabled individuals lack the flexibility and hand function required to manage bowel emptying.

Digital stimulation can be performed with the patient on the commode or recumbent in right sidelying. Inserting the finger with stimulation of the anus will result in an increase in the electrophysiologic activity of the rectum (Roman & Gonella 1987) and will stimulate the distal propulsion of fecal material. When a suppository is used, digital stimulation should be applied after the suppository dissolves and should be repeated every 10 minutes thereafter until emptying is completed.

In some patients, local defecation reflexes may be aberrant, resulting in a failure of sphincter relaxation in response to increased rectal pressures (Stone et al. 1990). This may be analogous to the uncoordinated activity of bladder and urinary sphincter known as detrusor-sphincter dyssynergia. Other patients with sacral nerve lesions or chronic overdistension of the rectum may not possess any discernible reflex activity. In such instances, digital removal of stool is necessary.

The same reflex mechanisms outlined above are stimulated by the use of suppositories and enemas. These agents act to soften and lubricate the stool for passage, but their ability actually to flush the bowel is minimal. In fact, these agents act primarily by providing an artificial irritant to the anorectal mucosa, which serves to promote motility in this region. Suppositories are inserted at the start of the bowel program, followed in most cases by digital stimulation. This route of chemical delivery is usually preferable to the use of enemas because most patients with sphincter paralysis will be unable to retain the enema fluid long enough for it to exercise its irritant effect. In addition, the insertion of hard plastic enema tips into the anus of an insensate patient may be dangerous, especially if the patient has hemorrhoids. Glycerin suppositories, which provide a mild irritant and osmotic effect on the rectum, are the first choice. Bisacodyl suppositories (Dulcolax) provide more irritation to the rectal mucosa and therefore are more likely to promote gas and secretion of mucus. These disadvantages usually are outweighed by the increased speed of emptying when this agent is used. If these techniques are not successful, carbon dioxide–releasing suppositories or small-volume minienema preparations (e.g., Therevac) can be employed. For patients with impaired hand function, special equipment for anal suppository self-insertion is available, but these devices must be used with care to guard against mucosa damage.

The chronic abuse of the anus and rectum for artificial bowel emptying no doubt promotes the formation of hemorrhoids; 57% of patients more than 5 years after their SCI complain of symptomatic hemorrhoids (Stone et al. 1990). Usually bleeding is the problem, but rectal mucosal prolapse may also result in chronic external secretion of fluid and result in skin breakdown in the perianal region. Most small hemorrhoids in this population will respond to hydrocortisone suppositories inserted after the completion of the bowel program. Sclerotherapy, elastic band ligation, and photocoagulation may be indicated when internal hemorrhoids prolapse or bleed persistently. Rectal bleeding should not be attributed to hemorrhoids until an anorectal examination is done. Conventional studies used in screening for GI neoplasms are often inadequate when used in this population, and the relative risk of GI neoplasms compared with the nondisabled population is a subject of debate.

FECAL IMPACTION

An obstruction of the colon with stool is a serious matter because it can quickly lead to life-threatening complications. Spontaneous colonic perforation is always a threat, while the patient is presented with even more risk during disimpaction when a damaged colonic mucosa is subjected to chemical and physical injury. In addition, chronic fecal distension of the rectum can result in stercoral ulcers of the rectal mucosa, which are essentially pressure sores of the bowel. Overfilling of the colon with stool is known to have a deleterious effect on proximal function of the GI tract and is no doubt the most frequent cause of nausea in this population (Youle & Read 1984). Most important, the promotion of autonomic dysreflexia secondary to rectal distension is potentially life threatening.

Most patients with SCI have some degree of fecal impaction upon admission to the rehabilitation hospital from the acute care setting. The diagnosis is not difficult. Those with mild degrees of impaction will complain of loss of appetite and nausea. Often these patients are mistakenly given antinausea preparations, most of which have anticholinergic and constipating properties, and the problem is exacerbated. On examination, abdominal distension and fecal masses may be noted. Factitious diarrhea may be present when liquid waste is propelled around a blockage of inspissated stool. Plain films of the abdomen may show a remarkable amount of stool in the colon, and air patterns in the intestines may be abnormal.

The treatment of this condition must take into account the special circumstances of these patients. In patients with new SCI, the impaction is usually of short duration and will usually be remediable by simple and noninvasive measures. If the patient is not experiencing vomiting or abdominal pain, and if bowel sounds are preserved, the impaction can be approached gradually from the rectum only. Many SCI centers automatically perform rectal evacuations with suppositories or enemas for the first three to four consecutive days after admission.

Patients with chronic spinal cord conditions and fecal impaction may not respond to such an approach. Because parasympathetic input (from the vagus nerve) is normal up to the transverse colon in these patients, chronic motility deficits may be most striking in the left colon (Menardo et al. 1987). Thus fecal impactions may develop in the proximal colon as a result of poor distal propulsion. In many cases severe dehydra-

tion is present, and stool will be extremely hard. The distal colon may be chronically damaged by longstanding stretching and chemical damage and may not respond to simple pharmacologic stimulation. Not uncommonly, intestinal pseudoobstruction will be present with vomiting, abnormal bowel sounds, and dilation of small bowel loops on radiography.

Efforts to remove a chronic fecal impaction from above by the use of oral cathartics usually are not successful and often will worsen the situation. If vomiting and ileus are present, decompression of the upper GI tract by nasogastric suction may be necessary. The use of oral agents in this setting would only add to abdominal pain and distension and might contribute to serious complications. If the stool can be reached digitally, fragmentation and extraction of the stool should be carried out using lidocaine jelly as a lubricant. In persons prone to autonomic dysreflexia, spinal anesthesia may be necessary. Suppositories are usually of little use in this setting. Sodium phosphate or tap water enemas can be tried with volumes limited to 1 pint per application. Soap-suds enemas should be avoided because they may be injurious to the rectal mucosa and may precipitate serum electrolyte disturbances.

When the impaction is proximal, a colonoscopically directed lavage using a water-soluble contrast medium (Gastrografin or Hypaque) in a 20% to 50% solution may be necessary. These substances are high in osmolality and stimulate emptying by drawing water into the gut lumen and stimulating peristalsis (Wrenn 1989). It must be remembered that another process may be responsible for the development of these obstructions. In light of this, it is not unreasonable to perform endoscopic or radiologic evaluation of the colon to determine whether tumors or other local pathology is present. Patients with recurrent, severe fecal impactions may be candidates for surgical decompression and, ultimately, colostomy. As secondary benefits, bowel care may be more convenient with a colostomy, and healing of pressure sores in the perianal region can be accelerated.

Ultimately, the best approach to the problem of recurrent fecal impactions is prevention. Clinicians are now faced with a growing number of persons who have survived for decades after injury, many of whom are noting increasing difficulty in maintaining a successful bowel-emptying schedule after years of artificial bowel stimulation. Some of these individuals ultimately will need to use oral laxatives regularly to prevent impaction. In addition to the risk of producing fecal incontinence, as noted above, the use of oral laxatives carries a number of additional risks.

Most oral laxatives have little primary effect on bowel motility; they exert action by changing the net water and ion transport across the bowel mucosa. The chronic use of irritant laxatives, including bisacodyl, phenolphthalein, senna, and cascara, will cause damage to the mucosa and ultimately may produce abnormal intestinal motor function (Tedesco & DiPiro 1985). The so-called bulk-forming laxatives, containing polysaccharide or cellulose, are among the safest preparations to use on a chronic basis. Many of these are derived from psyllium seed, and often they are combined with the irritant compounds listed above. Despite the fact that these agents are often considered benign fiber supplements, in actuality they augment the secretory function of the gut and downplay its absorptive function. Adequate hydration is crucial to the success of this type of therapy, and use of these agents must be monitored in diabetics because most have a high sugar content.

If this therapy is not successful in preventing recurrent impaction, then regular use of a hyperosmotic laxative such as milk of magnesia or lactulose is probably justified. Therapy is instituted with the knowledge that it may worsen cramping and produce electrolyte abnormalities (especially in patients with renal disease) when used on a chronic basis. Lactulose is metabolized in the colon to low–molecular weight compounds that lower the pH of the colon and stimulate peristalsis. Use of lactulose should be reserved in light of the fact that it is considerably more expensive than the other osmotic cathartics. In addition, although peristalsis may improve, actual waste removal from the rectum may be more difficult because the stool will be poorly formed.

DIARRHEA

For the person with a physical impairment, an increase in stool volume, liquidity, and frequency is more than an uncomfortable nuisance. Diarrhea can predispose the patient to the development of pressure sores and may become a dangerous medical condition for those who are unable physically to manage their replacement oral fluid intake. An exhaustive discussion of the potential causes of diarrhea is beyond the scope of this chapter, but there are a number of special considerations relevant to patients with SCI.

Initial consideration must be given to fecal impaction as the probable cause in these patients. Fecal stasis in the proximal colon may allow only liquid waste to pass, and treatment of this presumed diarrhea will certainly aggravate the real problem. Because impaction may not be evident by examination, a single plain radiograph of the abdomen to assess for fecal blockage obtained early on is usually the most efficient approach to an SCI patient with diarrhea.

A great percentage of patients seen in the rehabilitation setting will have been treated with antibiotics during their acute hospitalizations, and development of pseudomembranous

Exhibit 4–2 Steps to a Successful Bowel-Emptying Program

1. Evaluate and treat bowel impaction.
2. Promote physical mobilization and allow for basic mechanics of defecation.
3. Keep accurate records of bowel output.
4. Allow formation of a normal column of stool in the colon.
5. Regulate stool consistency from above (e.g., by dietary fiber manipulation).
6. Control bowel emptying from below (e.g., by suppositories, digital stimulation).
7. Do not insist upon daily bowel emptying.
8. Avoid oral cathartic medication.

colitis is not uncommon. Most often, *Clostridium difficile* is the responsible pathogen, especially in persons who have been treated with ampicillin, clindamycin, and cephalosporins. Institutionalized patients with secretory diarrhea without visible blood should be evaluated for the presence of *C. difficile* toxin immediately and placed on enteric precautions until results are available. Metronidazole, 500 mg four times daily, usually is sufficient in the treatment of those with confirmed colonization. Of course, stool examination for other pathogens is indicated in selected clinical situations, especially on pediatric rehabilitation units, where rotavirus outbreaks can have devastating effects.

The high incidence of polypharmacy in these patients should alert the physician to the use and abuse of various drugs with the potential for producing diarrhea. Surreptitious laxative abuse or overuse of chewing gum, candy, or ethanol should be considered, while drugs such as magnesium antacids, diuretics, and a host of antibiotics are common offenders.

In the great majority of instances, as in the nondisabled population, episodes of diarrhea are self-limited. After correctable causes are eliminated, the treatment focus should be body fluid replacement and protection of the perianal skin; an emollient ointment (Desitin or A&D Ointment) without antifungal compounds should be used. Once diarrhea is resolved, acidophilous preparations and yogurt may assist in reestablishing the normal bacterial flora of the intestinal tract. These products, widely used in Europe, contain dried but viable lactobacilli cultures appropriate for oral administration. These bacteria produce lactic acid and create an environment that favors the establishment of a normal acid bacterial flora. A 2- or 3-day course of treatment is helpful. The initial increase in flatus associated with this therapy will resolve spontaneously.

Exhibit 4–2 summarizes the steps in a successful bowel-emptying program.

REFERENCES

Albert, T., et al. 1990. Gastrointestinal complications in spinal cord injury. *Am. Spinal Inj. Assoc. Abstr. Dig.* 16:116.

Apple, D., and L. Hudson. 1990. "Spinal cord injury: The model." In *Proceedings of the National Consensus Conference on Catastrophic Illness and Injury,* 66–71, Atlanta, Ga: The Georgia Regional Spinal Cord Injury Care System. Shepherd Center for Treatment of Spinal Injuries, Inc.

Binnie, N., et al. 1988. The action of a cisapride on the chronic constitution of paraplegia. *Paraplegia* 26:151–158.

Bowen, J., et al. 1974. Increased gastrin release following penetrating central nervous system injury. *Surgery* 75:5:720–724.

Bracken, M.B., et al. 1990. A randomized, controlled trial of methylprednisolone or naloxone in the treatment of acute spinal cord injury. *N. Engl. J. Med.* 322:1405–1411.

Brindley, G., et al. 1982. Sacral anterior root stimulation in paraplegia. *Paraplegia* 20:365–381.

Cannon, L.A., et al. 1987. Prophylaxis of upper gastrointestinal tract bleeding in mechanically ventilated patients. A randomized study comparing the efficacy of sucralfate, cimetidine, and antacids. *Arch. Intern. Med.* 147:2101–2106.

Chapman, R., et al. 1985. Effect of oral dioctyl sodium sulfosuccinate on intake–output studies of the human small and large intestine. *Gastroenterology* 89:489–493.

Charney, K.J., et al. 1975. General surgery problems in patients with spinal cord injuries. *Arch. Surg.* 110:1083–1088.

Chassin, S.L., et al. 1988. Gallbladder dysmotility in spinal cord injury. *Am. Spinal Inj. Assoc. Abstr. Dig.* 14:5–6.

Claus-Walker, J., and L. Halstead. 1981. Metabolic and endocrine changes in spinal cord injury. *Arch. Phys. Med. Rehabil.* 62:595–601.

Connell, A.M., et al. 1963. The motility of the pelvic colon following complete lesions of the spinal cord. *Paraplegia* 1:98–115.

Cooper, I., et al. 1950. Metabolic consequences of spinal cord injury. *J. Clin. Endocrinol.* 10:858–870.

Cosman, B.C., et al. 1991. Gastrointestinal complications of chronic spinal cord injury. *J. Am. Paraplegia Soc.* 14:175–181.

Devroede, G., and J. LaMarche. 1974. Functional importance of extrinsic parasympathetic innervation to the distal colon and rectum in man. *Gastroenterology* 66:273–280.

Fadul, C., et al. 1988. Perforation of the gastrointestinal tract in patients receiving steroids for neurologic disease. *Neurology* 38:348–352.

Fealey, R., et al. 1984. Effect of traumatic spinal cord transection on human upper-gastrointestinal motility and gastric emptying. *Gastroenterology* 89:69–75.

Gelfand, D. 1980. Complications of gastrointestinal radiologic procedures. *Gastrointest. Radiol.* 5:293–315.

Glick, M., et al. 1984. Colonic dysfunction in patients with thoracic spinal cord injury. *Gastroenterology* 86:287–294.

Goligher, J.C., et al. 1955. The surgical anatomy of the anal canal. *Br. J. Surg.* 43:51–56.

Gore, R., et al. 1981. Gastrointestinal complications of spinal cord injury. *Spine* 6:538–544.

Greenfield, J. 1948. Abdominal operations on patients with chronic paraplegia. *Arch. Surg.* 59:1077–1087.

Greenway, R., et al. 1969. Long-term changes in gross body composition of paraplegia and quadriplegia patients. *Paraplegia* 7:301–318.

Hanson, R.W., and M.R. Franklin. 1976. Sexual loss in relation to other functional losses for spinal cord injured males. *Arch. Phys. Med. Rehabil.* 57:291–293.

Humphries, T., and D. Castell. 1981. Effect of oral bethanechol on parameters of esophageal peristalsis. *Dig. Dis. Sci.* 26:129–132.

Kaufman, P.N., et al. 1988. Role of opiate receptors in the regulation of colonic transit. *Gastroenterology* 94:1351–1356.

Kewalramani, L. 1979. Neurogenic gastroduodenal ulceration and bleeding with spinal cord injuries. *J. Trauma* 19:1:259–265.

Kiwerski, J. 1986. Bleeding from the alimentary canal during the management of spinal cord injury patients. *Paraplegia* 24:92–96.

Koch, T.R., et al. 1988. Idiopathic chronic constipation associated with decreased colonic vasoactive intestinal peptide. *Gastroenterology* 94:300–310.

Logeman, J. 1990. Swallowing disorders following spinal cord injury. Presented at the American Congress of Rehabilitation Medicine annual meeting, Phoenix, Arizona, October.

Longhurst, J.C. 1988. Gastrointestinal reflexes. *Gastroenterology* 85:524–533.

McCallum, R., et al. 1977. A controlled trial of metoclopramide in symptomatic gastroesophageal reflux. *N. Engl. J. Med.* 296:354.

Menardo, G., et al. 1987. Large bowel transit in paraplegic patients. *Dis. Colon Rectum* 30:924–928.

Messer, J., et al. 1983. Association of corticosteroid therapy and peptic ulcer disease. *N. Engl. J. Med.* 309:21–24.

Moses, F.M. 1988. Colonic perforation due to oral mannitol. [letter] *J.A.M.A.* 260:640.

Peiffer, S., et al. 1981. Nutritional assessment of the spinal cord injured patient. *J. Am. Diet. Assoc.* 78:501–505.

Peschiera, J., and S. Beerman. 1990. Intestinal dysfunction associated with acute thoracolumbar fractures. *Orthop. Rev.* 19:284–288.

Pollack, L., and I. Finkelman. 1954. The digestive apparatus in injuries to the spinal cord and cauda equina. *Surg. Clin. North Am.* 34:259–268.

Richardson, R., and L. Cerullo. 1979. Transabdominal neurostimulation in the treatment of neurogenic ileus. *Appl. Neurophysiol.* 42:375–382.

Ring, J., et al. 1974. Elimination rate of human serum albumin in paraplegic patients. *Paraplegia* 12:139–144.

Roman, C., and J. Gonella. 1987. *Physiology of the gastrointestinal tract.* 2d ed. New York, N.Y.: Raven.

Roth, E., et al. 1991. Superior mesenteric artery syndrome in spinal cord injury. *Arch. Phys. Med. Rehabil.* 72:417–420.

Rousseau, P. 1988. Treatment of constipation in the elderly. *Postgrad. Med.* 83:349–389.

Segal, J., et al. 1985. Decreased theophylline bioavailability and impaired gastric emptying in spinal cord injury. *Curr. Ther. Res.* 38:831–846.

Shuster, M. 1981. Motor disorders of the stomach. *Med. Clin. North Am.* 65:1269–1289.

Smout, A., et al. 1985. Effects of cisapride, a new gastrointestinal prokinetic substance, on interdigestive and postprandial motor activity of the distal esophagus in man. *Gut* 26:246–259.

Stone, J.M., et al. 1990. Chronic gastrointestinal problems in spinal cord injury patients: A prospective analysis. *Am. J. Gastroenterol.* 85:114–119.

Tanaka, M., et al. 1979. Gastroduodenal disease in chronic spinal cord injuries. *Arch. Surg.* 114:185–187.

Tedesco, F., and J. DiPiro. 1985. Laxative use in constipation. *Am. J. Gastroenterol.* 80:303–309.

Wattchow, D.A., et al. 1988. Distribution and coexistence of peptides in nerve fibers of the external muscle of the human gastrointestinal tract. *Gastroenterology* 95:32–41.

Weber, J., et al. 1985. Effect of brain stem lesions on colonic and anorectal motility. *Dig. Dis. Sci.* 30:419–425.

Wrenn, K. 1989. Fecal impaction. *N. Engl. J. Med.* 321:658–662.

Youle, M., and N. Read. 1984. Effects of painless rectal distension on gastrointestinal transit of a solid meal. *Dig. Dis. Sci.* 29:902–906.

Chapter 5

Managing the Neurogenic Bladder in Spinal Cord Injury

Yeongchi Wu and David Chen

Management of the neurogenic bladder has evolved from advances in the understanding of the physiology of micturition and care techniques during the past decades. Because there are many readily available textbooks on the anatomy and neurophysiology of the urinary bladder, it is the intention of this chapter to provide a framework for care of bladder dysfunction. In dealing with this longstanding problem and its potential life-threatening sequelae to the disabled, the following theoretical care model might prove to be simple and useful. The physiological phenomena follow simple physical principles.

NEUROGENIC SPHINCTER AS THE CAUSE FOR BLADDER DYSFUNCTION

The term *neurogenic bladder* refers to bladder dysfunction after involvement of neurocontrol of the urinary bladder. In fact, the bladder and urethral sphincter need to function in a coordinated fashion to achieve two totally opposite functions: retention and expulsion of the urine (Figure 5-1). Under normal conditions, the bladder functions as a reservoir to retain and expel the urine at will. After spinal cord injury (SCI), both retention and expulsion of urine may be affected (i.e., inability to hold urine until preparation for urination is made or inability to urinate completely when ready). Inability to retain urine results in incontinence, which can be managed by a collecting device, frequently timed voiding, or the use of anticholinergic agents. On the other hand, inability to expel urine results in

urinary retention, which causes medical complications such as urinary infection or renal dysfunction and therefore requires careful management.

Under normal conditions, there are three steps involved in micturition (Figure 5–2): Sensory feedback is required to inform the individual whether the bladder is full; when the bladder is full and voiding is desired, the detrusor muscle contracts; and while the detrusor muscle contracts, the external urethral sphincter is relaxed. At this moment, the urine in the bladder will be pushed out through the relaxed outlet.

For a person with SCI, awareness of bladder fullness may be impaired but could be compensated for by suprapubic palpation. The necessary bladder pressure from detrusor contraction might be produced by the Credé maneuver. Unfortunately, in severe SCI a substitute for relaxing the external urethral sphincter to achieve an opening of the outlet structure often is absent.

Inability to relax the external sphincter muscle during micturition will cause an increased outlet resistance, which in turn produces an increased intravesical pressure and high residual urine. The increased intravesical pressure is responsible for dilatation of the upper urinary tracts, and the high residual urine is the main cause for bacteriuria (Hinman 1971; Figure 5–2). The primary problem in bladder dysfunction, therefore, is not impaired detrusor function but mainly altered external urethral sphincter function. Practically, the impaired urethral sphincter rather than the detrusor should be blamed for the urinary bladder dysfunction. Therefore, in managing the neurogenic bladder, efforts should be aimed at solving the two prob-

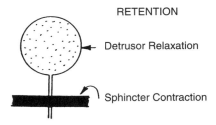

RETENTION

Detrusor Relaxation

Sphincter Contraction

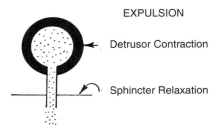

EXPULSION

Detrusor Contraction

Sphincter Relaxation

Figure 5–1 Detrusor-sphincter synchrony. Normally the detrusor muscle relaxes while the sphincter muscle contracts to retain the urine. During voiding, the detrusor contracts to push urine through the relaxed outlet.

lems of high intravesical pressure and high residual urine due to the impaired sphincter function.

RESIDUAL URINE, SAFE EMPTYING INTERVAL, AND THE WU BLADDER GRAPH

Urinary Tract Infection and Residual Urine

The reason for the higher incidence of urinary tract infection after SCI is the breakdown of natural defense mecha-

nisms. Dilution of the residual urine and intermittent evacuation of urine from the bladder protect it from infection. When one has a high volume of infected residual urine, there is a high starting total bacterial population that leads to rapid overgrowth of the bacteria. Delaying bladder emptying allows the residual bacteria more time to multiply in the bladder. This basic model for understanding the natural defense mechanism of the bladder against infection has been explained with a mathematical model (Boen & Sylwester 1965; Cox & Hinman 1961; Hinman & Cox 1966; O'Grady & Cattell 1966; Wu 1983; Figure 5–3).

Critical Voiding Period (Safe Emptying Interval)

Assuming that the bladder is simply a container after voiding, urine from the kidneys is added to the residual urine in the bladder (Hinman & Cox 1967; Wu 1983) at a linear rate, and the remaining bacteria increase in number at an exponential rate (Figure 5–4, left curve). This results in an initial reduction of the bacterial concentration, which is then followed by a rapid return to and surpassing of the original concentration (Figure 5–4, right curve). The time period from the previous emptying to the time when the bacterial concentration returns to the original level is clinically important and is defined (Wu 1983) as the safe emptying interval (SEI). Within this SEI, the bacterial concentration is lower than its level at the previous emptying. After the SEI, the bacterial concentration becomes higher than its original level. Therefore the decrease and increase of the bacterial concentration in the urine are determined by whether the bladder is emptied within or after the SEI (Figure 5–5). The same voiding interval may result in an increased bacterial concentration in one patient but a decreased concentration in another (Figure 5–6).

SEI Obtained by the Wu Bladder Graph

The Wu bladder graph (Figure 5–7), a slidelike graph developed from a mathematical equation (Figure 5–3), can be used

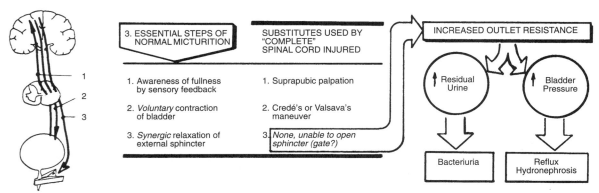

Figure 5–2 Dysfunction and complications in spinal neurogenic bladder. *Source:* From "Total Bladder Care for the Spinal Cord Injured Patient" by Y.C. Wu, 1983, *Annals of the Academy of Medicine,* 12(3), p. 388. Copyright 1983 by Academy of Medicine, Singapore. Reprinted by permission.

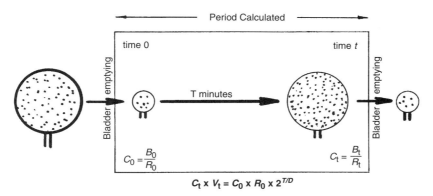

Figure 5–3 Mathematical model for analyzing the bladder defense mechanism. C_0, bacterial concentration at time 0; C_t, bacterial population at time t; R_0, residual urine; V_t, urine volume at time t; D, bacterial doubling time; T, time interval, in minutes between two consecutive bladder emptyings.

to determine the SEI by tracing from the residual urine amount (R_0) to the estimated urine volume (V_t) in the bladder at next voiding, thence to the bacterial doubling time (D), and finally to the SEI (Figure 5–7). For example, if patient A has a residual urine of 40 mL, a bladder capacity (or urine volume at the time of the next voiding) of 300 mL, and an infection with a bacterial doubling time of 60 minutes, the SEI will be about 3 hours. This is obtained by tracing on the Wu bladder graph

from point A (R_0 = 40), to A′ (V_t = 300), to A″ (D = 60), and finally to A‴ (SEI = 3 hours).

Significance of the Wu Bladder Graph

To maintain sterile urine or to eliminate bacteriuria, the bladder must always be emptied within the SEI. Therefore, it is favorable to void more frequently so that the actual bladder-emptying interval is shorter than the SEI or to increase the SEI so that it is longer than the actual bladder-emptying interval. Emptying the bladder more frequently is a matter of willingness by the patient, but increasing the SEI can be achieved by

Figure 5–4 Urine bacterial concentration with bladder emptying. As urine is drained from the kidneys into the bladder at a linear rate, the remaining bacteria increase at an exponential rate. This results in an initial dilution and then a return to the original bacterial concentration. The time interval from the previous emptying to the time when the bacterial concentration returns to the original level is defined as the SEI. *Source:* From "Total Bladder Care for the Spinal Cord Injured Patient" by Y.C. Wu, 1983, *Annals of the Academy of Medicine,* 12(3), p. 388. Copyright 1983 by Academy of Medicine, Singapore. Reprinted by permission.

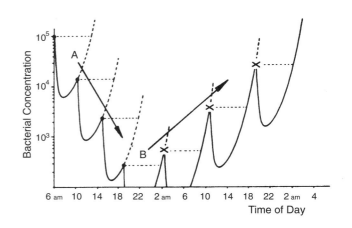

Figure 5–5 SEI and bacterial concentration. When the bladder is emptied within the SEI, the bacterial concentration will be lowered gradually until bacteria are eliminated (A). On the other hand, if the bladder is emptied after the SEI (x), each time significant bacteriuria will be inevitable (B). *Source*: From "Total Bladder Care for the Spinal Cord Injured Patient" by Y.C. Wu, 1983, *Annals of the Academy of Medicine,* 12(3), p. 389. Copyright 1983 by Academy of Medicine, Singapore. Reprinted by permission.

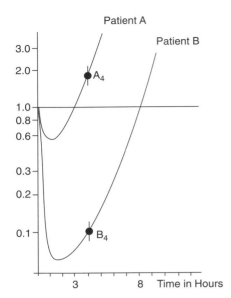

Figure 5–6 Differences in SEI and bacterial concentration. The same voiding interval (4 hours) can result in a higher bacterial concentration for patient A (A₄) but a lower concentration for patient B (B₄), who has a longer SEI.

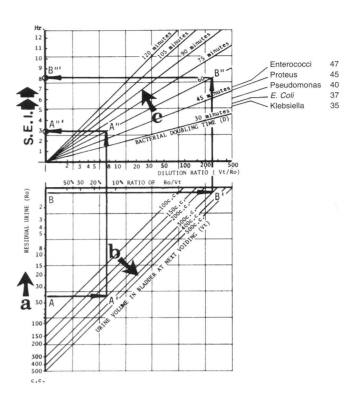

Figure 5–7 Wu bladder graph. The bladder graph is used to determine the SEI. By use of residual urine volume (a), bladder urine volume (b), and bacterial doubling time (c), the SEI can be obtained. Reducing the residual urine, increasing the bladder capacity, and/or prolonging the doubling time will extend the SEI. *Source*: From "Total Bladder Care for the Spinal Cord Injured Patient" by Y.C. Wu, 1983, *Annals of the Academy of Medicine*, 12(3), p. 389. Copyright 1983 by Academy of Medicine, Singapore. Reprinted by permission.

manipulation of the variables (i.e., reduction of the residual urine, increase of the bladder urine volume, and prolongation of the bacterial doubling time; Figure 5–9).

Each of the variables affects the SEI differently. Assuming that the bladder urine volume (V_t) and bacterial doubling time (D) remain constant, there will be an inverse parabolic relationship between the residual urine (R_0) and the SEI. In other words, a patient with low residual urine can void less frequently, whereas another patient with high residual urine must void more frequently to avoid bladder infection. Consequently, it is incorrect to assume that any certain volume is the acceptable residual urine without at the same time taking into account the frequency of the actual bladder emptying (Figure 5–8).

Components of the Bladder Defense Mechanism against Infection

The bladder graph in Figure 5–9 shows two components of the bladder defense mechanism: The upper part is the intrinsic component, and the lower part is the mechanical component. The intrinsic component consists of factors that affect the bacterial doubling time (D), such as the type of organism, urine pH, urea concentration, osmolality, antibacterial effect of the bladder mucosa, and the use of antibacterial agents. The mechanical component is the ratio of residual urine (R_0) to the bladder urine volume at the next voiding (V_t). Because the change in bacterial concentration is related to the time relationship between actual bladder emptying and the SEI, any

clinical study to determine the effectiveness of a given antibacterial agent (which will affect only the bacterial doubling time) for bladder infection will be theoretically inadequate if residual urine and the bladder urine volume (both of which are mechanical components) as well as the frequency of voiding are not controlled. From the bladder graph in Figure 5–9, one can appreciate that reduction of residual urine, increase of the bladder volume, and prolongation of the bacterial doubling time all result in an extension of SEI.

BLADDER PRESSURE

Assuming that the bladder works as a fluid container, the urethra as an outlet, and the urethral sphincter as the valve or gate for the water bag, one can understand a simple physical phenomenon: Whether the urine is to be drained or retained depends upon the equilibrium between the pressure in the bladder and the resistance at the outlet sphincter (Figure 5–10).

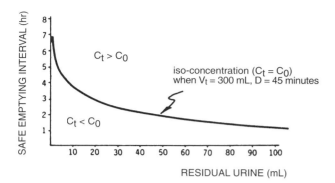

Figure 5–8 Inverse parabolic relationship between the residual urine volume (R_0) and the SEI when the bladder urine volume (V_t) and bacterial doubling time (D) remain unchanged. The higher the residual urine one has, the more frequently one needs to void to prevent or eliminate urinary infection. C_0, original bacterial concentration after the previous voiding; C_t, bacterial concentration at time t. *Source*: From "Total Bladder Care for the Spinal Cord Injured Patient" by Y.C. Wu, 1983, *Annals of the Academy of Medicine*, 12(3), p. 390. Copyright 1983 by Academy of Medicine, Singapore. Reprinted by permission.

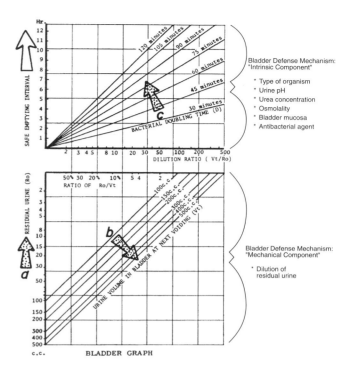

Figure 5–9 Bladder graph showing two components of bladder defense mechanisms: intrinsic and mechanical. The SEI can be prolonged by one or a combination of the following: reduction of residual urine volume (a), larger bladder capacity (b) for larger mechanical dilution of residual urine, and prolongation of the bacterial doubling time (c). *Source*: From "Total Bladder Care for the Spinal Cord Injured Patient" by Y.C. Wu, 1983, *Annals of the Academy of Medicine*, 12(3), p. 390. Copyright 1983 by Academy of Medicine, Singapore. Reprinted by permission.

When the pressure in the bladder exceeds the outlet resistance, urine is drained (Figure 5–10, a and d). When the outlet resistance remains higher than the bladder pressure, urine will be retained (Figure 5–10b). In spastic bladder with detrusor-sphincter dyssynergia, a high-pressure system may exist in the bladder (Figure 5–10c) that interferes with free urine flow from the kidneys to the bladder (Figure 5–10e). Prolonged functional obstruction leads to vesicoureteral reflux and/or hydronephrosis.

CLASSIFICATION OF NEUROGENIC BLADDER

Many classifications have been used to group bladder dysfunctions. Each has its merits and clinical values. Based on the level of motor neuron involvement, the neurogenic bladder can be classified as an upper motor neuron (UMN) type bladder, complete or incomplete, and a lower motor neuron (LMN) type bladder, complete or incomplete.

Another classification is based somewhat on the function of the urinary bladder; it includes the following types:

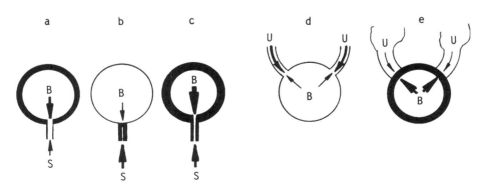

Figure 5–10 Bladder pressure and urine flow. The direction of urine flow is determined by the differential between the pressure in the bladder (B) and the resistance at the urethral sphincter (S). This relationship also exists between the ureters (U) and bladder.

- spinal shock bladder
- uninhibited bladder
- reflex bladder, coordinated and uncoordinated
- autonomous bladder
- motor paralytic bladder
- sensory paralytic bladder
- mixed UMN and LMN bladder

From a management viewpoint, bladder dysfunction is analogous to motor impairment of the limbs. The patient's potential to ambulate is determined by the presence of residual motor control in key gait muscles rather than by the level of SCI or the presence of involuntary muscle contraction. Similarly, whether the bladder is to function depends not on the involuntary detrusor contraction but on the residual function of the external urethral sphincter. Therefore, the classification of the spinal neurogenic bladder will be more practical if it is based on the patient's ability to achieve external urethral sphincter opening during the event of voiding (Figure 5–11):

- by voluntary control of the external urethral sphincter through the residual intact cerebrospinal pathway
- by inducing synergic reflexic opening of the external urethral sphincter at the spinal cord level using cutaneous or other stimulation

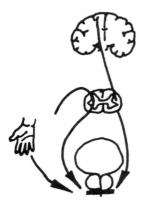

| | BLADDER TYPE | | | |
SPHINCTER CONTROL	C	S	Q	P
1. Cerebral Cortical	+	–	–	–
2. Spinal Synergic	.	+	–	–
3. Manual	.	.	–	+

Figure 5–11 Neurogenic bladder after SCI is classified based on the methods of achieving urethral sphincter opening. There are four types: C, S, Q, and P. *Source*: From "Total Bladder Care for the Spinal Cord Injured Patient" by Y.C. Wu, 1983, *Annals of the Academy of Medicine,* 12(3), p. 391. Copyright 1983 by Academy of Medicine, Singapore. Reprinted by permission.

- by intermittent self-catheterization with normal hand function

Based on this concept, the neurogenic bladder in patients with SCI can be classified into four groups (Figure 5–11):

- *Group C*: The patients in this group will have voluntary cortical control to relax the external urethral sphincter during micturition (Figure 5–12). This is often seen in patients with incomplete SCI, with Brown-Séquard syndrome, or central cord syndrome. Voluntary contraction and relaxation of the external urethral sphincter can be observed during the electromyographic (EMG) study. Almost all the patients with voluntary contraction and relaxation of the anal sphincter during rectal examination and voluntary movement of toes on one or two sides will have coordinated detrusor-sphincter function and are expected to regain normal bladder function.
- *Group S*: About 10% to 15% of patients with complete SCI and loss of cortical control of the external urethral sphincter may achieve synergic reflexic sphincter relaxation using Credé, Valsalva, or tapping maneuver (Figure 5–13). A coordinated detrusor-sphincter pattern can be observed during the urodynamic study.
- *Group Q*: This group of patients, with complete quadriplegia, does not have cortical control or spinal synergic relaxation of the external urethral sphincter (Figure 5–15). In addition, they do not have normal hand function for self-catheterization. Bladder emptying cannot be achieved by voluntary means or by perineal stimulation. Urethral catheterization can only be done by the caregiver. In some patients anal stretch (Figure 5–14) and the Credé maneuver resolve in bladder emptying (Figure 5–15).
- *Group P*: These patients have lost both cortical and spinal synergic control of the external urethral sphincter, but they have normal hand function to perform intermittent self-catheterization or anal stretch for bladder emptying. Most of the complete paraplegic patients have this type of neurogenic bladder.

BLADDER CARE ALGORITHM

With this classification based on residual sphincter function, one can match the commonly used methods of bladder management for each type of sphincter dysfunction (Figure 5–16). Because no single management method can be used for all types of bladder dysfunction, it would be logical to apply one of the most suitable methods to the particular type of bladder disorder after taking into consideration medical, social, and economic factors. For example, for a patient with incomplete SCI and partial voluntary control of the toes and anal sphincter, the care method may be an external catheter initially until normal bladder function returns. For a patient with no

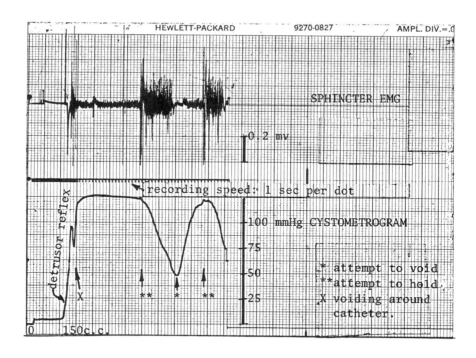

Figure 5–12 Cystometrogram/sphincter EMG recording from a patient with C5–6 incomplete SCI. The patient had voluntary control of bilateral toes and urethral sphincter. He was also able to void (*) or hold (**) the urine upon command. Voiding around the catheter was noted when the bladder pressure increased and the urethral sphincter activity reduced. *Source:* From "Total Bladder Care for the Spinal Cord Injured Patient" by Y.C. Wu, 1983, *Annals of the Academy of Medicine,* 12(3), p. 397. Copyright 1983 by Academy of Medicine, Singapore. Reprinted by permission.

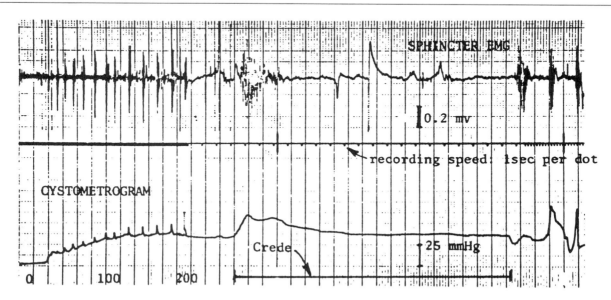

Figure 5–13 Cystometrogram/sphincter EMG recording from a patient with a T4–5 complete SCI. Note the gradual build-up of intravesical pressure with intermittent bursts of sphincter activity. Credé maneuver induced a transient increase followed by a prolonged (18-second) silent period of sphincter activity, suggesting detrusor-sphincter synergia. This phenomenon is rarely seen in patients with complete SCI. *Source:* From "Total Bladder Care for the Spinal Cord Injured Patient" by Y.C. Wu, 1983, *Annals of the Academy of Medicine,* 12(3), p. 397. Copyright 1983 by Academy of Medicine, Singapore. Reprinted by permission.

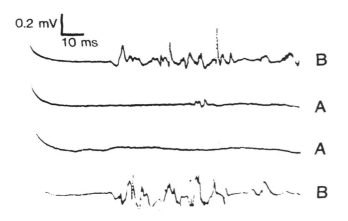

Figure 5–14 Sacral reflex latency study with single-sweep recording of the sphincter responses showing the off-and-on phenomenon of sacral reflex with (A) and without (B) the application of anal stretch. *Source:* From "Inhibition of the External Urethral Sphincter and Sacral Reflex by Anal Stretch in Spinal Cord Injured Patients" by Y.C. Wu, J.B. Nanninga, and B.B. Hamilton, 1986, *Arch. Phys. Med. Rehabil., 67,* p. 136.

volitional control of the urethral sphincter but who has detrusor-sphincter synergia, cutaneous stimulation may be used to induce voiding, and the external catheter may be needed to prevent incontinence. With complete quadriplegia and a dyssynergic sphincter function, one of three approaches may be considered: long-term indwelling catheterization, external sphincterectomy, or suprapubic cystostomy. Complete paraplegic patients may use long-term frequent intermittent catheterization, anal stretch, or external sphincterectomy.

WHAT TO LOOK FOR DURING A PHYSICAL EXAMINATION

Comprehensive history taking and physical examination can reveal much useful information important to the care of neurogenic bladder. The following areas are particularly essential.

Awareness of Bladder Fullness

Normally one prepares to empty the bladder when it is full. Awareness of bladder fullness is an important part of the mic-

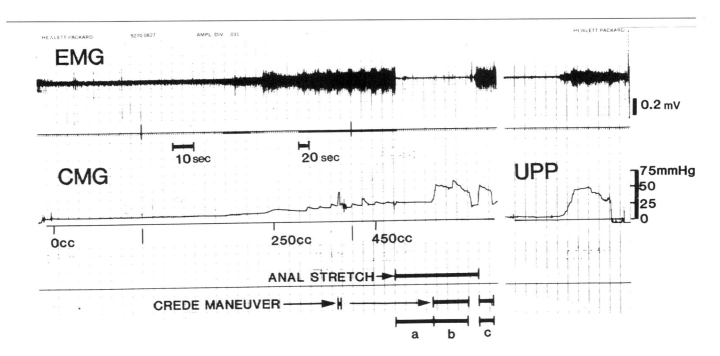

Figure 5–15 Cystometrogram (CMG)/sphincter EMG study of a patient with C-8 paraplegia revealing detrusor-sphincter dyssynergia. The Credé maneuver alone (c) increased the sphincter activity and intravesical pressure; anal stretch alone (a) significantly reduced the sphincter activity. The combination of anal stretch and Credé maneuver resulted in favorable conditions for bladder emptying: relaxation of the urethral sphincter and increase of intravesical pressure (b). *Source:* From "Inhibition of the External Urethral Sphincter and Sacral Reflex by Anal Stretch in Spinal Cord Injured Patients" by Y.C. Wu, J.B. Nanninga, and B.B. Hamilton, 1986, *Arch. Phys. Med. Rehabil., 67,* p. 136.

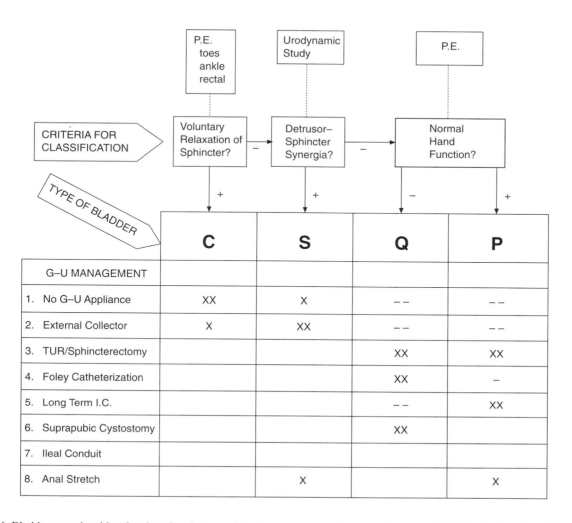

Figure 5–16 Bladder care algorithm for choosing the type of bladder management based on the type of bladder dysfunction. XX, recommended care methods. *Source:* From "Total Bladder Care for the Spinal Cord Injured Patient" by Y.C. Wu, 1983, *Annals of the Academy of Medicine,* 12(3), p. 392. Copyright 1983 by Academy of Medicine, Singapore. Reprinted by permission.

turition event. It tells the patient when to void or catheterize the bladder or whether to change a plugged catheter. The presence of sacral sensation to pin prick is an indication of incomplete cord injury and often is associated with intact sensation of bladder fullness.

Voluntary Control of the Toes or Anal Sphincter Muscle

The ability to move the toes or voluntarily contract/relax the anal sphincter during rectal examination is a positive indicator for bladder recovery. Because of the proximity of the cerebrospinal tract to the motor neurons of the urethral sphincter muscles and to the toe flexors or anal sphincter, preservation of toe or anal sphincter function often indicates intact volun-

tary control of the external urethral sphincter and a coordinated detrusor-sphincter pattern. This is true from clinical experience that patients with Brown-Séquard syndrome, central cord syndrome, or incomplete SCI almost always have normal bladder function.

Anal Tone or Bulbocavernosus Reflex

Routine rectal examination for anal tone or the presence of bulbocavernosus reflex has been used for a long time. The presence of the bulbocavernosus reflex or anal tone indicates the preservation of the reflex arc but does not correlate with a coordinated detrusor-sphincter function or bladder recovery. It sometimes becomes misleading information in the care of the neurogenic bladder. During rectal examination, it is more useful to check for voluntary contraction and relaxation of the anal sphincter muscle.

Anal Stretch and Anal Sphincter Relaxation

If the patient is not able to relax the spastic anal sphincter muscle, anal stretch with two fingers should be tried. In patients with complete thoracic paraplegia and a spastic anal sphincter, anal stretch will gradually reduce the anal tone, which often coincides with relaxation of the external urethral sphincter (Figures 5–14 and 5–15; Wu et al. 1986). This technique is useful for patients with spastic sphincter and difficulty inserting a catheter. For them, anal stretch can induce urethral sphincter relaxation and make catheterization easier (Donovan et al. 1977; Gans et al. 1975).

Voiding during Bowel Movement

There are patients who have high postvoid residual urine but urinate freely during bowel movement. This is due to simultaneous relaxation of the anal and urethral sphincters during defecation, a condition similar to when anal stretch and the Valsalva maneuver are applied simultaneously. When this is reported by the patient, one can measure the residual urine after a bowel program with or without anal stretch to determine the effectiveness of bladder emptying. If the residual urine is less than 30 mL, urethral catheterization is not needed at the time of the bowel program.

URODYNAMIC STUDY OF THE NEUROGENIC BLADDER

Urodynamic study of the neurogenic bladder records the neurophysiological function of the detrusor and external urethral sphincter. This study is of value for patients with impairment of storage and/or discharge of urine. The urinary bladder functions as a container, a system that involves orthodromic pressure in the bladder and antidromic resistance at the urethral outlet level. The difference between the orthodromic pressure and the antidromic resistance as well as the external urethral sphincter activity determines whether the urine is stored in or discharged by the intravesical pressure. The urodynamic study consists of the following procedures:

- documentation of bladder-filling sensation
- routine EMG study of the external urethral sphincter
- cystometrogram/sphincter EMG during:
  1. gradual bladder filling
  2. Credé or Valsalva maneuver or abdominal tapping
  3. anal stretch

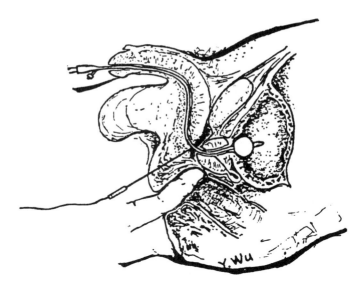

Figure 5–17 Measurement of motor action potentials. In male patients, the needle electrode is inserted through the perineal floor about 2 cm anterior to the anus and toward the apex of the prostate, guided by a finger in the rectum. Insertion activities can be observed on the EMG monitor when the needle electrode penetrates the external urethral sphincter. In female patients, the needle electrode is inserted about 0.5 cm to 1.0 cm lateral to the urethral meatus. The sphincter is encountered about 1 cm from the surface. *Source:* From "Total Bladder Care for the Spinal Cord Injured Patient" by Y.C. Wu, 1983, *Annals of the Academy of Medicine,* 12(3), p. 395. Copyright 1983 by Academy of Medicine, Singapore. Reprinted by permission.

- urethral pressure profile
- sacral reflex latency

Documentation of Bladder-Filling Sensation

The sensation of bladder fullness alerts the individual to prepare for bladder emptying. It is important because bladder emptying is part of an individual's daily activities. During the urodynamic study, it is necessary to document whether there is bladder-filling sensation and at what capacity the patient experiences urgency.

EMG Study of the External Urethral Sphincter

Besides looking for spontaneous activity and motor action potentials of the external urethral sphincter (Figure 5–17), it is more important to document the patient's ability for voluntary contraction and relaxation of the urethral sphincter upon command (Figure 5–12). One should not be confused by the involuntary EMG activity induced by cutaneous stimulation. The presence of volitional contraction or relaxation of the external urethral sphincter indicates an intact connection between the cerebral cortex and the urethral sphincter. This voluntary control of the sphincter muscle is a favorable sign for regaining normal bladder function and is often seen in patients with incomplete SCI (e.g., Brown-Séquard syndrome and central cord syndrome).

Cystometrogram/Sphincter EMG Study

This procedure documents the time relationship between the intravesical pressure and the sphincter EMG activity. It shows whether the detrusor muscle and external sphincter muscle are acting coordinately (synergia) or against each other (dyssynergia). While the bladder is filled with normal saline (drip speed, 300 mL in 15 to 20 minutes) to a maximal amount of 500 mL, the pressure in the bladder and the EMG activity of the external urethral sphincter are recorded simultaneously (Figures 5–12, 5–13, and 5–15). During the study, several responses are observed (Diokno et al. 1974).

Detrusor Contraction during Gradual Bladder Filling

Detrusor contraction is indicated by a sudden rise of the intravesical pressure. It occurs voluntarily in normal individuals during voiding as well as involuntarily in patients after noxious stimulation. It occurs at 300- to 400-mL capacity in normal conditions and 50- to 200-mL capacity in the spastic bladder and is absent in patients during spinal shock or with LMN lesions. Three factors are important in analyzing the detrusor reflex:

1. *Bladder capacity at the time when detrusor reflex occurs:* This indicates the amount of urine that can be held in the bladder before involuntary voiding (incontinence) occurs.

2. *Maximal pressure in the bladder during detrusor contraction:* This is the maximal orthodromic pressure produced in the bladder, to be compared with the antidromic resistance at the external urethral sphincter (measured from the urethral pressure profile, discussed below). The difference between the intravesical pressure and the urethral resistance determines the direction of urine flow.

3. *Sphincter EMG activity during detrusor contraction:* This shows whether there is detrusor-sphincter synergia or dyssynergia. In the presence of increased sphincter activity in patients with detrusor-sphincter dyssynergia, voiding will be incomplete and potentially harmful to the upper urinary tracts because of back pressure from high outlet resistance (Hinman 1971).

Credé, Valsalva Maneuver, or Abdominal Tapping

Because these techniques often are used by patients for bladder evacuation, it is important to document whether these techniques are achieving a favorable condition: relaxation of the external urethral sphincter muscle and increased pressure in the bladder (Figure 5–13). In most of the patients with com-

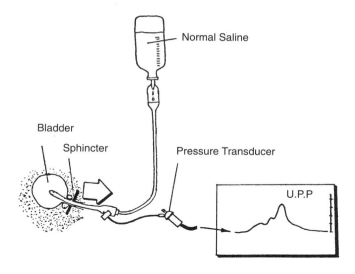

Figure 5–18 Set up for recording the urethral pressure profile (U.P.P.). *Source:* From "Total Bladder Care for the Spinal Cord Injured Patient" by Y.C. Wu, 1983, *Annals of the Academy of Medicine,* 12(3), p. 396. Copyright 1983 by the Academy of Medicine, Singapore. Reprinted by permission.

plete UMN lesions these maneuvers tend to induce both increased intravesical pressure and increased sphincter activity.

Anal Stretch Response

Anal stretch, rather than anal stimulation, inhibits both detrusor and urethral sphincter contraction in many patients with complete SCI. If this is present, the patient with normal hand function can be taught to do anal self-stretch and to apply the Valsalva maneuver simultaneously to achieve bladder emptying (Figure 5–15). Anal stretch can effectively inhibit the bulbocavernosus reflex and relax the urethral sphincter. It should be tried when one encounters difficulty catheterizing patients with spastic sphincters (Figures 15–14 and 15–15; Donovan et al. 1977; Gans et al. 1975; Wu et al. 1986).

Urethral Pressure Profile

The change of pressure (outlet resistance) in the urethra is recorded during slow withdrawal of a water-filled catheter that is connected to a pressure transducer (Figure 5–18). Comparison of the peak pressure in the urethra with the intravesical pressure recorded on the cystometrogram provides information about the possibility of bladder emptying (Figure 5–15).

Sacral Reflex Latency

The bulbocavernosus reflex has been utilized widely as a part of the clinical evaluation, but its presence only suggests an intact reflex arc. More precisely, it can be tested by the sacral reflex latency study. Abnormally prolonged or absent latency of the sacral reflex suggests involvement somewhere along the reflex arc. The sacral latency study is done by stimulating the glans penis and recording the response from the external urethral sphincter.

BLADDER MANAGEMENT

Several methods of bladder management are described below. It is important to incorporate these techniques into the patient's life style. Consideration must be given to the patient's resources, physical abilities, and social situation in choosing a method of bladder management.

Indwelling Catheterization

Indwelling catheterization is commonly used during the acute phase of SCI when accurate fluid intake and output are carefully monitored. Attempts to remove the catheter should be made to minimize the inevitable bacteriuria; removal of an indwelling catheter, however, does not guarantee elimination of urinary complications if the outlet obstruction is not overcome. Proper care of the indwelling catheter is essential to prevent potential urinary problems from plugging and kinking

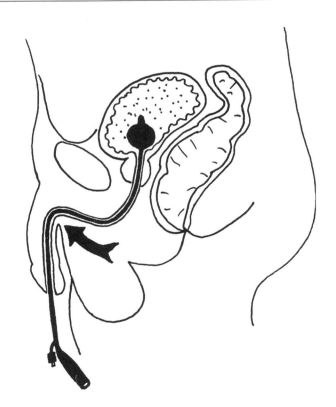

Figure 5–19 Indwelling catheterization. The indwelling catheter should be taped to the abdominal wall to prevent pressure at the penoscrotal angle and to avoid accidental traction injury of the urethra.

of the catheter. Increase fluid intake and urine output to maintain free urinary flow and to reduce the sediment in the catheter. The leg bag should be emptied frequently to avoid overdistension of and back pressure on the bladder. Taping the catheter to the abdominal wall will help prevent a pressure sore from occurring at the penoscrotal angle (Figure 5–19) and accidental traction injury to the urethra. Many patients who like the convenience of an indwelling catheter but would like to avoid urethral catheterization choose a suprapubic catheter. This technique is described Chapter 6.

Bladder Training

Bladder training is a commonly used term, although it is not clearly defined. There is controversy as to whether the bladder can be trained at all. Eventual return of bladder function still relies on ultimate recovery of the spinal cord neurophysiology. To some degree, bladder training using the intermittent catheterization technique may be considered a range of motion exercise of the bladder. As in range of motion exercise to the paralyzed legs, the intermittent catheterization alone cannot be expected to change the uncoordinated detrusor-sphincter function to a coordinated pattern; if there is a chance for the eventual return of bladder function, however, avoiding bladder contracture by intermittent catheterization is desirable.

Intermittent Catheterization

For anyone requiring urethral catheterization because of inadequate bladder emptying, intermittent catheterization must be done *every 4 to 6 hours to prevent infection or whenever the bladder is full to prevent high intravesical pressure and incontinence.* In the presence of bacteriuria, the frequency of intermittent catheterization should be increased by following the principle of the SEI mentioned earlier. In other words, by frequent intermittent catheterization, the bladder is emptied completely within the SEI, and both bacteriuria and bladder overdistension can be avoided. As a rule of thumb, there is no need for patients on intermittent catheterization to increase fluid intake; anticholinergic agents are useful to reduce contractibility and to increase the bladder capacity, however, so that there will be no incontinence between catheterizations.

RIC-Wu (Touchless®) Disposable Catheter

The RIC-Wu Catheter Kit (Figure 5–20) is a regular rubber catheter encapsulated in a long transparent plastic tube that is sealed at its two ends. The top chamber is opened to cover the glans penis so that the inner catheter can be guided into the urethra. The inner catheter is lubricated before being inserted into the meatus by the lubricant deposited in the bottom of the top chamber. There is no need to wear sterile gloves because the catheter is handled from the outside of the plastic tube

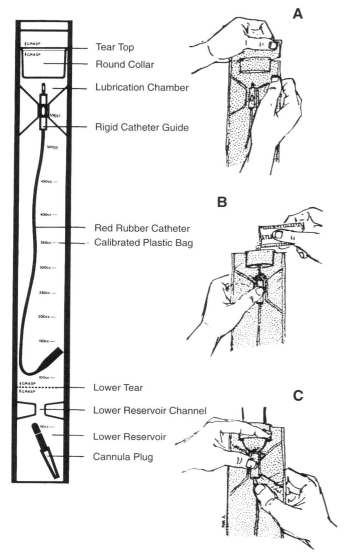

Figure 5–20 Design and use of the RIC-Wu Catheter (Touchless®). The regular rubber catheter is encapsulated in a long transparent plastic tube with its two ends sealed to maintain sterility. In using the catheter kit, the top chamber first is opened (A), lubricant is deposited onto the catheter guide (B), and then the top chamber is applied over the glans penis after cleansing preparation of the urethral meatus and glans (C). The inner catheter then is grasped from outside the bag and is pushed into the bladder. *Source*: From "Total Bladder Care for the Spinal Cord Injured Patient" by Y.C. Wu, 1983, *Annals of the Academy of Medicine*, 12(3), p. 393. Copyright 1983 by Academy of Medicine, Singapore. Reprinted by permission.

(Figure 5–21). The long plastic tube serves also as a container for collecting the catheterized urine. The opening between the urethral meatus and the catheter is minimal (Figure 5–22), thus reducing the chance of contamination during the procedure (Wu et al. 1980). This catheter kit currently is distributed by the C.R. Bard Company.

Wu Reusable Catheter

The Wu Reusable Catheter (Figure 5–23) is a special catheter that can be resterilized; it is inexpensive for long-term sterile intermittent catheterization. It has the advantage of being sterile compared with the clean intermittent catheterization technique (Lapides et al. 1976) and less expensive compared with the disposable catheter tray. It can be assembled with materials available on the market (Figure 5–24). The catheter is kept sterile because the Penrose tube is connected end to end after resterilization with povidone-iodine or hydrogen peroxide solution (Wu et al. 1981). This catheter has not been manufactured for distribution but is potentially useful in developing countries.

Clean Intermittent Catheterization

Long-term intermittent catheterization (Lapides et al. 1976) using nonsterile clean technique is an accepted procedure and is used by patients with SCI. It achieves complete bladder emptying and thus an increased SEI. It also avoids the high intravesical pressure often found in patients with detrusor-sphincter dyssynergia. It must be remembered that *intermittent catheterization using clean technique should be done frequently—every 4 to 6 hours—and within the SEI to prevent urinary infection*. There is a high risk of recurrent urinary infection and bladder overdistension if the bladder is catheterized infrequently.

URINARY TRACT INFECTION VS. BACTERIAL COLONIZATION

Urinary infection in the population with SCI is an important problem because the high morbidity and mortality rates in SCI are related in part to urinary complications. Frequent infection, reinfection, and relapse infection as well as the development of antibiotic-resistant organisms lead to difficulty in deciding whether to treat urinary infection in SCI patients. Questions often raised are urinary infection vs. urinary colonization, the definition of significant bacteriuria, localization of urinary infection, and short-term vs. long-term antibacterial therapy.

Urinary Infection vs. Urinary Colonization

The presence of bacteria in the urine is different from tissue invasion by the organisms in the urinary tract. The former is considered bacteriuria, and the latter often is accompanied by the presence of increased WBCs in the urinary tract infection. With the presence of an indwelling catheter, the patient inevitably will acquire bacteriuria no matter what kind of preventive measures are taken. Because catheterized urine specimens rather than spontaneous midstream specimens often are used in SCI patients, the conventional criteria for significant bacteriuria in neurologically intact individuals as originally

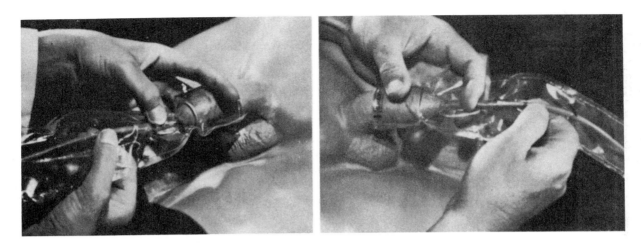

Figure 5–21 Position of the hands for staff (left) and self (right) catheterization using the RIC-Wu (Touchless®) Catheter Kit. *Source*: From "RIC-Wu Catheter Kit: New Device for an Old Problem" by Y.C. Wu, R. King, B.B. Hamilton, and H.B. Betts, 1980, *Arch. Phys. Med. Rehabil. 61*, p. 456.

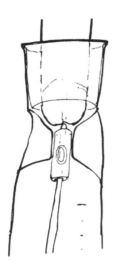

Figure 5–22 RIC-Wu Catheter Kit application. The catheter is introduced into the urethra through a small opening between the urethra and the catheter guide. *Source*: From "RIC-Wu Catheter Kit: New Device for an Old Problem" by Y.C. Wu, R. King, B.B. Hamilton, and H.B. Betts, 1986, *Arch. Phys. Med. Rehabil. 61*, p. 456.

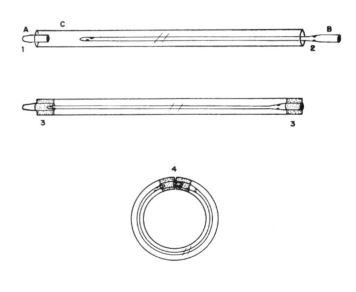

Figure 5–23 Wu Reusable Catheter. To assemble, the first catheter (A) is cut at its tapering section next to the wide end to form the connector (1); the long end is discarded. The opening of the connector must be slightly larger than the shaft of the second catheter (B), so that the tip of the catheter can pass through. Two holes (2) in the tapered section of the second catheter (B) aid in rising and sterilization and permit exit of air trapped in the Penrose tube. Contact cement is used to fasten the connector (A) and the second catheter (B), as shown by the stippled areas (3). End-to-end assembly (4) permits retention of the catheter in aseptic condition. Source: From "Reusable Catheter for Long-Term Sterile Intermittent Catheterization" by Y.C. Wu, B.B. Hamilton, M.A. Boyink, and J.B. Nanninga, 1981, *Arch. Phys. Med. Rehabil. 62*, p. 40.

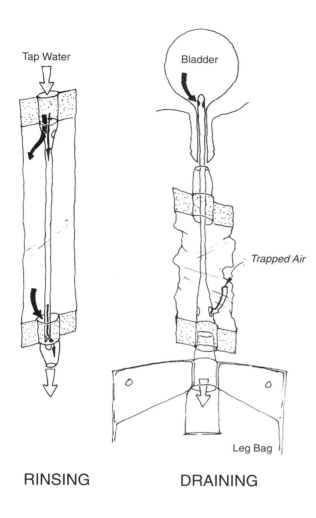

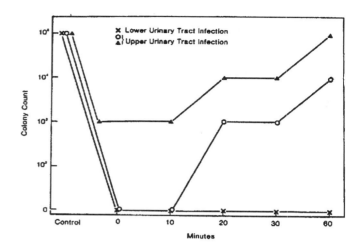

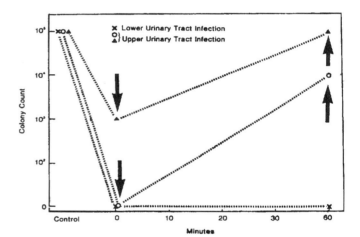

Figure 5–24 Wu Reusable Catheter application. When the tip of the catheter enters the bladder (right), the urine is drained through the inner catheter while air trapped in the Penrose tube escapes through the two holes into the leg bag. For rinsing, tap water is run through the unit (left). Source: From "Reusable Catheter for Long-Term Sterile Intermittent Catheterization" by Y.C. Wu, B.B. Hamilton, M.A. Boyink, and J.B. Nanninga, 1981, *Arch. Phys. Med. Rehabil., 62,* p. 40.

Figure 5–25 (Top) Fairley washout test (modified from Merritt & Keys 1982). Elase, neomycin, and 2,000 mL of normal saline are used to prepare the bladder. Six urine specimens are collected for bacterial counting. (Bottom) Wu modified washout procedure. The bladder is irrigated 20 times with 50 mL of normal saline with or without initial instillation of diluted povidone-iodine solution. Three urine specimens (preirrigation, immediate postirrigation, and 90-minute postirrigation) are collected for bacterial counting using the semiquantitative dip-slide method.

defined (Kass 1956, 1963) have been modified for these patients. With impaired sensation, the classic symptoms of dysuria, frequency, urgency and suprapubic pain are not reliable in the population with SCI, and gross pyuria indicates an increased risk of morbidity due to untreated urinary infection (Peterson & Roth 1989).

Localization of Urinary Tract Infection

Once bacteriuria is confirmed, distinction between upper and lower urinary tract infection is clinically important be-

cause of the potential renal damage in upper tract infections. For patients with renal infection, conventional short courses in antibacterial therapy for 1 or 2 weeks are associated with a high frequency of relapse. Repetitive and insufficient antibiotic therapies also cause selection of highly resistant organisms, which are another problem in the hospital.

The Fairley bladder washout procedure for localizing the site of urinary infection (Fairley et al. 1966) and the modified Fairley test (Giroux & Perkash 1985) are too complicated for routine clinical application. They also pose the difficulty of

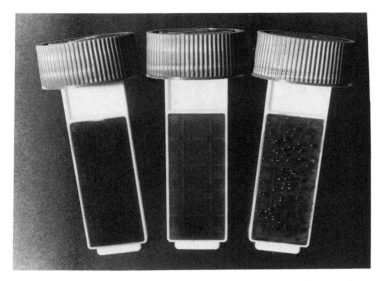

Figure 5–26 Modified washout procedure. The three urine specimens show a confluent growth (>10⁶ colonies per milliliter) in the preirrigation specimen on dip-slide (left), no growth in the immediate postirrigation specimen (middle), and a density of 10,000 colonies per milliliter in the 90-minute postirrigation specimen (right).

achieving an ideal bladder preparation for the washout study. The antibody-coated bacteria screening test is not accepted as a useful procedure for the population with SCI (Merritt & Keys 1982).

A simplified method with some diagnostic and therapeutic value using modified bladder irrigation and dip-slide semiquantitative bacterial counting is being tested at this center (Figure 5–25; Cohen & Kass 1967; Guttmann & Naylor 1967). In our modified washout test, the bladder is irrigated 20 times with 50 mL of normal saline with or without initial instillation of diluted povidone-iodine solution (1:1 dilution with normal saline). Three urine specimens (preirrigation, immediate postirrigation, and 90-minute postirrigation) are collected for semiquantitative bacterial counting using the dip-slide procedure (Figure 5–26). In addition to the change in bacterial concentration, the change in total bacterial population also is compared with the postirrigation bacterial concentration and population. Because the bladder irrigation is expected to suppress the growth of residual bacteria during the lag phase of growth for at least 2 hours, any dramatic increase

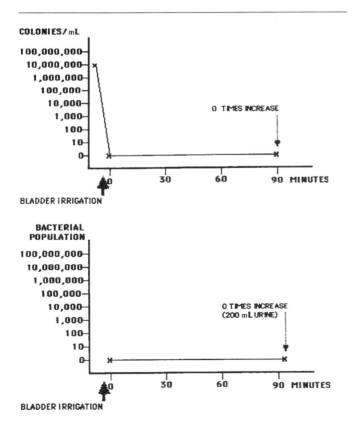

Figure 5–27 Changes in the bacterial concentration and bacterial population in patients with bacteriuria limited to the bladder.

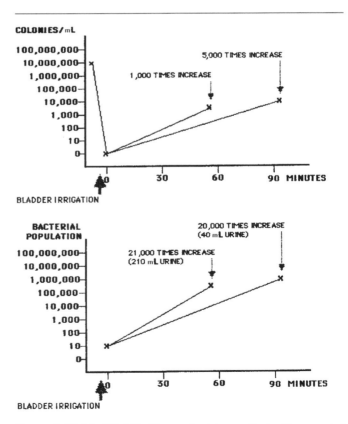

Figure 5–28 Modified bladder washout in a patient with suspected upper urinary tract infection. There is a 1,000- to 2,000-fold increase in bacterial concentration and a 20,000- to 21,000-fold increase in total bacterial population.

in the total bacterial population would indicate migrating of the bacteria from either the upper urinary tracts or the prostate. Further clinical data are being collected to define the usefulness of this procedure (Figures 5–27 and 5–28).

Monitoring Bacteriuria

The high incidence of recurrent urinary infection requires frequent monitoring to reduce the morbidity rate from untreated urinary infection. Home monitoring of bacteriuria and pyuria will be important for the prevention of secondary complications after SCI. Possible methods for such home monitoring are the use of dip-slide for semiquantitative bacterial counting and dip-stick for detection of nitrite and leukocyte esterase. Dip-slide culture and the dip-stick method are simple procedures and can be taught to most patients with SCI. Long-term use could be part of a self-care program to monitor and adjust the bladder care program, indicating for example the need for increased frequency of intermittent catheterization when bacteriuria is detected.

REFERENCES

Boen, J.R., and D.L. Sylwester. 1965. The mathematical relationship among urinary frequency, residual urine and bacterial growth in bladder infection. *Invest. Urol.* 2:468–473.

Cohen, S.N., and E.H. Kass. 1967. A simple method for quantitative urine culture. *N. Engl. J. Med.* 277:176–180.

Cox, C.E., and F. Hinman, Jr. 1961. Experiments with induced bacteriuria, vesical emptying and bacterial growth on the mechanism of bladder defense to infection. *J. Urol.* 86:739–748.

Diokno, A.S., et al. 1974. Periurethral striated muscle activity in neurogenic bladder dysfunction. *J. Urol.* 112:743–749.

Donovan, W.H., et al. 1977. Anal sphincter stretch: A technique to overcome detrusor-sphincter dys-synergia. *Arch. Phys. Med. Rehabil.* 58:320–324.

Fairley, K.F., et al. 1966. The site of infection in pregnancy bacteriuria. *Lancet* 1:939.

Gans, B.M., et al. 1975. Urinary catheterization in severe sphincter spasticity: Report of two cases. *Arch. Phys. Med. Rehabil.* 56:498.

Giroux, J., and I. Perkash. 1985. Limited value of the Fairley test in urological infections in patients with neuropathic bladders. *J. Am. Paraplegia Soc.* 8:10–12.

Guttmann, D., and G.R.E. Naylor. 1967. Dip-slide aid to quantitative urine culture in general practice. *Br. Med. J.* 3:343–345.

Hinman, F., Jr. 1971. Obstruction: Back pressure or residual volume and laminar flow. *J. Urol.* 105:702–708.

Hinman, F., Jr. 1977. Intermittent catheterization and vesical defense. *J. Urol.* 117:57–60.

Hinman, F., Jr., and C.E. Cox. 1966. The voiding vesical defense mechanism: The mathematical effect of residual urine, voiding interval and volume on bacteriuria. *J. Urol.* 96:491–498.

Hinman, F., Jr., and C.E. Cox. 1967. Residual urine volume in normal male subjects. *J. Urol.* 96:641–645.

Kass, E.H. 1956. Asymptomatic infection of urinary tract. *Trans. Assoc. Am. Physicians* 69:56.

Kass, E.H. 1963. The meaning of significant bacteria. *J.A.M.A.* 184:727–729. (Letter to the editor.)

Lapides, J., et al. 1976. Further observation on self-catheterization. *J. Urol.* 116:169–171.

Merritt, S.L., and T.F. Keys. 1982. Limitation of the antibody-coated bacteria test in patients with neurogenic bladder. *J.A.M.A.* 247:1723–1725.

O'Grady, F., and W.R. Cattell. 1966. Kinetics of urinary tract infection. *Br. J. Urol.* 38:156–162.

Peterson, J.R., and E.J. Roth. 1989. Fever, bacteriuria and pyuria in spinal cord injured patients with indwelling urethral catheters. *Arch. Phys. Med. Rehabil.* 70:839–842.

Wu, Y. 1983. Total bladder care for the spinal cord injured patient. *Ann. Acad. Med. Singapore* 12:387–399.

Wu, Y., et al. 1980. RIC-Wu Catheter Kit: New device for an old problem. *Arch. Phys. Med. Rehabil.* 61:455–459.

Wu, Y., et al. 1981. Reusable catheter for long-term sterile intermittent catheterization. *Arch. Phys. Med. Rehabil.* 62:39–42.

Wu, Y., et al. 1986. Inhibition of the external urethral sphincter and sacral reflex by anal stretch in spinal cord injured patients. *Arch. Phys. Med. Rehabil.* 67:135–136.

Chapter 6

Surgical Management of the Neurogenic Bladder

John B. Nanninga

Surgical intervention is considered often in the management of patients with neurogenic bladder dysfunction. Surgical procedures are designed either to improve the bladder as a storage organ or to reduce resistance to drainage of urine. There are several techniques that are used to provide more effective emptying.

SPHINCTEROTOMY

Male patients who demonstrate striated sphincter dyssynergy are candidates for division of the sphincter, provided that they can use an external collector. The abnormality in sphincter function can be demonstrated by voiding cystourethrography, preferably with fluoroscopic monitoring. Also, the study combining a cystometrogram with sphincter electromyography will aid in documenting the detrusor contraction and abnormal burst of sphincter activity. The division of the sphincter usually is performed at the 12-o'clock position (anterior) with a Collings blade and cutting current or a standard resectoscope loop electrode (Barrett et al. 1990; Nanninga et al. 1977). The incision should pass through the urethral mucosa into the sphincter tissue. Electrocoagulation is performed on the bleeding points. An indwelling catheter is left in place for 7 to 10 days. At times, the bladder neck also may be resected if it does not open well on the radiographic studies mentioned above. Some residual urine may remain when only sphincterotomy is done (Nanninga et al. 1977).

TRANSURETHRAL RESECTION

In instances where the bladder neck (internal sphincter) fails to open during a bladder contraction, it may be desirable to resect the bladder neck and some degree of prostatic tissue. As an alternative, an incision of the bladder neck can be performed at 5 and 7 o'clock. The incision should carry through the full thickness of bladder muscle (Barrett et al. 1990). There seems to be less chance of retrograde ejaculation with the incision technique.

PUDENDAL NEURECTOMY OR BLOCK

Here the sectioning or chemical block is aimed at reducing sphincter resistance by eliminating neural input to the striated sphincter. There is some danger of impotence and fecal incontinence with this procedure (Engel & Schirmer 1974).

SUPRAPUBIC CATHETERIZATION

Here the urethra is simply bypassed because a catheter is placed in the bladder by cystotomy over the bladder. This can be performed by percutaneous technique using a relatively small catheter and subsequently dilating the tract with catheter changes, or it can be performed as a cystotomy through a lower abdominal incision and with insertion of a tube of 24F to 28F size. The permanent use of the suprapubic tube will, over time, lead to a contracted bladder with resultant leaking of urine around the tube or through the urethra. Recurrent calculi may also occur with the use of the permanent tube.

URINARY DIVERSION

In rare instances, patients have not adapted to various other means of emptying the urinary bladder. There may be anatomic reasons, such as previous trauma to the urethra or bladder that has made catheterization difficult. There may also be loss of bladder compliance, so that incontinence occurs from lack of low-pressure storage. There may be upper tract changes as well. In these circumstances, construction of an ileal or colon conduit may offer a reasonable solution to urinary drainage. The patient or some dependable aide does have to acquire the ability to change the collection appliance. In the past, the ileal conduit has been associated with upper tract changes (Pitts & Muecke 1979); recent advances in antibiotics and stone management, however, have provided better means of treating urinary infections and renal calculi. Improvements in urinary collection applications have reduced the complication from stomal stenosis, but the threat of long-term complications remains: ureteroileal stricture, stomal problems, calculi formation, and bowel obstruction from adhesions. In recent years, neobladders fashioned from bowel, which can be intermittently catheterized, have been developed (King et al. 1987). Time will tell whether these also carry the risk of infections, calculi, or other as yet unrecognized problems.

PROCEDURES TO PROMOTE BLADDER STORAGE AND CONTINENCE

Leakage between catheterizations is a troublesome problem not infrequently encountered in the care of patients with spinal cord injury. Several techniques are available that can aid in reducing or eliminating the problem.

Denervation

Patients with hyperreflexic bladders often are bothered by incontinence despite anticholinergic medications that they may have been taking. Trying to perform intermittent catheterization more often than every 4 hours is frustrating and at times impossible. Consequently, decreasing the nerve input to the bladder will decrease the frequency of contractions. Denervation can be accomplished with chemical agents (phenol or 50% alcohol) or actual rhizotomy of sacral nerves (Barrett et al. 1990). The effect of the chemical agents usually wears off after 12 months. Surgical denervation is directed at sectioning of S-3 roots and possibly S-2 or S-4 if stimulation indicates that they play a role in bladder contraction. In men, impotence may occur, and some degree of fecal incontinence may follow.

Cystoplasty

Here, in an effort to achieve larger bladder capacity, a segment of colon or ileum is excised with its mesentery intact and is detubularized so as to prevent high-pressure (>40 cm H_2O) contractions. This segment is anastomosed to the bladder, which is bivalved so as to provide for a wide anastomotic line. With this augmented bladder, the patient can perform intermittent catheterization from a reservoir of 500 mL or greater. If there is sphincter incompetence, a fascial sling, Stamey suspension of the bladder neck (for women), or artificial sphincter can be inserted to aid in retention. Details of various procedures for augmenting or substituting the bladder are available in surgical texts (King et al. 1987).

RENAL CALCULI

Calculi may occur in the kidney, ureter, or urinary bladder. Treatment of stones has changed considerably over the past 5 years (Chaussy & Fuchs 1989). It is now unusual to have to perform open surgical removal of calculi, whether in the upper or lower tract.

Urinary bladder calculi are easily removed by use of electrohydraulic lithotripsy. The probe through which the electrical energy is delivered is passed into the bladder through the cystoscope. The stones are then pulverized with a series of electrical shocks, and the fragments are washed out through the cystoscope.

Renal calculi are now treated with extracorporeal shock wave lithotripsy (ESWL) or percutaneous ultrasonic lithotripsy. In some instances both methods are used consecutively to treat large, branched calculi. For stones less than 2 mL in volume, ESWL is effective in fragmenting the stones. The patient does have to be partially submerged in a water-filled tub, and some degree of anesthesia, or at least sedation, is required. New lithotripter models offer relatively pain-free treatment and may replace the older, bulkier models. At times, a urethral stent may be inserted to facilitate passage of calculous fragments after ESWL. The stent is removed several days or even weeks later, when radiography demonstrates that most or all of the fragments have passed.

Ureteral calculi can now be treated by several methods. One technique involves passing a ureteral catheter up to the stone and injecting viscous fluid such as anesthetic jelly, which forces the stone back to the kidney, where it can be treated with ESWL. With the development of the ureteroscope, direct visualization of the stone is possible, and the stone can be grasped and pulled out. For larger ureteral stones, an ultrasonic probe can be passed and used to fragment the stone. Recently, a laser (tuned dye) has been developed that can be used directly on the stone to pulverize it (Dretler 1990). After the removal of the ureteral calculus by whatever means, a stent may have to be passed and left in place until the edema has subsided and fragments have passed.

IMPOTENCE

Loss of erectile ability commonly accompanies spinal lesions of the sacral cord or cauda equina. During the past few years, pharmacologic management of impotence by injection of vasodilating agents directly into the corpora cavernosum has increased in use; there are patients, however, in whom penile prostheses provide for adequate sexual performance or facilitate placement of an external urinary collector (Goldstein & Krane 1992). For sexual function, the inflatable devices offer a more realistic and cosmetically acceptable solution. The malleable types are more effective in holding an external collector in place. New prostheses have the reservoir contained in the corporal component, thus reducing potential problems with tubing and valves in older models.

Risks in the use of penile prostheses in the population with spinal cord injury include erosion, often because the patient cannot feel excess pressure on the penis, and infection, which often is related to urinary tract infection. Either problem requires removal of the prosthesis. These risks are far greater in men with new spinal cord injury and penile prostheses.

PRIAPISM

This condition sometimes is seen in the acutely injured patient, usually one with a high cervical injury. If the erection persists for several hours, detumescence should be performed. Initially, this may be done with a 16- to 18-gauge needle inserted into the corpora followed by irrigation with normal saline. If the erection recurs, an attempt should be made to create a shunt between the corpora cavernosum and spongiosum. This can be done with a biopsy needle (Winter 1978), or a surgical procedure can create such a shunt (Wendel & Grayhack 1981).

FUTURE CONSIDERATIONS

Electrostimulation

The development of implantable stimulators, similar to the type used for control of chronic pain, has enabled surgeons to couple nerves to the bladder with stimulating electrodes (Brindley et al. 1986; Schmidt 1986). The devices are battery powered and programmable, and the electrodes are coupled to the nerve by one of several types of couplers. The bladder is emptied by activating the stimulator. It appears that in the next few years the system will be refined and establish respectable dependability.

Intrathecal Pumps

The development of implantable infusion systems has enabled surgeons to control, or at least alter, certain aspects of nervous system function. The use of implantable infusion systems has allowed baclofen to be delivered closer to the targeted sites in the CNS. The baclofen pump is used to control skeletal muscle spasticity but also has certain benefits in bladder management. In regard to the urinary system, a reduction in bladder hyperreflexia with increased bladder capacity and decreased sphincter activity has been noted, and this has enabled the patient to be free of an indwelling catheter (Nanninga et al. 1989). However, normal voiding may not occur with the pump. There are undoubtedly other potential pharmacological agents that can be used to provide effective bladder storage and emptying.

REFERENCES

Barrett, D., et al. 1990. Surgery for the neurogenic bladder. *Am. Urol. Assoc. Update Ser.* 9:38.

Brindley, G., et al. 1986. Sacral anterior root stimulation for bladder control in paraplegia: The first 50 cases. *J. Neurol. Neurosurg. Psychiatry* 49:1104–1114.

Chaussy, C., and G. Fuchs. 1989. Current state and future development of noninvasive treatment of human urinary stones with extracorporeal shock wave lithotripsy. *J. Urol.* 141:782.

Dretler, S. 1990. Evaluation of ureteral laser lithotripsy: 225 patients. *J. Urol.* 143:267.

Engel, R., and H. Schirmer. 1974. Pudendal neurectomy in neurogenic bladder. *J. Urol.* 112:57.

Goldstein, I., and R. Krane. 1992. "Diagnosis and therapy of erectile dysfunction." In *Campbell's Urology,* eds. P. Walsh et al., 6th ed., 3033–3066. Philadelphia, Pa.: Saunders.

King, L., et al. 1987. *Bladder construction and continent urinary diversion.* Chicago, Ill.: Year Book Medical.

Nanninga, J., et al. 1977. An explanation for the persistence of residual urine after external sphincterotomy. *J. Urol.* 118:821.

Nanninga, J., et al. 1989. Effect of intrathecal baclofen on bladder and sphincter function. *J. Urol.* 142:101.

Pitts, W., and E. Muecke. 1979. A 20-year experience with ileal conduits: The fate of the kidneys. *J. Urol.* 122:154.

Schmidt, R. 1986. Advances in genitourinary neurostimulation. *Neurosurgery* 18:1041.

Wendel, E., and J.T. Grayhack. 1981. Corpora cavernosa–glans penis shunt for priapism. *Surg. Gynecol. Obstet.* 153:586.

Winter, C. 1978. Priapism cured by creation of fistulas between glans penis and corpora cavernosa. *J. Urol.* 119:227.

Chapter 7

Sexual Function after Spinal Cord Injury

Gary M. Yarkony

Sexual functioning after a spinal cord injury (SCI) is an area of great concern during the rehabilitation process. It is common for patients to request information during the rehabilitation phase, but this issue may arise during the acute care period. Although women generally maintain their fertility after injury, the impact on sexual functioning is a major problem for both sexes. Past attitudes of the woman as the passive partner with minimal sexual problems after SCI must be discarded. This chapter reviews sexual dysfunction in individuals with SCI and addresses management techniques.

MALE SEXUAL DYSFUNCTION

Several investigators have attempted to define the importance of sexual dysfunction in individuals with SCI in comparison with their other losses. Hanson and Franklin (1976) reported that paraplegic veterans chose legs and bowel and bladder return before sexual function and that quadriplegic veterans ranked upper extremities, bowel and bladder return, and leg return before sexual function. In a mixed rehabilitation population, Spergel et al. (1976) reported that improved sexual functioning ranks low in importance to other rehabilitation variables. In a series of 50 veterans, Phelps et al. (1987) reported that general medical condition and bowel and bladder control ranked higher as important concerns for living than sexual ability.

Other sources differ. Reports in the nonmedical literature have suggested that many individuals with SCI mourn the loss of sexual function more than the loss of walking (Cole et al.

1973). Comarr (1970) has stated that most patients without genital sensation sublimate their sexual gratification into that of their mates, which becomes a substitute for their own absent orgasm. These observations have not been substantiated by scientific study.

Physiology of Erection and Ejaculation

Management of sexual dysfunction requires an understanding of the vascular mechanisms and neurophysiology involved in erection and ejaculation. Erections can be classified as reflexogenic and psychogenic (Weiss 1972). Psychogenic stimuli can be both facilitory or inhibitory, and the degree of tactile stimulation necessary to produce a reflex erection can be diminished by psychic stimulation.

Supraspinal mechanisms (Krane & Siroky 1981; Weiss 1972) for facilitation and inhibition of erection are complex. The limbic system and hypothalamus play a key role. Lesions in the ansa reticularis may cause impotence. The visceral efferent pathways connecting the brain and spinal cord descend in the lateral columns in the area of the pyramidal tracts. The spinal centers related to erection are in the sympathetic preganglionic fibers from T-11 to L-2 and the parasympathetic fibers from S-2 through S-4 (Benson et al. 1980; Krane & Siroky 1981; Weiss 1972). The parasympathetic system acts synergistically with the sympathetic system to produce erections.

Erections no longer are considered due purely to parasympathetic cholinergic stimuli (Guyton 1986) and involve noncholinergic/nonadrenergic mechanisms of both systems, which is known as cotransmission. Nitric oxide is now known to be the neurotransmitter for erections. The phenomenon of psychogenic erections in paraplegics with complete lower motor neuron (LMN) lesions and abolished reflexogenic erections indicates that pathways for erection from the sympathetic outflow exist. Reflex erections are mediated via the sacral parasympathetics with sensory input from the pudendal nerve. Sacral parasympathetic fibers are involved in neurologically intact individuals with psychogenic erections as well. T-10 is the critical level for perception of gonadal pain in paraplegic men (Bors 1950). Emission is primarily under sympathetic control; it is followed by closure of the bladder neck and then somatic relaxation and contraction of the bulbourethral muscles for ejaculation.

Erection is a vascular phenomenon (Guyton 1986; Weiss 1972). The penis contains vascular potential spaces between the arteries and veins, which are collapsed when the penis is flaccid. Polsters, valvelike structures containing smooth muscle, were considered the primary control of this mechanism. Recent evidence casts doubt on their existence and proposes that they may represent a degenerative phenomenon.

Erection and Ejaculation after SCI

The ability to have erections, to ejaculate, and to have successful coitus after SCI has been the subject of numerous investigations and reviews (Comarr 1971; Griffith et al. 1973; Higgins 1979; Tarabulcy 1972). Munro et al. (1948) first reported 74% of subjects to have erections unrelated to level and 7% to 8% to have ejaculation as well as two pregnancies in 84 subjects. Kuhn's (1950) study was the only one to include observation. He noted that erections could invariably be induced if there was reflex activity below the level of the lesion and that a sharply circumscribed reflexogenic area existed that included the corona of the glans and the penile frenulum. Twenty-two of 25 patients with lesions from T-2 to T-12 had erections; the other 3 patients developed incomplete erections but reported they had full erections at other times.

In a series of 200 patients, Talbot (1949) reported 42.5% with reflex erections, 21.0% with psychic erections, and 36.5% without erections. Of those who regained sexual function, 76% did so within 6 months and almost all within a year. Erections were more common with lesions above T-11 and in incomplete lesions. Twenty-three percent (46) of the 200 patients had successful intercourse, and 10% of the whole group ejaculated. In a second study in 1955, Talbot estimated a 5% rate of fertility and noted that if erections returned 76% began to do so within the first 6 months and 94% in the first year.

Bors and Comarr (1960) reported findings in 529 patients, and Comarr (1970) reported on an additional 150 patients a decade later; Comarr summarized the data from these studies

in 1977: They showed 93% reflexogenic erections in upper motor neuron (UMN) complete lesions, 98% reflex erections in UMN incomplete lesions, 26% psychogenic erections in LMN complete lesions, and 83% psychogenic erections in LMN incomplete lesions. Comarr stated that patients' final answers were reported in these studies even if he doubted their validity (Comarr 1970, 1977).

Zeitlin et al. (1957) noted similar findings in 100 patients 1 year after injury. In 638 patients, Tsuji et al. (1961) noted erections in 54% overall, 50% of the complete injured, and 67% of the incomplete injured. Other studies with similar results include those by Cibeira (1970), Joacheim and Wahle (1970), Fitzpatrick (1974), Sjogren and Egberg (1983), and Lamid (1985). The last four studies had fewer than 60 subjects, and Cibeira's had poor documentation of methodology. Lamid used nocturnal penile tumescence monitors in a small sample with various postonset times, making his results difficult to interpret. Because individuals with SCI may have nocturnal erections or reflex erections that are unreliable or too brief for intercourse, the utility of these studies is limited.

The ability to ejaculate (Higgins 1979) is reported to be low in all studies. For complete lesions, it is less than 10%. Reports for incomplete lesions are as high as 32%. Ejaculation generally is more common with LMN lesions and with more caudal lesions. Orgasms are defined poorly in the available studies (Higgins 1979). Extragenital responses include headache, warm sensation, physical pleasure, and sexual excitement (Comarr 1970; Higgins 1979; Kuhn 1950; Zeitlin et al. 1957).

These studies generally relied on patient report, which is a serious methodological flaw. This limits the value of the data but does give a good idea of general trends. Kuhn's (1950) study in a small series of paraplegics was the only study to include actual observation. The data must also be considered in light of the fluctuation in erectile function pointed out by several investigators. Erections may not occur when desired, may not be satisfactory for penetration, or may not last sufficiently to satisfy the partner. It is important to note that the statistical reports do not allow for an accurate prognosis for any one patient. All persons with SCI must be evaluated individually.

Testicular Biopsy Specimens and Hormonal Function

There are numerous reports of testicular biopsies after SCI. The first reports (Horne et al. 1948) showed abnormalities in five of seven patients, and one patient had one abnormal and one normal biopsy specimen. There were various degrees of spermatogenic arrest and one case of Leydig hypertrophy. Stemmermann et al. (1950) reported on specimens in 4 cases sampled by necropsy and 16 volunteers sampled by biopsy. The 3 trauma patients in the 4 autopsy reports all had serious medical complications that may have affected testicular function. Of the 16 young paraplegic men in good general health, 6 were normal and 10 had evidence of maturation arrest. This did not correlate with level, duration, epididymitis, or sexual potency. Bors et al. (1950) reported on 34 biopsy specimens, of which 3 were normal. The main finding was tubular atrophy with no disturbance of Leydig cells. The investigators stated that the specimens had less abnormal pathology with lesions below T-11 and that abnormal pathology correlated with impaired sweating.

Leriche et al. (1977–78) concluded after studying 57 patients that a neurogenic testicle does exist. They noted active spermatogenesis in 50% of their series, sclerosis at the interstitial tissue in 64%, and constant anomalies of tubes. They noted improved spermatogenesis at lower levels. Perkash et al. (1985) reported on 13 biopsy specimens, 6 of which were normal. Tubular atrophy and spermatogenic activity were reduced mildly in 6 cases and were markedly reduced in 1 case. Specimens were not related to years after injury. Testosterone and luteinizing hormone levels were higher in paraplegics than in controls. Morely et al. (1979) reported on 7 biopsy specimens: 4 abnormal, 2 with decreased spermatogenesis and normal Leydig cells with atrophy of seminiferous-thickened basement membranes and increased Leydig cells, and 1 with normal spermatogenesis and increased Leydig cells. Marked hyperplasia of Leydig cells has been reported by Keye (1956) on autopsy of a severely debilitated incomplete paraplegic.

Abnormalities of scrotal temperature have been proposed as an etiologic factor causing abnormal testicular morphology. Morales and Hardin (1958) indicated no differences between paraplegics and controls. This study did not indicate the subjects' positions during recording, which is now known to be particularly relevant. Scrotal temperatures (Brindley 1982) increase in paraplegics who are sitting in wheelchairs, and this may be a contributing factor to these abnormalities. Temperatures are not significantly different in bed, and paraplegics can lower scrotal temperature by sitting with the thighs apart and using scrotal slit underpants. Because paraplegics cannot walk or run, they lose the advantage of these activities, which lower scrotal temperatures.

In spite of the numerous testicular biopsy specimens reported in the literature, insufficient data exist to correlate the abnormalities with potential contributing factors such as level, urologic management, history of urologic complications, and medications. Abnormalities of hormonal production and control clearly are not contributing factors. Numerous studies (Morely et al. 1979; Phelps et al. 1987; VerVoort 1987) indicate normal levels of testosterone and an intact hypothalamic–pituitary–testicular axis. Acutely, postinjury plasma testosterone levels may drop, particularly in quadriplegics (VerVoort 1987). Further study is needed to determine the etiologic factors predisposing to testicular abnormalities. The etiology of these abnormalities is probably multifactorial.

Techniques To Restore Erections

Intracavernous Injections of Vasoactive Substances

Virag (1982) and colleagues (1984) first reported the use of intracavernous injections of papaverine to restore erections, stating that its use was discovered accidentally during a surgical procedure (Michal et al. 1977). Further studies of its therapeutic effects led to the conclusion that penile prosthesis and revascularization procedures could be avoided if a proper nonsurgical therapy was available. This technique bypasses psychological, neurological, and hormonal influence by acting locally on the penile vasculature (Lue & Tanagho 1987). Brindley (1983, 1984a) described the use of intracavernous injection of phenoxybenzamine, which is not available in an injectable form in the United States. Further studies by Brindley (1986a) showed that seven drugs that relax smooth muscle can cause an erection to some degree and that papaverine and phenoxybenzamine are used therapeutically. He suggested that short-acting substances such as thymoxamine, phentolamine, and verapamil, which cause brief erection, can be used for teaching purposes or for brief assessment of the erect penis.

The majority of studies of this technique have used combinations of papaverine and phentolamine. Zorgniotti and Lefleur (1985) described injection at the posterolateral aspect of the base of the penis with a 28.5-gauge needle without aspiration. Sidi et al. (1986) studied 100 men of whom 17 had SCI, with response in all 17. The dose ranged from 0.1 to 1.0 mL of a combination of 25mg/mL papaverine plus 0.83 mg/mL phentolamine. Two patients with SCI had sustained erections requiring treatment. Sidi et al. (1986) recommended papaverine alone in neurogenic patients.

Nellans et al. (1987) studied 69 patients with SCI of mixed etiology and noted side effects in 14.5% and a good response in 14 of 15 with neurological impotence. Wyndaele et al. (1986) studied 12 patients with SCI, beginning with 2 mg phentolamine and 10 mg papaverine and progressing to 10 mg phentolamine and 80 mg papaverine. Girdley et al. (1988) studied 78 patients, giving 0.3 mL of a solution of 5 mg phentolamine dissolved in 10 mL phentolamine (30 mg/mL) initially. Up to 2 mL of this solution was given. Some patients noted decreased effectiveness of the medication with time. Lue and Tanagho (1987) recommend injection with a 25-gauge needle with a rubber band at the base of the penis followed by pressure for 2 minutes. Although doses as high as 120 mg papaverine have been used, these investigators recommend starting with 3 mg (0.1 mL) in neurogenic impotence and progressing at 3-mg increments. Satisfactory responses at low doses such as this have been consistent in the clinical experience at our center (Rehabilitation Institute of Chicago), particularly in patients with partial or inconsistent reflex erections that were neither sufficient nor reliable for intercourse.

Minor side effects include transient pain and paresthesias, ecchymosis, and fibrotic changes at the site of injection. Infection, although not reported to be a risk in the general population (Abramowicz 1987), has been reported in two individuals with SCI using injection techniques and external catheters (Lue & Tanagho 1987). The most serious complication is priapism. There is a higher risk of priapism with the combination of papaverine and phentolamine in neurologic patients (Lee & Sharifi 1987). Stief and Watterauer (1988) recommend the combination because papaverine alone has caused fibrosis of intracavernous tissue after repeated doses in monkeys. There are numerous treatment options to manage priapism (Brindley 1984a; Lue & Tanagho 1987; Lue et al. 1986). The treatment depends on the duration. Aspiration both removes the drug and decreases intracavernous pressure; it is considered by many the first-line treatment. Adrenergic agents may be added, but their judicious use is recommended because of hypertensive episodes and the danger of cardiac ischemia. Surgical shunting procedures may be necessary in severe cases.

It should be noted that neither papaverine nor phentolamine is FDA approved for these purposes (Abramowicz 1987). Signed informed consent should be obtained before their use. Unreliable patients may perform multiple injections, resulting in priapism (Watters et al. 1988). Papaverine (Juenemann et al. 1986; Weiner 1985), a nonspecific smooth muscle relaxant, acts by decreasing resistance to arterial inflow and increasing resistance to venous outflow. The filling of sinusoids passively obstructs venous outflow. Phentolamine (Juenemann et al. 1986; Weiner 1985), an α–adrenergic blocker, acts by decreasing resistance to arterial inflow. Its effectiveness is less than that of papaverine, and it does not increase resistance to venous outflow. The combination of the two drugs is stable in solution for 40 days (Benson & Seifert 1988).

Prostaglandins currently are being studied as an alternative to these medications. Prostaglandins may be injected alone or in combination with papaverine (Gerber & Levine 1991).

Vacuum Techniques

Vacuum tumescence constriction therapy (Witherington 1987) describes the use of external devices that create a vacuum and cause an erectionlike state that is maintained by a constricting band. The penis is placed in a rigid tube; a pump creates the vacuum needed, filling the corpora with blood, and a constricting band at the base of the penis maintains the erection for up to 30 minutes. The ErecAid (Osbon Medical Systems, Augusta, Ga.; Figure 7–1), originally marketed as the Youth Equivalent Device, has been available since 1917. The device generally is effective but results in decreased blood flow while the rubber band is in place (Nadig et al. 1986). The erections also differ in that the penile temperature falls, there is congestion of extracorporeal penile tissue, and the penis may not pivot because it is only rigid distal to the constrictive

band. The ejaculation may be trapped proximal to the band as well. Many similar devices are available, some with mechanisms to limit the degree of vacuum created. Examples are the Response System (Smith-Collins Pharmaceuticals, Westchester, Penn.) and the Post-T-Vac (EKC Corporation, Dodge City, Kan.; Figure 7–1).

Intracavernous injections of papaverine, phentolamine, and vacuum tumescence constriction therapy have been combined to augment partial erections (Marmar et al. 1988). The time to produce an erection was diminished, and blood flow increased during the constriction interval. There were no patients with SCI in this study.

Penile Prostheses

Many types of penile prostheses are available. The two basic designs are semirigid and inflatable. Semirigid prostheses can be hinged, malleable, or articulating. Inflatable penile prostheses can be multicomponent or self-contained.

The Small-Carrion prosthesis (Cole 1988; Small 1976) is a paired silicone device and adds length, width, and firmness. It is not adjustable in any way. The Finney Flexirod (Finney 1977) is hinged and allows the penis to hang in a more normal manner. The Jonas silicone silver penile prosthesis (Jonas & Jacob 1980; Tawil & Gregory 1986) allows for various positions with improved function. There are two articulating designs. The Duraphase (Krane 1988) is an articulating device that is always activated and is therefore similar in function to a malleable prosthesis. The Omniphase (Krane 1986, 1988) has an activating mechanism that shortens the device, making it rigid. This is accomplished by bending via rotation of the penis.

Multicomponent inflatable prostheses have a pumping mechanism, a reservoir, and paired penile prostheses. These

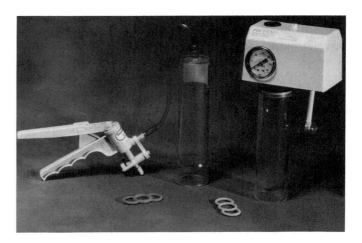

Figure 7–1 Vacuum constriction tumescence therapy devices: ErecAid (left) and Post-T-Vac (right).

are far more expensive than the semirigid rod (Krauss 1987). Although they are more physiologic, mechanical breakdown has been a major problem, although this should be diminished by new designs (Furlow 1979; Joseph et al. 1984; Juenemann et al. 1986; Malloy et al. 1980; Merrill 1988). Newer designs with more uniform dilatation and improved performance may be more difficult to operate, an important consideration in patients with SCI (Mulcahy 1988a). Sexual partners may be more satisfied with this design (Beutler et al. 1984; Gerstenberger et al. 1979). New self-contained inflatable devices (Flexiflate and Hydroflex) eliminate the separate reservoir and pumping mechanism. There is no change in length or girth during erection. The inflation/deflation mechanism of the Hydroflex is the most difficult to use. Girth and rigidity are less than with the original multicomponent designs (Mulcahy 1988b).

These devices may be used in individuals with SCI for both impotence (Golgi 1979; Green & Sloan 1986; Light & Scott 1981; Rossier & Fam 1984) and maintenance of external catheters (Hanson & Merritt 1985; Rossier & Fam 1984; Smith et al. 1980; Van Arsdalen et al. 1981). Melman and Hammond (1978) first reported use of the Small-Carrion prosthesis primarily for maintaining a condom catheter. Dangers of these devices include a high erosion rate in some series as well as risk of infection and mechanical problems (Collins & Hackler 1988; Golgi 1979; Hanson & Merritt 1985; Rossier & Fam 1984).

Golgi (1979) reported follow-up of 25 of 30 men with SCI with Small-Carrion implantation used solely for external catheters. Extrusion occurred in 2 secondary to infection, and a wound infection occurred in 2 others. Smith et al. (1980) implanted 33 penile prostheses, 27 rigid and 6 inflatable, for neurogenic bladders. Eight of the 11 patients with SCI in the study had regular intercourse, satisfying their partners, and 4 of these reported some sensation of climax. The study noted that 8 patients performed intermittent catheterization more easily because the penis was more accessible. No erosions were reported in a 3- to 36-month follow-up. Light and Scott (1981) placed 18 inflatable penile prostheses: Eight required revision (5 surgical and 3 mechanical), and 3 required removal, 2 of these because of erosion. The majority of female partners interviewed expressed satisfaction.

Van Arsdalen et al. (1981) implanted 20 noninflatable prostheses in patients with SCI. The erosion rate was 25%. The prostheses were implanted to maintain condom catheters; skin problems were decreased in 14 patients. Rossier (in Perkash et al. 1985) reported a series of 36 semirigid prostheses for men with SCI. Postoperative complications resulted in removal of 7 (19.5%), 6 of these because of extrusion and 1 because of surgical error; infection occurred in 4 (11%). Prostheses were more successful for intercourse if the patient had some erectile capacity. Hanson and Franklin (1976) reported erosion with 22% of semirigid rods as opposed to 8% of inflat-

able prostheses. Nine of the 29 inflatable prostheses required minor surgical repairs.

Green and Sloan (1986) stressed the importance of combining psychosexual counseling with surgical treatment. They recommend implantation of prostheses when there is a stable bladder program, a recent radiographic urological evaluation, sterile urine, and no decubiti. Results were reported in 40 patients: Six patients had inflatable prostheses, and 34 had semirigid rods. Thirty-five patients were available for follow-up. Of these, 31 reported satisfactory intercourse, and 4 stated that their semirigid prostheses were not rigid enough for intercourse.

Iwatsubo et al. (1986) implanted a Shirai type semirigid prosthesis in 37 patients with SCI; 86% reported better condom fitting, and 41% reported improved sexual function. The erosion rate of only 5% (which was due to wound infection) was attributed to the flat rib shape, which the prosthesis designers consider more physiologic. Collins and Hackler (1988) reported placement of 53 semirigid devices with a 33% extrusion rate and 10 inflatable prostheses, of which 4 were lost. After reimplantation, 52 of 63 patients had functional prostheses.

Penile prostheses should be used judiciously in the population with SCI. The rate of infection in the general population is 2%, but it is 7% in the population with SCI. The erosion rate in the general population is 1% but is reported to be 11% in the population with SCI (Collins & Hackler 1988). Clearly defined criteria must be developed for their usage.

Other Methods

Sacral anterior root stimulators (Brindley et al. 1982, 1986) were developed as a means of obtaining urinary continence. These devices may produce erection as well, which can last the duration of the electrical stimulation. It is doubtful that this device will be implanted solely for erectile dysfunction.

Yohimbine (Morales et al. 1987; Reid et al. 1987), an α-adrenoreceptor given orally, has been studied for the treatment of impotence. Reid et al. (1987), in a placebo-controlled double-blind partial crossover study, showed yohimbine to be as effective as sex and marital therapy in psychogenic impotence. This beneficial effect was proposed to be due to its enhancement of sympathetic outflow. Morales et al. (1987) studied yohimbine in patients with organic impotence. There was no statistically significant difference between yohimbine and placebo. Despite this, the investigators stated that because of safety and ease of administration it may be used in patients who reject more invasive methods. There is no documentation of its benefits in SCI. Further study of this agent is needed.

Methods To Obtain Semen

Guttmann and Walsh (1971) described the use of intrathecal neostigmine methylsulfate in 1947 to obtain semen for sperm analysis; to check sperm motility, concentration, and cytology after hormone treatment; or for artificial insemination. Neostigmine is a reversible acetylcholine esterase inhibitor. The drug was given via lumbar puncture. The test was positive in 58.2% of patients. The majority of negative results occurred with lesions between T-10 and L-4. Side effects included headache, sweating, vomiting, and one death, which occurred at a previously tolerated dosage. Pregnancies using this technique have been reported by Spira (1956), Chapelle et al. (1976), and Otoni et al. (1985). Chapelle et al. stated that two segments of T-11, T-12, and L-1 must be intact for the technique to be successful. This technique largely has been abandoned (Francois & Maury 1987).

Chapelle et al. (1983) have reported the use of subcutaneous physostigmine, which differs from neostigmine in that it can cross the blood-brain barrier and can be given by subcutaneous injection. Peripherally acting parasympathetic blockers are used to inhibit the peripheral effects of nausea and vomiting. The investigators state that this technique is as effective as intrathecal neostigmine but has fewer side effects. Francois and Maury (1987) reported that Chapelle et al. (1983) achieved 27 pregnancies in 80 paraplegics using this technique. Two milligrams of physostigmine sulfate are injected subcutaneously followed by masturbation 15 minutes later. This may be followed by an additional 1 mg of physostigmine after 30 minutes. For side effects, metoclopramide was used, if necessary, with atropine. For the technique to be successful, T-12, L-1, and L-2 must be intact. The most common side effects are orthostatic hypotension, tachycardia, nausea, and vomiting. Autonomic dysreflexia has not been observed.

Vibratory stimulation of the penis may induce reflex ejaculation, and pregnancies have been reported from this technique. Comarr (1970) described a patient using a "Swedish massager" to obtain sperm and inseminate his wife with the condom-collected ejaculate. Tarabulcy (1972) reported the use of a vibrator to obtain semen from men with SCI, but no details of the technique were reported. Brindley (1981b) studied this technique further and reported success in 12 of 21 men using the Ling 201 vibrator (Figure 7–2), which originally was designed for industrial use, or the Pifco vibrator for home use. He refined this technique further and in 1984 reported positive results in 48 of 81 men with mostly complete SCI using the Ling vibrator at 80 Hz and 2.5 mm (Brindley 1984b). This technique was rarely successful before 6 months and failed in all patients without reflex hip flexion after stroking of the bottom of the foot. Brindley reported 11 pregnancies in eight couples. Vibratory ejaculation was felt to produce better sperm quality than electroejaculation, which improved with successive attempts.

Sarkarati et al. (1987) used the Ling vibrator and were successful in 8 of 33 patients, 1 within the first 6 months after injury. Vibratory ejaculation was accompanied by rhythmic reflex contraction of anal and genital muscles and abdominal contractions. Szasz (1986), using a vibrator at 60 to 80 Hz, reported success in 14 of 17 men with lesions above T12–L1 and failure in 5 men with lesions below this level. The major side effect of this technique is autonomic dysreflexia, which may prevent successful completion of the clinical trial.

Electroejaculation, obtaining semen by electrical stimulation with electrodes in the rectum, may be successful where vibratory stimulation fails or autonomic dysreflexia prohibits its usefulness (Brindley 1984b). Brindley (1981a) describes the goal of electroejaculation to be stimulation of the proper nerve fibers and as few as possible of the wrong ones with the

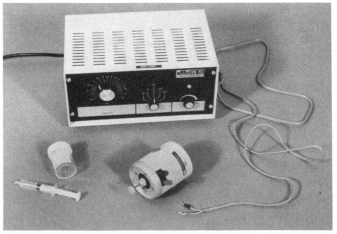

(A)

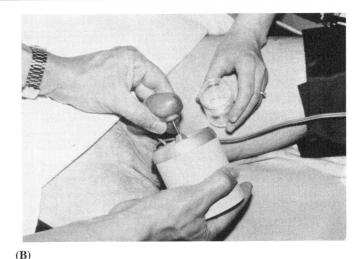

(B)

Figure 7–2 (A) The Ling 201 vibrator. **(B)** Vibratory stimulation being applied.

least possible risk of thermal and electrolytic damage to the rectal mucosa. The technique stimulates myelinated sympathetic efferent fibers of the hypogastric plexus (Brindley 1986b). Electroejaculation may be successful within the first 6 months. There have been numerous techniques described, and there is some debate in the literature as to the electrical safety of various methods used.

The first report in men with SCI was made by Horne et al. (1948), who obtained sperm by electroejaculation in 13 of 18 patients, 10 by electrical stimulation and 3 by masturbation. The 5 failures had lesions below T-11. A urethral sound was used and placed in the region of the seminal vesicles or prostate. Current was sinusoidal or faradic, 45 or 60 mA, and 90 V. Stimulation was followed by massage of the seminal vesicles and prostate. Massage without electrical stimulation was unsuccessful in all but 1 case. Potts (1957) and Rowan et al. (1962) reported unsuccessful attempts at electroejaculation. Bensman and Kottke (1966) reported successful electroejaculation using a rectal diathermy probe in 3 patients, 2 with cervical lesions and 1 with a T-12 lesion. All sperm was obtained from the urine and was nonmotile. Frankel et al. (1974) reported the hemodynamic effects of rectal electroejaculation and noted hypertensive headache and a rise in plasma noradrenaline and prostaglandin E.

The first reported pregnancy using semen obtained by electroejaculation from a T-12 paraplegic of 3 years' duration was reported by Thomas et al. (1975). A live birth occurred, but the neonate died within 24 hours. David et al. (1977–78) used a Grass stimulator and a custom-designed rectal probe and obtained specimens in 4 of 6 patients with UMN lesions, of whom 3 had incomplete lesions. Sperm motility was poor with a high percentage of abnormal cells. Francois et al. (1978–79) reported the next live birth in 1977 after electroejaculation; they also reported successful electroejaculation in

13 of 31 patients. Brindley used an electroejaculation device (Figure 7–3) and reported a pregnancy in 1980, reported results in 84 men in 1981a, and summarized his results with 73 additional men, totaling 154 subjects in 1984b. Sixty-nine patients had external success (spermatozoa at the meatus but not necessarily motile), and 28 had retrograde success with sperm in the next urine. Semen was obtained by electroejaculation in 21 of the 34 men for whom the vibrator failed. Brindley (1984b) reported 11 pregnancies in eight couples, 3 by electroejaculation, 7 by vibration, and 1 by masturbation.

Martin et al. (1983) and Warner et al. (1986) refer to their technique of electroejaculation as rectal probe electrostimulation (RPE). These investigators state that their technique is safer than Brindley's because their current density is lower and their sinusoidal waveform is safer than the rectangular waveform. They described a modified Foley catheter with a port in the prostatic urethra to prevent retrograde ejaculation. Success was reported in 22 patients. They reported retrograde ejaculation in 6 patients, antegrade ejaculation in 4, both in 10, and neither in 2. Nine patients with lesions below L-2 could not tolerate the stimulation.

Halstead et al. (1987) used RPE in 12 subjects with antegrade success in 9 and retrograde success in 1. Sperm suitable for insemination was obtained in 4 subjects. The investigators used their own equipment as well. Repeated attempts yielded an improvement in sperm quality. Sarkarati et al. (1987) used the equipment developed by Brindley and had success in 8 of 22 subjects with lesions from C-6 to T-12, but with no improvement in repeated attempts and low-quality samples. Bennett et al. (1988) at the University of Michigan reported positive results in 7 of 13 cervical lesions, all of 14 thoracic lesions, 1 in 3 lumbar lesions, and 13 of 20 complete and 8 of 17 incomplete lesions. They reported pregnancies in 4 of 10 patients and stated that the best results were obtained in men with lesions at the thoracic level. Recurrent urinary tract infections or epididymitis appeared to affect negatively the ability to have an ejaculation.

These studies are difficult to compare because of the various methods used, although the many reported pregnancies make this procedure promising. Electroejaculation appears to succeed with a large proportion of men because it requires survival of the T-10 to L-2 segments. Reflex function in the lumbar cord is not necessary. Pregnancies that are confirmed by paternity testing are a concern in evaluating techniques reported to enhance fertility. Further study is needed to compare the various devices available for safety and efficacy.

Counseling

Thorough physical evaluation is an important adjunct to a counseling program (Comarr & Vique 1978a; 1978b). The patient and the staff dealing with the patient should be aware of the physiological changes that occur and of the probable

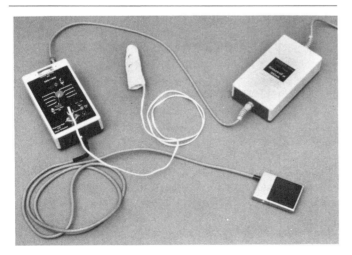

Figure 7–3 Brindley's electroejaculation device.

functional outcomes. Awareness on the part of the patient should greatly enhance community reintegration. It is unclear at what time after injury a counseling program is most effective. The rehabilitation phase has been reported to be the time at which patients are most likely to desire information regarding sexual functioning (Miller 1988). A sexual counseling program is a mandatory part of any rehabilitation program and can be accomplished through both individual and group therapy (Cole et al. 1973; Eisenberg & Rustad 1976; Melnyk et al. 1979).

Rehabilitation Institute of Chicago Male Sexual Dysfunction Clinic

Management of sexual dysfunction is an integral part of rehabilitation of individuals with SCI. The first step is counseling of the patient and his partner. The individual with SCI should be provided both general information in regard to sexual functioning after SCI and more specific guidelines based on the physical examination and experience with other individuals at that level. Written or audiovisual materials may assist in this process. It is important to note that erectile functioning may not return for 6 to 12 months and that aggressive intervention should be limited initially. The individual with SCI should be aware of the possibilities to restore both erectile functioning and fertility before discharge. Services in our center generally are initiated 6 months after injury. This allows for natural recovery and avoids the disappointment of vibratory ejaculation failing during the initial trial. Patients are shown videos of the techniques to restore erection and are allowed to decide which technique they prefer unless specific medical conditions prevent its use. A medical work-up is required of patients who do not have SCI as an obvious cause of sexual dysfunction. They must be aware of the risks of each technique, particularly scarring and priapism from intracavernous injections and the decreased blood flow from constrictive rings around the penis with vacuum tumescence constriction therapy. Informed consent is obtained before penile injections. Patients generally choose the technique they consider the most natural or safest.

For fertility, we begin with the Ling vibrator 6 months after injury and then try commercially available vibrators. The Ling is used initially because of the good response reported in the literature, allowing for the best initial results. Patients may be given vibrators for home use, although autonomic dysreflexia is a limiting factor. Electroejaculation with the equipment developed by Seager and Halstead (Halstead et al. 1987; Figure 7–4) is then used if there is no response or if autonomic dysreflexia develops. This may become the first choice if home units become available. Evaluation for sexually transmitted disease is required when fertilization is requested. Consultation with a gynecologist may be needed for insemination, especially when a low sperm count is involved.

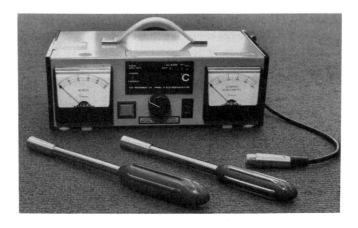

Figure 7–4 Electroejaculation equipment developed by Seager.

Recent advances have improved the possibilities for sexual rehabilitation after SCI. Further study is needed to determine the long-term risks and benefits of these techniques and to provide adaptive devices that the individual with SCI can manage independently.

FEMALE SEXUAL FUNCTIONING

Recent studies have acknowledged that sexual adjustment is an important part of the rehabilitation process for women with SCI (Stirt et al. 1979). Women reportedly have less impairment in sex role functions and identification after disability than men (Weiss & Diamond 1966), although the adjustment may take several years after injury. Disability also may lead to postinjury divorce, further complicating adjustment (DeVivo & Fine 1985).

The woman's self-concept and degree of perceived independence after injury may affect her participation as a sexual partner (Guttmann et al. 1965). Counseling (Cole 1975; Fitting et al. 1978; Griffith & Trieschmann 1975; Romano 1981; Thornton 1979) may play an important part in the adaptation process. Women must acknowledge that sexuality is an integral part of their being and be encouraged to experiment with their sexual expression. Counseling may be needed on a short- or long-term basis. Issues in counseling may be related to problems such as positioning, contractures, management of menstrual periods, or dealing with bladder and bowel incontinence. Other areas that may require long-term counseling include presentation and perception of self and social skills, communication and cueing during sexual activity, and the impact of the injury on marriage and family (Romano 1981). Counseling may be helpful before conception to help the woman with SCI prepare for the difficulties she may encounter in caring for the child.

In spite of the absence of genital sensation, other erogenous areas such as the breasts, shoulders, neck, or mouth may enhance the sexual experience (Thornton 1979). Women report orgasm in spite of evidence that it is not possible with complete lesions of the spinothalamic tracts (Ohry et al. 1978). Phantom orgasms have been reported in the dreams of paraplegics (Money 1960). Orgasm (Geiger 1979) may be described as similar to that of able-bodied women or as a wide variety of psychological experiences, such as pleasant, relaxed, glowing feelings (Bregman & Hadley 1976). Vaginal lubrication may occur reflexively with lesions above T-9 and not at all with lesions between T-10 and T-12, and psychogenic lubrication may occur in lesions below T-12 (Berard 1989).

Amenorrhea may result from SCI, although its occurrence is not uniform, and menstruation generally returns within 1 year (Cole 1975). Reports of secondary amenorrhea after SCI range from 50% to 60% (Axel 1982; Griffith & Trieschmann 1975). Comarr (1966) reported that the majority of women with SCI will have return of menses within 6 months, although one woman's delay was 30 months. Women at or near the climacteric may lose their menses. Axel (1982) reported a mean return in 5 months. Axel's report contradicted Comarr's (1966) report that dysmenorrhea will cease. Galactorrhea may occur with or without loss of menstruation. If associated with hyperprolactinemia, a pituitary lesion must be considered.

Birth control is a complex issue after SCI (Cole 1975). Intrauterine device usage is limited by the woman's lack of pain sensation. The use of a diaphragm is limited by dexterity. Oral contraceptive use may further increase the risk of deep venous thrombosis.

Pregnancy, Labor, and Delivery

There are numerous reports of pregnancy occurring in women with SCI. These reports date back to 1906, noting painless labor and cesarean section without anesthesia. Unfortunately, these generally are in the form of case studies (Abouleish 1980; Bradley et al. 1957; Daw 1973; Ferguson & Catanzorite 1984; Gimovsky et al. 1985; Goller & Paeslack 1970; Guttmann et al. 1965; Hardy & Worrell 1965; Letcher & Goldfine 1986; McCunniff & Dewon 1984; McGregor & Meeuwsen 1985; Mulla 1957; Nath et al. 1979; Oppenheimer 1971; Romano 1981; Saunders & Yeo 1968; Spielman 1984; Stirt et al. 1979; Verduyn 1989; Ware 1934; Watson & Downey 1980) and reviews (Berard 1989; Ciliberti et al. 1954; Turk et al. 1983; Verduyn 1986). There are no controlled studies resulting in guidelines for optimum management at the present time.

Women may sustain an SCI during pregnancy. They may not be aware that they are pregnant or may be unable to inform the staff of this because of associated brain injury. Pregnancy during the acute phase may limit radiological evaluation and surgical treatment of the injured spine, necessitating conservative spine management.

Goller and Paeslack (1970) have reported two cases in which the fetus may have sustained cranial injuries at the time of the accident in which the mother was rendered paraplegic. This may have been due to direct trauma, anorexia, or hypoxemia. In a second series (Goller & Paeslack 1972) based on a questionnaire of 45 women at the time of injury, there were 31 healthy newborns. Five children were born with malformations or disability. There were five miscarriages, two abortions, one death due to lung immaturity and one stillbirth due to placenta previa. Insufficient data exist to analyze the abnormalities in these births, which probably were multifactorial. The investigators also reported 130 women with SCI and 147 normal children born to women who became pregnant after their spinal cord injury, including 10 miscarriages, 3 abortions, and 5 stillbirths. They noted an increase in premature and small-for-date children in this group but no problems with malformations.

Robertson (1972) and Robertson and Guttmann (1963) reported their experience with 25 women with SCI giving birth to 33 children. Several of their observations generally are well accepted. It is well known that the uterus can contract with the nerve supply severed. Because labor will be painless with lesions above T-10, examination may be necessary to determine the onset of labor. Premature labor is more common, and premature delivery may occur in unfavorable surroundings without competent medical care. These investigators recommended that the examination begin at week 28, with hospital admission if the cervix is effaced, and routine admission by week 35. Home tokodynamometry and patient instruction in uterine palpation may be helpful as well (Greenspoon & Paul 1986). Nonabsorbable sutures are recommended to repair the episiotomy because of the risk of sterile abscess from buried catgut.

Greenspoon and Paul (1986) noted that SCI is not by itself an indication for cesarean section. Indications are no different from those in women without SCI. Breastfeeding is successful as well, although there is a case report of it stimulating autonomic dysreflexia (Devenport & Swenson 1983).

Greenspoon and Paul (1986) recommend a team approach in dealing with these pregnancies; ideally, the team would consist of the primary care physician, neurologist, rehabilitation personnel, obstetrician, anesthesiologist, and urologist. The delivery facility should be able to perform invasive hemodynamic monitoring, and the neonatal unit should be ready to care for a premature infant. The management of the patient includes recognition and treatment of autonomic dysreflexia, the ability to support respiration in cervical lesions, prevention of unsupervised delivery, surveillance for urinary tract infections, treatment of anemia, skin care to prevent pressure ulcers, maintenance of normal bowel function, counseling, and contraception and sterilization.

Autonomic dysreflexia during labor has generated numerous reports and much controversy. Obviously the first step is awareness of this condition by the labor and delivery team of physicians and nurses. There are recent reports of intraventricular hemorrhage with resultant neurological deficits (McGregor & Meeuwsen 1985; Verduyn 1989) and death (Abouleish 1980; Verduyn 1989), indicating that unrecognized autonomic dysreflexia still results in morbidity and mortality.

Although autonomic dysreflexia generally occurs in lesions at T-6 and above, there was a case of dysreflexia in the postpartum period in a woman with a T-10 lesion (Gimovsky et al. 1985). Monitoring the situation may require an intraarterial catheter, cardiac monitoring, the ability to administer antihypertensive medication, fetal monitoring (because maternal hypotension may cause fetal hypoperfusion), and appropriate anesthesia. Cardiac dysrhythmias may occur in the mother as a result of the dysreflexia, although they are not considered a general manifestation of the dysreflexia or solely due to the pregnancy (Guttmann et al. 1965).

Reserpine 2 weeks before the expected date of delivery has been recommended as a means to prevent autonomic dysreflexia (Saunders & Yeo 1968). It has been suggested that cystometrograms can predict dysreflexia during delivery, but guidelines are lacking. Nitroglycerin has been given intravenously during cesarean section in hypertensive women but has not been studied in women with SCI. Nitroprusside has been used, but epidural anesthesia is required, and concerns exist about the metabolic effects of cyanide, which has been detected in fetal blood after maternal exposure to nitroprusside (Ravindran et al. 1981). Young et al. (1983) reported the use of diazepam (Valium), diphenhydramine (Benadryl), and promethazine (Phenergan). None of these drugs is used commonly to treat dysreflexia. This report resulted in numerous letters suggesting that continuous epidural anesthesia or spinal anesthesia would have been more appropriate (McCunniff & Dewon 1984; Spielman 1984). This suggestion was based on reports of its success by Stirt et al. (1979), Ciliberti et al. (1954), and Abouleish (1980). Many believe epidural anesthesia to be the method of choice because it blocks the reflex arc. It is considered easy to perform and control and beneficial in that it prevents rather than treats the syndrome. Epidural anesthesia has been reported to improve patient comfort (Watson & Downey 1980) and to be preferable to spinal anesthesia because of difficulties in controlling the level of block and the

increased risk of hypotension (Stirt et al. 1979). One case has been reported of epidural anesthesia failing and spinal anesthesia succeeding. This was due to catheter placement difficulties. Nath et al. (1979) suggested that, if autonomic dysreflexia cannot be controlled, prompt delivery by cesarean section may be the most expedient method of management.

Other suggestions to prevent autonomic dysreflexia include avoidance of external restraints, an indwelling catheter to prevent bladder distension (particularly during the later stages of pregnancy), and use of anesthetic ointments during examination and catheter manipulation.

Labor may be associated with uterine hyperactivity, which is corrected by oxytocin (Young et al. 1983). Spasms of abdominal muscles may massage the uterus between contractions. Early mobilization after delivery is encouraged to prevent deep venous thrombosis. Physical therapy for lower extremity passive range of motion should be available.

Urologic complications have been noted as a result of pregnancy. Although ileal conduits are used less frequently, obstruction may occur (Guttmann et al. 1965). Urinary infection may lead to pyelonephritis or septicemia (Bradley et al. 1957; Wanner et al. 1987). It should not be assumed that normal patterns of voiding will resume after delivery. Increased residual urines have resulted, and the loss of reflex bladder function has occurred with a corresponding need for indwelling catheters (Wanner et al. 1987). An indwelling catheter may facilitate bladder management as pregnancy progresses.

Management of anemia with oral iron may exacerbate constipation and require modification of the bowel program. Folate deficiencies may be present in women being treated for seizure disorders.

The rehabilitation team may be helpful to the obstetrician. Consultation may be obtained in regard to positioning for comfort and treatment of pressure ulcers. The rehabilitation facility may be an appropriate site to manage the patient during pregnancy (Letcher & Goldfine 1986). After delivery, our center has admitted the mother and child to the same room. This facilitates bonding and allows the mother to learn to care for the infant as part of her rehabilitation.

Summary

Pregnancy associated with SCI represents a challenge to the obstetrician. A team approach to caring for these women may result in the best outcomes. Further studies are needed to determine optimal management during pregnancy and delivery.

REFERENCES

Abouleish, E. 1980. Hypertension in a paraplegic parturient. *Anesthesiology* 53:348–349.

Abramowicz, M., ed. 1987. Intracavernous injections for impotence. *Med. Lett. Drugs Ther.* 29:95–96.

Axel, S.J. 1982. Spinal cord injured women's concerns: Menstruation and pregnancy. *Rehab. Nurs.* 7:10–15.

Bennett, C.J., et al. 1988. Sexual dysfunction and electroejaculation in men with spinal cord injury: Review. *J. Urol.* 139:453–457.

Bensman, A., and F.J. Kottke. 1966. Induced emission of sperm utilizing stimulation of the seminal vesicles and vas deferens. *Arch. Phys. Med. Rehabil.* 47:436–443.

Benson, G.S., and W.E. Seifert. 1988. Is phentolamine stable in solution with papaverine? *J. Urol.* 140:970–971.

Benson, G.S., et al. 1980. Neuromorphology and neuropharmacology of the human penis. *J. Clin. Invest.* 65:506–513.

Berard, E.J.T. 1989. The sexuality of spinal cord injured women: Physiology and pathophysiology, a review. *Paraplegia* 22:99–112.

Beutler, L.E., et al. 1984. Women's satisfaction with partners' penile implant, inflatable vs. non-inflatable prosthesis. *Urology* 14:552–558.

Bors, E. 1950. Perception of gonadal pain in paraplegic patients. *Arch. Neurol. Psychol.* 63:713–718.

Bors, E., and A.E. Comarr. 1960. Neurological disturbances of sexual function with special reference to 529 patients with spinal cord injury. *Urol. Surv.* 10:191–222.

Bors, E., et al. 1950. Fertility in paraplegic males: A preliminary report of endocrine studies. *J. Clin. Endocrinol.* 10:381–398.

Bradley, W.S., et al. 1957. Pregnancy in paraplegia: A case report with urologic complication. *Obstet. Gynecol.* 10:573–575.

Bregman, S., and R.G. Hadley. 1976. Sexual adjustment and feminine attractiveness among spinal cord injured women. *Arch. Phys. Med. Rehabil.* 57:448–450.

Brindley, G.S. 1980. Electroejaculation and the fertility of paraplegic men. *Sex. Disabil.* 3:223–229.

Brindley, G.S. 1981a. Electroejaculation: Its technique, neurological implications and uses. *J. Neurol. Neurosurg. Psychiatry* 44:9–18.

Brindley, G.S. 1981b. Reflex ejaculation under vibratory stimulation in paraplegic men. *Paraplegia* 19:299–302.

Brindley, G.S. 1982. Deep scrotal temperature and the effect on it of clothing, air temperature activity, posture and paraplegia. *Br. J. Urol.* 54:49–55.

Brindley, G.S. 1983. Cavernosal α-blockage: A new technique for investigating and treating erectile impotence. *Br. J. Psychiatry* 143:332–337.

Brindley, G.S. 1984a. New treatment for priapism. *Lancet* 2:220–221.

Brindley, G.S. 1984b. The fertility of men with spinal injuries. *Paraplegia* 22:337–348.

Brindley, G.S. 1986a. Pilot experiments on the action of drugs injected into the human corpus cavernosum penis. *Br. J. Pharmacol.* 87:495–500.

Brindley, G.S.. 1986b. "Sexual and reproductive problems of paraplegic men." In *Oxford reviews of reproductive biology,* ed. J.R. Clark, 214–221. Oxford, England: Clarendon.

Brindley, G.S., et al. 1982. Sacral anterior root stimulators for bladder control in paraplegia. *Paraplegia* 20:365–381.

Brindley, G.S., et al. 1986. Sacral anterior root stimulators for bladder control in paraplegia: The first 50 cases. *J. Neurol. Neurosurg. Psychiatry* 49:1104–1114.

Chapelle, P.A., et al. 1976. Pregnancy of the wife of a complete paraplegic by homologous insemination after an intrathecal injection of neostigmine. *Paraplegia* 14:173–177.

Chapelle, P.A., et al. 1983. Treatment of anejaculation in the total paraplegic by subcutaneous injection of physostigmine. *Paraplegia* 21:30–36.

Cibeira, J.B. 1970. Some conclusions on a study of 365 patients with spinal cord lesions. *Paraplegia* 7:249–254.

Ciliberti, B.J., et al. 1954. Hypertension during anesthesia in patients with spinal cord injuries. *Anesthesiology* 15:273–279.

Cole, H.M., ed. 1988. Penile implants for erectile impotence. *J.A.M.A.* 260:997–1000.

Cole, T.M. 1975. Sexuality and physical disabilities. *Arch. Sex. Behav.* 4:389–403.

Cole, T.M., et al. 1973. A new programme of sex education and counseling for spinal cord injured adults and health care professionals. *Paraplegia* 11:111–124.

Collins, K.P., and R.H. Hackler. 1988. Complications of penile prosthesis in the spinal cord injury population. *J. Urol.* 140:984–985.

Comarr, A.E. 1966. Observations on menstruation and pregnancy among female spinal cord injury patients. *Paraplegia* 3:263–272.

Comarr, A.E. 1970. Sexual function among patients with spinal cord injury. *Urol. Int.* 25:134–168.

Comarr, A.E. 1971. Sexual concepts in traumatic cord and cauda equina lesions. *J. Urol.* 106:375–378.

Comarr, A.E. 1977. "Sexual function in patients with spinal cord injury." In *The total care of spinal cord injury,* ed. P.S. Pierce and V.H. Nickel, 171–185. Boston, Mass.: Little, Brown.

Comarr, A.E., and M. Vique. 1978a. Sexual counseling among male and female patients with spinal cord and/or cauda equina injury, part 1. *Am. J. Phys. Med.* 57:107–122.

Comarr, A.E., and M. Vique. 1978b. Sexual counseling among male and female patients with spinal cord and/or cauda equina injury, part 2. *Am. J. Phys. Med.* 57:215–227.

David, A., et al. 1977–78. Spinal cord injuries: Male infertility aspects. *Paraplegia* 15:11–14.

Daw, E. 1973. Pregnancy problems in a paraplegic patient with an ileal conduit bladder. *Practitioner* 211:781–784.

Devenport, J.K., and J.R. Swenson. 1983. An unusual cause of autonomic dysreflexia. *Arch. Phys. Med. Rehabil.* 64:485 (abstract).

DeVivo, M.J., and P.R. Fine. 1985. Spinal cord injury: Its short-term impact on marital status. *Arch. Phys. Med. Rehabil.* 66:501–504.

Eisenberg, M.G., and L.C. Rustad. 1976. Sex education and counseling program on a spinal cord injury service. *Arch. Phys. Med. Rehabil.* 57:135–140.

Ferguson, J.E., and V.A. Catanzorite. 1984. Clinical management of spinal cord injury. *Obstet. Gynecol.* 64:588–589.

Finney, R.P. 1977. New hinged silicone penile implant. *J. Urol.* 118:585–587.

Fitting, M.D., et al. 1978. Self-concept and sexuality of spinal cord injured women. *Arch. Sex. Behav.* 7:143–156.

Fitzpatrick, W.F. 1974. Sexual function in the paraplegic patient. *Arch. Phys. Med. Rehabil.* 55:221–227.

Francois, N., and M. Maury. 1987. Sexual aspects in paraplegic patients. *Paraplegia* 25:289–292.

Francois, N., et al. 1978–79. Electroejaculation of a complete paraplegic followed by pregnancy. *Paraplegia* 16:248–251.

Frankel, H.L., et al. 1974. Blood pressure, plasma catecholamines and prostaglandins during artificial erection in a male tetraplegic. *Paraplegia* 12:205–211.

Furlow, W.L. 1979. Inflatable penile prosthesis: Mayo Clinic experience with 175 patients. *Urology* 13:166–171.

Geiger, R.L. 1979. Neurophysiology of sexual response in spinal cord injury. *Sex. Disabil.* 2:257–266.

Gerber, G.S., and L.A. Levine. 1991. Pharmacological erection program using prostaglandin E_1. *J. Urol.* 146:786–789.

Gerstenberger, D.L., et al. 1979. Inflatable penile prosthesis, follow-up study of patient-partner satisfaction. *Urology* 14:583–587.

Gimovsky, M.L., et al. 1985. Management of autonomic hyperreflexia associated with a low thoracic spinal cord lesion. *Obstet. Gynecol.* 153:223–224.

Girdley, F.M., et al. 1988. Intracavernous self-injection for impotence: A long-term therapeutic option? Experience in 78 patients. *J. Urol.* 140:972–974.

Golgi, H. 1979. Experience with penile prosthesis in spinal cord injury patients. *J. Urol.* 121:288–289.

Goller, H., and V. Paeslack. 1970. Our experiences about pregnancy and delivery of the paraplegic woman. *Paraplegia* 8:161–166.

Goller, H., and V. Paeslack. 1972. Pregnancy, damage and birth complications in the children of paraplegic women. *Paraplegia* 10:213–217.

Green, B.G., and S.L. Sloan. 1986. Penile prostheses in spinal cord injured patients: Combined psychosexual counseling and surgical regimen. *Paraplegia* 24:167–172.

Greenspoon, J.S., and R.H. Paul. 1986. Paraplegia and quadriplegia: Special considerations during pregnancy and labor and delivery. *Am. J. Obstet. Gynecol.* 155:738–741.

Griffith, E.R., and R.B. Trieschmann. 1975. Sexual functioning in women with spinal cord injury. *Arch. Phys. Med. Rehabil.* 56:18–21.

Griffith, E.R., et al. 1973. Sexual function in spinal cord injured patients: A review. *Arch. Phys. Med. Rehabil.* 54:539–543.

Guttmann, L., and J.T. Walsh. 1971. Prostigmin assessment test of fertility in spinal man. *Paraplegia* 9:39–50.

Guttmann, L., et al. 1965. Cardiac irregularities during labour in paraplegic women. *Paraplegia* 3:144–151.

Guyton, A.C. 1986. *Textbook of medical physiology.* 7th ed. Philadelphia, Pa.: Saunders.

Halstead, L.S., et al. 1987. Rectal probe electrostimulation in the treatment of anejaculatory spinal cord injured men. *Paraplegia* 25:120–129.

Hanson, R.W., and M.R. Franklin. 1976. Sexual loss in relation to other functional losses for spinal cord injured males. *Arch. Phys. Med. Rehabil.* 57:291–293.

Hanson, T.J., and J.L. Merritt. 1985. Penile prostheses in spinal cord injured patients. Presented at the International Medical Society of Paraplegia annual scientific meeting. Edinburgh, September 2–5, 1985.

Hardy, A.G., and D.W. Worrell. 1965. Pregnancy and labour in complete tetraplegia. *Paraplegia* 3:182–186.

Higgins, G.E. 1979. Sexual response in spinal cord injured adults: A review of the literature. *Arch. Sex. Behav.* 8:173–196.

Horne, H.W., et al. 1948. Fertility studies in the human male with traumatic injuries of the spinal cord and cauda equina. *N. Engl. J. Med.* 239:959–961.

Iwatsubo, E., et al. 1986. Noninflatable penile prosthesis for the management of urinary incontinence and sexual disability of patients with spinal cord injury. *Paraplegia* 24:307–310.

Joacheim, K.A., and H. Wahle. 1970. A study on sexual function in 56 male patients with complete irreversible lesions of the spinal cord and cauda equina. *Paraplegia* 8:166–172.

Jonas, O., and G.H. Jacob. 1980. Silicone-silver penile prosthesis: Description, operative approach and results. *J. Urol.* 123:865–867.

Joseph, D.B., et al. 1984. Long-term evaluation of the inflatable penile prosthesis. *J. Urol.* 131:670–673.

Juenemann, K.P., et al. 1986. Hemodynamics of papaverine- and phentolamine-induced penile erection. *J. Urol.* 136:158–161.

Keye, J.D., Jr. 1956. Hyperplasia of Leydig cells in chronic paraplegia. *Neurology* 6:68–72.

Krane, R.J. 1986. Omniphase penile prosthesis. *Semin. Urol.* 4:247–251.

Krane, R.J. 1988. Penile prostheses. *Urol. Clin. North Am.* 15:103–109.

Krane, R.J., and M.B. Siroky. 1981. Neurophysiology of erection. *Urol. Clin. North Am.* 8:91–102.

Krauss, D.T. 1987. Management of impotence II—Selected surgical procedures: Penile prostheses. *Clin. Ther.* 9:149–156.

Kuhn, R.A. 1950. Functional capacity of the isolated human spinal cord. *Brain* 73:1–51.

Lamid, S. 1985. Nocturnal penile tumescence studies in spinal cord injured males. *Paraplegia* 23:26–31.

Lee, M., and M. Sharifi. 1987. Information and treatment with intracavernous injections of papaverine and phentolamine. *J. Urol.* 137:1008–1110 (letter).

Leriche, A., et al. 1977-78. Histological and hormonal testicular changes in spinal cord patients. *Paraplegia* 15:274–279.

Letcher, J.C., and L.J. Goldfine. 1986. Management of a pregnant paraplegic patient in a rehabilitation center. *Arch. Phys. Med. Rehabil.* 67:477–488.

Light, J.K., and F.B. Scott. 1981. Management of neurogenic impotence with inflatable penile prosthesis. *Urology* 17:341–343.

Lue, T.F., and E.A. Tanagho. 1987. Physiology of erection and pharmacological management of impotence. *J. Urol.* 137:829–835.

Lue, T.F., et al. 1986. Priapism: A refined approach to diagnosis and treatment. *J. Urol.* 136:104–108.

Malloy, T.R., et al. 1980. Comparison of the inflatable penile and the Small-Carrion prostheses in the surgical treatment of erectile impotence. *J. Urol.* 123:678–679.

Marmar, J.L., et al. 1988. The use of a vacuum constrictor device to augment a partial erection following an intracavernous injection. *J. Urol.* 140:975–979.

Martin, D.E., et al. 1983. Initiation of erection and semen release by rectal probe electrostimulation. *J. Urol.* 129:637–642.

McCunniff, D.E., and D. Dewon. 1984. Pregnancy after spinal cord injury. *Obstet. Gynecol.* 63:757.

McGregor, J.A., and J. Meeuwsen. 1985. Autonomic hyperreflexia: A mortal danger for spinal cord damaged women in labor. *Am. J. Obstet. Gynecol.* 151:330–333.

Melman, A., and G. Hammond. 1978. Placement of the Small-Carrion penile prosthesis to enable maintenance of an indwelling condom catheter. *Sex. Disabil.* 1:292–298.

Melnyk, R., et al. 1979. Attitude changes following a sexual counseling program for spinal cord injured persons. *Arch. Phys. Med. Rehabil.* 60:601–605.

Merrill, D.C. 1988. Clinical experience with the Mentor inflatable penile prosthesis in 301 patients. *J. Urol.* 140:1424–1427.

Michal, V., et al. 1977. Arterial epigastricocavernous anastomosis for the treatment of sexual impotence. *World J. Surg.* 1:515–520.

Miller, S.B. 1988. Spinal cord injury: Self-perceived sexual information and counseling needs during the acute, rehabilitation and post-rehabilitation phases. *Rehabil. Psychol.* 33:221–226.

Money, J. 1960. Phantom orgasm in the dreams of paraplegic men and women. *Arch. Gen. Psychol.* 3:373–382.

Morales, A., et al. 1987. Is yohimbine effective in the treatment of organic impotence? Results of a controlled trial. *J. Urol.* 137:1168–1172.

Morales, P.A., and J. Hardin. 1958. Scrotal and testicular temperature studies in paraplegics. *J. Urol.* 79:972–975.

Morely, J.E., et al. 1979. Testicular function in patients with spinal cord damage. *Horm. Metab. Res.* 11:679–682.

Mulcahy, J.T. 1988a. The Hydroflex self-contained inflatable prosthesis: Experience with 100 patients. *J. Urol.* 140:1422–1423.

Mulcahy, J.T. 1988b. Use of ex-cylinders in association with AM5700 inflatable penile prosthesis. *J. Urol.* 140:1420–1421.

Mulla, N. 1957. Vaginal delivery in a paraplegic patient. *Am. J. Obstet. Gynecol.* 73:1346–1348.

Munro, D., et al. 1948. The effect of injury to the spinal cord and cauda equina on the sexual potency of men. *N. Engl. J. Med.* 239:904–911.

Nadig, P.W., et al. 1986. Non-invasive device to produce and maintain an erection-like state. *Urology* 27:126–131.

Nath, M., et al. 1979. Autonomic hyperreflexia in pregnancy and labor: A case report. *Am. J. Obstet. Gynecol.* 134:390–391.

Nellans, R.E., et al. 1987. Pharmacological erection: Diagnosis and treatment applications in 69 patients. *J. Urol.* 138:52–54.

Ohry, A., et al. 1978. Sexual function, pregnancy and delivery in spinal cord injured women. *Gynecol. Obstet. Invest.* 9:281–291.

Oppenheimer, W.M. 1971. Pregnancy in paraplegic women: Two case reports. *Am. J. Obstet. Gynecol.* 110:784–786.

Otoni, T., et al. 1985. A paraplegic fathering a child after an intrathecal injection of neostigmine: Case report. *Paraplegia* 23:32–37.

Perkash, I., et al. 1985. Reproductive biology of paraplegics: Results of semen collection, testicular biopsy and serum hormone evaluation. *J. Urol.* 134:284–288.

Phelps, G., et al. 1987. Sexual experience and plasma testosterone levels in male veterans after spinal cord injury. *Arch. Phys. Med. Rehabil.* 64:47–52.

Potts, I.F. 1957. The mechanism of ejaculation. *Med. J. Aust.* 1:495–497.

Ravindran, R.S., et al. 1981. Experience with the use of nitroprusside and subsequent epidural analgesia in a pregnant quadriplegic patient. *Anesth. Analg.* 60:61–63.

Reid, K., et al. 1987. Double-blind trial of yohimbine in treatment of psychogenic impotence. *Lancet* 2:421–423.

Robertson, D.N.S. 1972. Pregnancy and labour in the paraplegic. *Paraplegia* 10:209–212.

Robertson, D.N.S., and L. Guttmann. 1963. The paraplegic patient in pregnancy and labor. *Proc. R. Soc. Med.* 56:381–387.

Romano, M.D. 1981. "Counseling the spinal cord injured female." In *Human sexuality and rehabilitation,* ed. A. Sha'ked, 157–166. Baltimore, Md.: Williams & Wilkins.

Rossier, A.B., and B.A. Fam. 1984. Indication and results of semi-rigid penile prosthesis in spinal cord injury patients: Long-term followup. *J. Urol.* 131:59–62.

Rowan, R.L., et al. 1962. Electroejaculation. *J. Urol.* 87:726–729.

Sarkarati, M., et al. 1987. Experience in vibratory and electroejaculation techniques in spinal cord injury patients: A preliminary report. *J. Urol.* 138:59–62.

Saunders, D., and J. Yeo. 1968. Pregnancy and quadriplegia—The problem of autonomic dysreflexia. *Aust. N.Z. J. Obstet. Gynaecol.* 8:152–154.

Sidi, A.A., et al. 1986. Intracavernous drug-induced erections in the management of male erectile dysfunction: Experience with 100 patients. *J. Urol.* 135:704–706.

Sjogren, K., and K. Egberg. 1983. The sexual experience in younger males with complete spinal cord injury. *Scand. J. Rehabil. Med.* 9(suppl):189–194.

Small, M.P. 1976. Small-Carrion penile prosthesis, a new implant for management of impotence. *Mayo Clin. Proc.* 51:336–338.

Smith, A.D., et al. 1980. Penile prosthesis: Adjustment to treatment in patients with neurogenic bladder. *J. Urol.* 124:363–364.

Spergel, P., et al. 1976. Sex-rehabilitation issue: What priority and when? *Arch. Phys. Med. Rehabil.* 57:562 (abstract).

Spielman, F.J. 1984. Parturient with spinal cord transection: Complications of autonomic hyperreflexia. *Obstet. Gynecol.* 64:147.

Spira, R. 1956. Artificial insemination after intrathecal injection of neostigmine in a paraplegic. *Lancet* 1:670–671.

Stemmermann, G.N., et al. 1950. A study of the germinal epithelium in male paraplegics. *Am. J. Clin. Pathol.* 20:24–34.

Stief, C.G., and V. Watterauer. 1988. Erectile responses to intracavernous papaverine and phentolamine: Comparison of single and combined delivery. *J. Urol.* 140:1415–1416.

Stirt, J.A., et al. 1979. Obstetric anesthesia for a quadriplegic patient with autonomic hyperreflexia. *Anesthesiology* 51:560–562.

Szasz, G. 1986. Vibratory stimulation of the penis in men with spinal cord injury. Presented at the 12th annual scientific meeting, American Spinal Injury Association. San Francisco, March 13–15, 1986.

Talbot, H.S. 1949. A report on sexual function in paraplegics. *J. Urol.* 61:265–270.

Talbot, H.S. 1955. The sexual function in paraplegia. *J. Urol.* 73:91–100.

Tarabulcy, E. 1972. Sexual function in the normal and in paraplegia. *Paraplegia* 10:201–208.

Tawil, E.A., and J.G. Gregory. 1986. Failure of the Jones prosthesis. *J. Urol.* 135:702–703.

Thomas, R.J.S., et al. 1975. Electroejaculation of the paraplegic male followed by pregnancy. *Med. J. Aust.* 2:798–799.

Thornton, C.E. 1979. Sexual counseling of women with spinal cord injuries. *Sex. Disabil.* 2:267–277.

Tsuji, I., et al. 1961. The sexual function in patients with spinal cord injury. *Urol. Int.* 12:270–280.

Turk, R., et al. 1983. The female paraplegic and mother-child relations. *Paraplegia* 21:186–191.

Van Arsdalen, K.N., et al. 1981. Penile implants in spinal cord injury patients for maintaining external appliances. *J. Urol.* 126:331–332.

Verduyn, W.H. 1986. Spinal cord injured women, pregnancy and delivery. *Paraplegia* 24:231–240.

Verduyn, W.H. 1989. A deadly combination induction of labor with oxytocin/Pitocin in spinal cord injured women, T6 and above. *Proc. Am. Spinal Inj. Assoc.,* 15:3–9, 15th Annual Meeting, April 3-5, 1989.

VerVoort, S.M. 1987. Infertility in spinal cord injured male. *Urology* 29:157–165.

Virag, R. 1982. Intracavernous injection of papaverine for erectile failure. *Lancet* 2:938.

Virag, R., et al. 1984. Intracavernous injection of papaverine as a diagnostic and therapeutic method in erectile failure. *Angiology* 35:79–87.

Wanner, M.B., et al. 1987. Pregnancy and autonomic hyperreflexia in patients with spinal cord lesions. *Paraplegia* 25:482–490.

Ware, H.H., 1934. Pregnancy after paralysis—Report of three cases. *J.A.M.A.* 102:1833–1834.

Warner, H., et al. 1986. Electrostimulation of erection and ejaculation and collection of semen in spinal cord injured humans. *J. Rehabil. Res. Dev.* 23:21–31.

Watson, D.W., and G.O. Downey. 1980. Epidural anesthesia for labor and delivery of twins of a paraplegic mother. *Anesthesiology* 52:259–261.

Watters, G.R., et al. 1988. Experience in the management of erectile dysfunction using the intracavernosal self-injection of vasoactive drugs. *J. Urol.* 140:1417–1419.

Weiner, N. 1985. "Drugs that inhibit adrenergic nerves and block adrenergic receptors." In *The pharmacological basis of therapeutics,* ed. A.C. Gillman et al., 7th ed., 181–221. New York, N.Y.: Goodman & Gilman.

Weiss, A.J., and M.D. Diamond. 1966. Sexual adjustment, identification and attitudes of patients with myelopathy. *Arch. Phys. Med. Rehabil.* 47:245–250.

Weiss, H.D. 1972. The physiology of human penile erection. *Ann. Intern. Med.* 76:793–799.

Witherington, R. 1987. External aids for treatment of impotence. *J. Urol. Nurs.* 6:1–7.

Wyndaele, J.J., et al. 1986. Intracavernous injection of vasoactive drugs, an alternative for treating impotence in spinal cord injury patients. *Paraplegia* 24:271–275.

Young, B.K., et al. 1983. Pregnancy after spinal cord injury: Altered maternal and fetal response to labor. *Obstet. Gynecol.* 62:59–63.

Zeitlin, A.B., et al. 1957. Sexology of the paraplegic male. *Fertil. Steril.* 8:337–344.

Zorgniotti, A., and R. Lefleur. 1985. Auto-injection of the corpus cavernosum with a vasoactive drug combination for vasculogenic impotence. *J. Urol.* 133:39–41.

Chapter 8

Pressure Ulcers: Medical Management

Gary M. Yarkony

Pressure ulcers are complications of spinal cord injury (SCI) that should be prevented, not treated. They are known by numerous other names, including decubitus ulcers, bed sores, ischemic ulcers, and pressure sores. At one time, pressure ulcers were considered a natural and inevitable complication of SCI (Guttmann 1955). Pressure ulcers continue to be a major public health problem. Approximately 3% to 11% of hospitalized patients have pressure ulcers, and the prevalence in nursing homes is estimated to be 15% to 25% (National Pressure Ulcer Advisory Panel 1989a).

Data from the Model SCI Systems (Heinemann et al. 1989; Stover & Fine 1986) give an indication of the pressure ulcer problem after SCI during the initial acute care and rehabilitation phases. Of the patients admitted within 24 hours to a model system, only 4.2% develop ulcerations. Thirteen percent of those cases are severe. The majority of the severe ulcerations occur in the sacral region, which is the most common site of pressure ulcer formation. The next most common site is the heels, followed by the ischium. As individuals spend less time in bed and are mobile in wheelchairs, the ischium and trochanters become areas of greater risk.

ETIOLOGY

Pressure (Kosiak 1959) and shear (Reichel 1958) are considered the prime etiologic factors in pressure (presshear) ulcer formation. Pressures above capillary pressure cause ischemia of skin and other soft tissues. Larsen et al. (1979) determined that external pressures exceeding actual mean blood pressure will stop skin circulation. Skin in areas of bony prominences with diminished soft tissue such as the ischium, trochanters, and sacrum are most susceptible. Kosiak (1959) demonstrated the relationship between pressure and time in dogs. He described a hyperbolic curve demonstrating that with greater pressure less time was needed to induce a pressure ulcer and that prolonged time periods with lower pressure can result in ulceration, an inverse relationship. Daniel et al. (1981, 1985) studied normal and paraplegic swine and noted a similarly shaped curve with some important differences. Higher values of pressure and time were needed to produce ulceration. The skin of swine is considered a better experimental model than that of dogs, and this explains these differences. Initial pathological changes occurred in muscle and progressed upward toward the skin as opposed to changes at all levels equally, as described by Kosiak (1959).

There is a decrease in the threshold in the pressure-time curve for paraplegic animals (Figure 8–1). This may be related to several factors. SCI results in impaired mobility and increases the likelihood of periods of prolonged ischemia. This is further exacerbated by the loss of sensation, which removes the stimulus to change position. Incontinence may macerate the skin and facilitate skin breakdown. Wasting of tissue, particularly in the area of bony prominences, results in increased interface pressures between the support surface and soft tissues overlying the bony prominences.

Shearing (Bennett et al. 1979; Reichel 1958) is the second major external force that results in pressure (presshear) ulcers. Guttmann (1955) described shearing as having an effect that is

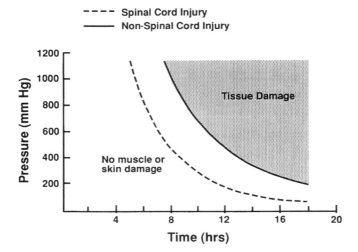

Figure 8–1 Pressure duration curves for normal and paraplegic animals. *Source:* From "Pressure Sores and Paraplegics: An Experimental Model" by R.K. Daniel, et al., 1985, *Annals of Plastic Surgery, 15*, p. 48. Copyright 1985 by Little, Brown and Co. Reprinted with permission.

much more disastrous than vertical pressure because it cuts off large areas of vascular supply. The undermining that is often observed in pressure ulcers is secondary to shearing forces. Shearing places blood vessels under stretch and results in extensive tissue dissection and cleavage. Elevating the head of the bed may increase shearing on the sacrum and increase the risk of pressure ulceration in a paraplegic. Shear, when sufficiently high (100 g/cm²), may reduce the pressure needed to produce blood flow occlusion by a factor of 2 (Bennett et al. 1979). Pressure is the primary force because it has a greater effect than shear and because its presence is required to stabilize the tissue and permit the development of shear.

Pressure and shear are the principal factors, but the problem is clearly multifactorial. Friction (Dinsdale 1974) applies the mechanical forces to the epidermis and is a factor in the pathogenesis of pressure ulcers that occur in the absence of an ischemic mechanism. Cigarette smoking (Lamid & El Ghatit 1983) may increase the risk of pressure ulceration as a result of its deleterious effects on the vascular system.

Hypoalbuminemia (Allman et al. 1986) and resultant interstitial edema impede adequate exchange of nutrients, oxygen, and waste products between the cells and circulation. Skin exposure to the bacteria and toxins in stool may be an important factor in pathogenesis of pressure ulcers beyond the effects of skin maceration from moisture. Pressure sites in septic individuals may be a nidus of infection and may increase susceptibility to ulceration. Skin areas with increased temperature have greater metabolic demands and may result in increased ischemia. Heterotopic ossification (Hassard 1975) may predispose to ulceration by causing asymmetry in seating and localized edema or compression of vasculature. Reduced tissue

perfusion may result from hypotension and increases the risk of pressure ulceration. An inverse relationship has been reported to exist between mean systolic blood pressure and ulcer development. Prolonged immobilization on a backboard during the immediate postinjury period may predispose to pressure ulcer development (Mawson et al. 1988). Patients with peripheral vascular disease may be more prone to ulceration of their extremities.

Psychosocial factors may have a major impact on pressure ulcer development (Anderson & Andberg 1979). There is a negative correlation between satisfaction with activities after SCI and days lost from major activities due to pressure ulcers. Individuals who become depressed or addicted or who are dissatisfied in spite of the ability to care for themselves often develop ulcerations. Pressure ulcers occurring during the initial phase after injury may have a negative impact on subsequent social adjustment. Pressure ulcers increase time in bed and delay the accrual of experience after injury, inhibiting adjustment during the initial rehabilitation phase (Gordon et al. 1982). The ulcers may stop the rehabilitation process, hike costs of rehabilitation, and frustrate the staff; goals are limited when seating time is limited.

Pressure ulcers do not occur with greater frequency in quadriplegics. In fact, in some series the incidence is higher in paraplegics. A false sense of security should not develop based on an individual's independence in self-care and ability to perform pressure reliefs and to turn in bed.

CLASSIFICATION

There are many classification systems for pressure ulcers (Moriarty 1988; Shea 1975; Yarkony et al. 1990). Shea's system is used widely and has resulted in significant variation in documentation among staff members. Studies from our center (Rehabilitation Institute of Chicago) (French et al. 1983) indicate that, in spite of a teaching session on the Shea classification, consistency of documentation declines at 6 months, which may relate to difficulties in identifying borders such as that between the epidermis and dermis on the Shea system.

A classification system developed at our center has been found to have greater interrater reliability than the Shea classification (Exhibit 8–1). This system has two advantages. First, it classifies a red area as a separate classification (grade 1) to encourage prevention. A healed ulcer is classified as PSH (pressure sore healed) to indicate a scarred area with potential for further background. The second advantage is that the ulcer is classified by the tissue at the base, thus eliminating the need to identify borders and decreasing confusion if a border such as deep fascia and muscle is identified in the same ulcer.

Exhibit 8–1 describes three commonly used classifications for pressure ulcers. The classification developed by the National Pressure Ulcer Advisory Panel is recommended in the clinical practice guidelines prepared by the Association for

Exhibit 8–1 Three Pressure Ulcer Classifications

Yarkony-Kirk Classification

1. Red area
   - Present longer than 30 minutes but less than 24 hours
   - Present longer than 24 hours
2. Epidermis and/or dermis ulcerated with no subcutaneous fat observed
3. Subcutaneous fat observed, no muscle observed
4. Muscle/fascia observed, no bone observed
5. Bone observed, but no involvement of joint space
6. Involvement of joint space
7. Pressure sore healed: Indicate PSH

Shea Classification

1. Limited to epidermis, exposing dermis; includes a red area
2. Full thickness of dermis to the junction of the subcutaneous fat
3. Fat obliterated, limited by the deep fascia, undermining of skin
4. Bone at the base of ulceration
5. Closed large cavity through a small sinus

National Pressure Ulcer Advisory Panel

- Stage 1: Nonblanchable erythema of intact skin (heralding lesion of skin ulceration)
- Stage II: Partial-thickness skin loss involving epidermis and/or dermis; ulcer is superficial and presents clinically as an abrasion, blister, or shallow crater
- Stage III: Full-thickness skin loss involving damage or necrosis of subcutaneous tissue that may extend down to, but not through, underlying fascia; ulcer presents clinically as a deep crater with or without undermining of adjacent tissue
- Stage IV: Full-thickness skin loss with extensive destruction, tissue necrosis, or damage to muscle, bone, or supporting structures (e.g., tendon, joint, capsule, etc.)

Healthcare Policy Research (National Pressure Ulcer Advisory Panel 1989b; Panel for the Prediction and Prevention of Pressure Ulcers in Adults 1992).

PREVENTION

Nursing care and patient/family education are the keys to pressure ulcer prevention. A well-educated patient who assumes responsibility for skin care is the ultimate goal (Rehabilitation Institute of Chicago 1990).

Proper bed positioning and frequent turns generally beginning every 2 hours are the first step in pressure ulcer prevention. Skin should be checked between turns, and turning time can be increased when hyperemia over bony prominences resolves within 30 minutes. The prone position gives rise to smaller high-pressure areas and larger low-pressure areas

(Lindan et al. 1965). All positions, including sidelying, should be used. Eventually the patients should be independent or able to direct a caregiver in skin checks, turning, and bed positioning.

Sitting is limited to 30 to 60 minutes initially and is slowly increased every few days if hyperemia resolves within 30 minutes. Pressure reliefs are performed or repeated for 1 minute every 15 to 30 minutes. Although studies have shown that individuals with SCI can sit for prolonged periods with pressures above capillary pressure (32 mm Hg), frequent pressure reliefs should be encouraged (Patterson & Fisher 1986; Redfern et al. 1973). This is not a consistent finding in all individuals.

Because rehabilitation seeks to discharge individuals, home equipment used in the hospital should be similar to the equipment they will use after discharge. Skin tolerance should be determined before discharge on a standard mattress and the wheelchair cushion that will be used at home. The costs of specialized beds is an important consideration. Air-flotation beds and air-fluidized beds should be used only temporarily in the initial phases of rehabilitation to heal or prevent ulcerations. They may also be used when positioning is a problem because of pain and other factors that make pressure ulceration inevitable without the use of the bed (Thomson et al. 1980). With an air-fluidized bed, the individual floats on a bed of air and beads, which is based on a process called fluidization in which powders or granules behave as a liquid. With air-flotation or low-airflow beds, the patient is supported on an air-permeable fabric. Air-flotation beds are more practical in the rehabilitation facility but should be used sparingly because they are not suitable for transfer training or home use. An eggcrate foam mattress pad atop a standard mattress generally is all that is needed. Occasionally an alternating air pressure mattress is recommended, but leaks and mechanical breakdown are common problems.

The appropriate wheelchair cushion should be considered in terms of positioning and impact on transfers in addition to pressure relief characteristics. It is important to stress to the patient that the wheelchair cushion is helpful in prevention of ulceration but will not eliminate the need for proper skin care and pressure reliefs. Wheelchair cushions can reduce pressure over bony prominences but do not decrease pressure below capillary pressure (Souther et al. 1974).

The majority of cushions available are made of foam or gel or are air or water filled. None of them is a panacea for pressure ulcers. Foam cushions generally will produce higher temperatures at the seating surface than the others. Gel cushions will maintain skin temperature, and water-filled cushions will decrease skin temperature. Cooling of gel cushions after 3 hours may be required to continue their ability to maintain skin temperature. Humidity increases less on foams than gels and increases the most on water-filled cushions. The ROHO cushion causes a significant increase in humidity and less of an increase in temperature than foam cushions (Seymour & Lacefield 1985; Stewart et al. 1980). The Jay cushion is a gel cushion that improves seating posture.

Air-filled cushions (ROHO and Bye-Bye Decubiti; Krouskop et al. 1986) require the individual to monitor the air pressure on a daily basis, which calls for a high degree of personal responsibility. The Bye-Bye Decubiti cushion will cause an increase in ischial pressures if seating is not proper (Seymour & Lacefield 1985). Foam cushions, which are used infrequently, need to be replaced every 6 months (Ferguson-Pell et al. 1986).

Body weight may have an impact on wheelchair seating pressure. Thin patients have higher pressures over bony prominences and a greater frequency of maximum pressures occurring in a bony location than average weight or obese patients (Garber & Krouskop 1982).

Many devices have been proposed to monitor or encourage pressure reliefs (Merbitz et al. 1985), including calculators or watches that beep periodically and monitoring devices that measure pressure reliefs. It is unclear whether these devices provide a major benefit in preventing skin ulceration. One unusual finding is that some individuals will not develop pressure ulcers in spite of extended time periods without pressure reliefs. Because these individuals cannot readily be identified, and because it is unknown whether this is a short- or long-term phenomenon, pressure reliefs should be encouraged.

Medical management plays an important role in pressure ulcer prevention. Maintenance of adequate nutrition is essential. Dietary intake must often be supplemented by parenteral or enteral hyperalimentation until the individual can maintain adequate nutrition voluntarily. Cigarette smoking should be avoided (Lamid & El Ghatit 1983). Adequate bowel and bladder management will prevent incontinence and the resultant skin maceration.

Electrical stimulation recently has been proposed as a means of preventing pressure ulcers. Electric muscle stimulation (Levine et al. 1990) produces changes in seating interface pressure distribution and changes the shape of the buttocks, which may assist in preventing pressure ulcers. Electrically stimulated muscles may benefit from an increase in mass. Patient compliance may be a major factor in determining the utility of these systems. Individuals with lower motor neuron lesions or those with severe atrophy may not respond to this technique.

TREATMENT OF PRESSURE ULCERS

There are as many proposed treatments for pressure ulcers as there are pressure ulcers. Often they are used without the principal ingredient in the treatment program: removal of the pressure. There is some truth to the adage that you can put anything on the pressure ulcer except the patient. Actually, one should be careful about what one puts on a pressure ulcer (of course, the patient should be the last thing one considers placing on it). Most ulcers can be treated cheaply and effectively without expensive dressings or various potions for débridement as long as the pressure is removed (Exhibit 8–2). The complete elimination of pressure serves several other purposes besides allowing the wound to heal. Individuals learn that if they get an ulcer they cannot sit or lie on it. It is hoped that they will avoid getting ulcers in the future to avoid the loss of sitting. It also teaches the key factor in treating ulcers at home: no sitting. Although ulcers may heal in spite of brief sitting periods, this is quite variable and often not possible. After discharge, individuals may have difficulty judging the minimal sitting that is possible.

Débridement of pressure ulcers is not complicated and does not require enzymatic preparations. There are two basic approaches. Surgical débridement is the simplest and quickest method. If it cannot be accomplished or if necrotic tissue remains after débridement, wet-to-dry saline dressings are recommended, which generally will clear up any local wound infection. Saline is the recommended preparation. Povidone-iodine (Betadine; Thomas 1988) may cause allergic reactions, thyroid suppression, and metabolic acidosis because it is absorbed into the skin. Povidone-iodine, hydrogen peroxide, and Dakin's solution should not be applied to pressure ulcers.

Wound healing is the next consideration after the wound is clean after débridement. Wounds should be managed in an environment that facilitates the growth of healthy tissue without constantly traumatizing the wound or removing or damaging new granulation tissue or epithelium. Winter (1962) was the first to demonstrate the value of wound healing in a moist environment. Moist wounds in domestic pigs epithelized twice as fast as dry wounds, which in turn led to an earlier appearance of new connective tissue. Experiments in humans confirmed the more rapid epithelialization in occluded wounds (Hinman & Maibach 1963). In an air-exposed wound, epithelium has to grow at right angles under a scab (eschar), whereas in a moist wound without eschar the epithelium can spread directly across the wound surface.

Many occlusive dressings create a hypoxic environment in the wound (Varghese et al. 1986). This environment fosters angiogenesis (Knighton et al. 1981) in the healing ulcer and does not inhibit wound healing because the oxygen required is carried through the local blood supply (Varghese et al. 1986). Bacterial growth is also not a problem under wounds occluded with DuoDERM, although bacteria have been recovered from wounds treated with Op-site or Vigilon (Mertz et al. 1985). Several studies demonstrate the benefits of occlusive dressing in animals (Alvarez et al. 1983) and humans (Yarkony et al. 1984). Hydrocolloid dressings (DuoDERM) in a controlled study were more efficacious than wet-to-dry Dakin's dressings (Gorse & Messner 1987).

Optimal medical management is essential to pressure ulcer healing. Hypoalbuminemia may be a predisposing factor or

Exhibit 8–2 Steps in Healing a Pressure Ulcer

1. Remove pressure
2. Débride wound
   - Surgical
   - Wet-to-dry saline dressing
3. Moist wound environment
   - Occlusive dressings
   - Nonadherent dressings
4. Nutrition
   - Protein calorie nutrition
   - Vitamin C (500 mg twice a day)
   - Zinc (220 mg twice a day)
   - Multivitamin with minerals
5. Anemia: evaluation and treatment

may result from protein loss through an ulcer. Supplementation with zinc (Norris & Reynolds 1971), vitamin C (Taylor et al. 1974), and a multivitamin with minerals in patients with adequate oral intake ensures that the necessary vitamins and trace elements are present for wound healing. Zinc levels should be checked before administration because high levels of zinc may interfere with wound healing. Proper evaluation and treatment of anemia are essential.

Numerous other treatments have been proposed to heal pressure ulcers. Electric current has been applied in two studies (Carley & Wainapel 1985; Kloth & Feedar 1988) that either had a small sample size or used inappropriate methods of treatment as controls. Most preparations for débridement are unnecessary, and many occlusive dressings available are not well studied. Air-fluidized beds are useful, although further study is needed to obtain a cost–benefit analysis (Allman et al. 1987; Thomson et al. 1980).

Surgical management (Herces & Harding 1978) of nonhealing wounds is addressed in Chapter 9. Postsurgical management of the pressure ulcer requires readmission to the rehabilitation facility. This allows for slowly increased sitting tolerance with careful wound observation and permits the nursing and therapy staffs to reeducate the patients about skin management and pressure ulcer prevention.

COMPLICATIONS

Pressure ulcers are a potentially fatal complication of SCI. Complications include local infection, pelvic abscess, osteomyelitis, sepsis, and malignant degeneration. They should not be accepted as inevitable. The teaching programs should make the patient and caregiver aware of these complications to serve as a stimulus for prevention activities.

Local infection (Sugarman 1985) may be present with grossly purulent exudate and/or extensive surrounding inflammation. The diagnosis may often be obscure and require computed tomography (CT), needle aspiration, or gallium scans. Spontaneous rupture of an abscess may occur without clinical suspicion. CT may be helpful in identifying intrapelvic and extrapelvic abscesses (Firooznia et al. 1982). Local infection is treated by débridement and wet-to-dry saline dressings. Povidone-iodine has been reported to be beneficial, but there are numerous problems associated with its use. Systemic antibiotics are rarely needed.

Osteomyelitis (Sugarman 1987; Thornhill-Joynes et al. 1986) cannot be identified by clinical examination or predicted by the length of time the ulcer is present. Recurrence of healed or surgically treated ulcer may be due to osteomyelitis. Although bone biopsy is the definitive test, a high index of suspicion may be generated by noninvasive testing. A positive plain film, a WBC greater than $15,000/mm^3$, or a sedimentation rate greater than 120 mm/h are suggestive but not conclusive (Lewis et al. 1988). Bone scans or gallium scans are only helpful if negative, in which case osteomyelitis is unlikely. Positive bone scans are common and generally reflect the presence of the soft tissue injury.

Bacteremia (Galpin et al. 1976) from pressure ulcers has been reported to occur in 3.49 episodes per 10,000 patient discharges. In one series, the mortality rate was as high as 55%. Common organisms are bowel flora (Gram-negative bacilli and anaerobes), *Staphylococcus aureus, Proteus mirabilis,* and *Escherichia coli* (Bryan et al. 1983). Treatment requires both surgical débridement and antimicrobial chemotherapy.

Amputations (Lawton & DePinto 1987) may result from recurrent ulcers that lead to severe osteomyelitis or extensive skin breakdown leaving little tissue for flap closure. Reconstruction with myocutaneous flaps is preferable to amputation. Amputation may lead to balance and seating problems that may cause further ulceration. There may also be a significant psychological impact from the loss of the extremity.

Malignant degeneration in a pressure ulcer, burn scar, stasis ulcer, or other chronic skin lesion is known as Marjolin's ulcer (Berkwits et al. 1986). As the life span of persons with SCI increases, this may become more prevalent. Repeated ulceration and healing in a poorly vascularized scar with a poor covering of epidermis may undergo discharge, foul odor, and bleeding. Ulcers are often present for more than 20 years before malignancy develops. Biopsy provides a definitive diagnosis.

REFERENCES

Allman, R.M., et al. 1986. Pressure sores among hospitalized patients. *Ann. Intern. Med.* 105:337–342.

Allman, R.M., et al. 1987. Air-fluidized beds or conventional therapy for pressure sores. *Ann. Intern. Med.* 107:641–648.

Alvarez, O.M., et al. 1983. Effect of occlusive dressings on collagen synthesis and reepithelialization in superficial wounds. *J. Surg. Res.* 35:142–148.

Anderson, T.P., and M.M. Andberg. 1979. Psychosocial factors associated with pressure sores. *Arch. Phys. Med. Rehabil.* 60:341–346.

Bennett, L., et al. 1979. Shear vs. pressure as causative factors in skin blood flow occlusion. *Arch. Phys. Med. Rehabil.* 60:309–314.

Berkwits, L., et al. 1986. Marjolin's ulcer complicating a pressure ulcer: Case report and literature review. *Arch. Phys. Med. Rehabil.* 67:831–833.

Bryan, C.S., et al. 1983. Bacteremia associated with decubitus ulcers. *Arch. Intern. Med.* 143:2093–2095.

Carley, P.T., and S.F. Wainapel. 1985. Electrotherapy for acceleration of wound healing: Low-intensity direct current. *Arch. Phys. Med. Rehabil.* 66:443–446.

Daniel, R.K., et al. 1981. Etiologic factors in pressure sores: An experimental model. *Arch. Phys. Med. Rehabil.* 62:492–498.

Daniel, R.K., et al. 1985. Pressure sores and paraplegics: An experimental model. *Ann. Plast. Surg.* 15:41–49.

Dinsdale, S.M. 1974. Decubitus ulcers: Role of pressure and friction in causation. *Arch. Phys. Med. Rehabil.* 55:147–152.

Ferguson-Pell, M., et al. 1986. Development of a modular wheelchair cushion for spinal cord injured persons. *J. Rehabil. Res. Dev.* 23:63–76.

Firooznia, H., et al. 1982. Computed tomography of pressure sores, pelvic abscess and osteomyelitis in patients with spinal cord injury. *Arch. Phys. Med. Rehabil.* 63:545–548.

French, E., et al. 1983. Improving reliability in assessment of skin breakdown. Presented at the Association of Rehabilitation Nurses annual conference, Houston, Texas, November 2–6, 1983, 8–9.

Galpin, J.E., et al. 1976. Sepsis associated with decubitus ulcers. *Am. J. Med.* 61:346–350.

Garber, S.L., and T.A. Krouskop. 1982. Body build and its relationship to pressure distribution in seated wheelchair patients. *Arch. Phys. Med. Rehabil.* 63:17–20.

Gordon, W.A., et al. 1982. The relationship between pressure sores and psychosocial adjustment in persons with spinal cord injury. *Rehabil. Psychol.* 27:185–191.

Gorse, G.T., and R.L. Messner. 1987. Improved pressure sore healing with hydrocolloid dressings. *Arch. Dermatol.* 123:766–771.

Guttmann, L. 1955. The problem of treatment of pressure sores in spinal paraplegics. *Br. J. Plast. Surg.* 8:196–211.

Hassard, G.H. 1975. Heterotopic bone formation about the hip and unilateral decubitus ulcers in spinal cord injury. *Arch. Phys. Med. Rehabil.* 56:355–358.

Heinemann, A.W., et al. 1989. Functional outcome following spinal cord injury: A comparison of specialized spinal cord injury center vs. general hospital short-term care. *Arch. Neurol.* 46:1098–1102.

Herces, S.J., and R.L. Harding. 1978. Surgical treatment of pressure sores. *Arch. Phys. Med. Rehabil.* 59:193–200.

Hinman, C.D., and H. Maibach. 1963. Effect of air exposure and occlusion on experimental human skin wounds. *Nature (London)* 200:377–378.

Kloth, L.C., and J.A. Feedar. 1988. Acceleration of wound healing with high voltage, monophasic, pulsed current. *Phys. Ther.* 68:503–508.

Knighton, D.R., et al. 1981. Regulation of wound-healing angiogenesis—Effect of oxygen gradients and inspired oxygen concentration. *Surgery* 90:262–270.

Kosiak, M. 1959. Etiology and pathology of ischemic ulcer. *Arch. Phys. Med. Rehabil.* 42:62–68.

Krouskop, T.A., et al. 1986. Inflation pressure effect on performance of air-filled wheelchair cushions. *Arch. Phys. Med. Rehabil.* 67:126–128.

Lamid, S., and A.Z. El Ghatit. 1983. Smoking, spasticity and pressure sores in spinal cord injured patients. *Am. J. Phys. Med.* 62:300–306.

Larsen, B., et al. 1979. On the pathogenesis of bedsores. *Scand. J. Plast. Reconstr. Surg.* 13:347–350.

Lawton, R.L., and V. DePinto. 1987. Bilateral hip disarticulation in paraplegics with decubitus ulcers. *Arch. Surg.* 122:1040–1043.

Levine, S.P., et al. 1990. Electric muscle stimulation for pressure sore prevention: Tissue shape variation. *Arch. Phys. Med. Rehabil.* 71:210–215.

Lewis, V.L., Jr., et al. 1988. The diagnosis of osteomyelitis in patients with pressure sores. *Plast. Reconstr. Surg.* 81:229–232.

Lindan, O., et al. 1965. Pressure distribution on the surface of the human body: I. Evaluation in lying and sitting positions using a "bed of springs and nails." *Arch. Phys. Med. Rehabil.* 46:378–385.

Mawson, A.R., et al. 1988. Risk factors for early occurring pressure ulcers following spinal cord injury. *Am. J. Phys. Rehabil.* 67:123–127.

Merbitz, C.T., et al. 1985. Wheelchair push-ups: Measuring pressure relief frequency. *Arch. Phys. Med. Rehabil.* 66:433–439.

Mertz, P.M., et al. 1985. Occlusive wound dressings to prevent bacterial invasion and wound infection. *J. Am. Acad. Dermatol.* 12:662–668.

Moriarty, M.B. 1988. How color can clarify wound care. *R.N.* 51:49–54.

National Pressure Ulcer Advisory Panel. 1989a. Pressure ulcers prevalence, cost and risk assessment: Consensus development conference statement. *Decubitis* 2:24–28.

National Pressure Ulcer Advisory Panel. 1989b. *Pressure ulcers: Incidence, economics, risk assessment* (consensus development conference statement). West Dundee, Ill.: S-N.

Norris, J.R., and R.E. Reynolds. 1971. The effect of oral zinc sulfate on decubitus ulcers. *J. Am. Geriatr. Soc.* 19:793–797.

Panel for the Prediction and Prevention of Pressure Ulcers in Adults. 1992. *Pressure ulcers in adults: Prediction and prevention: Clinical practice guideline number 3* (AHCPR Publication no. 92-0047). Rockville, Md.: Agency for Health Care Policy and Research, Public Health Service, U.S. Department of Health and Human Services.

Patterson, R.P., and S.V. Fisher. 1986. Sitting pressure-time patterns in patients with quadriplegia. *Arch. Phys. Med. Rehabil.* 67:812–814.

Redfern, S.J., et al. 1973. Local pressures with ten types of patient support systems. *Lancet* 2:277–280.

Rehabilitation Institute of Chicago, Division of Nursing. 1990. *Rehabilitation nursing procedures.* Gaithersburg, Md.: Aspen.

Reichel, S.M. 1958. Shearing force as a factor in decubitus ulcer in paraplegics. *J.A.M.A.* 166:762–763.

Seymour, R.J., and W.E. Lacefield. 1985. Wheelchair cushion effect on pressure and skin temperature. *Arch. Phys. Med. Rehabil.* 66:103–108.

Shea, J.D. 1975. Pressure sore classification and management. *Clin. Orthop.* 112:89–100.

Souther, S.G., et al. 1974. Wheelchair cushions to reduce pressure under bony prominences. *Arch. Phys. Med. Rehabil.* 55:460–464.

Stewart, S.F.C., et al. 1980. Wheelchair cushion effect on skin temperature, heat flux and relative humidity. *Arch. Phys. Med. Rehabil.* 61:229–233.

Stover, S.L., and P.R. Fine. 1986. *Spinal cord injury: The facts and figures.* Birmingham, Ala.: University of Alabama.

Sugarman, B. 1985. Infection and pressure sores. *Arch. Phys. Med. Rehabil.* 66:177–179.

Sugarman, B. 1987. Pressure sores and underlying bone infection. *Arch. Intern. Med.* 147:553–555.

Taylor, T.V., et al. 1974. Ascorbic acid supplementation in the treatment of pressure sores. *Lancet* 2:544–546.

Thomas, C. 1988. Wound healing halted with the use of povidone-iodine. *Ostomy/Wound Manage.* 17:30–33.

Thomson, C.W., et al. 1980. Fluidised-bead bed in the intensive therapy unit. *Lancet* 1:568–570.

Thornhill-Joynes, M., et al. 1986. Osteomyelitis associated with pressure ulcers. *Arch. Phys. Med. Rehabil.* 67:314–318.

Varghese, M.C., et al. 1986. Local environment of chronic wounds under synthetic dressings. *Arch. Dermatol.* 22:52–57.

Winter, G.D. 1962. Formation of scab and rate of epithelialization of superficial wounds in skin of young domestic pig. *Nature (London)* 193:293–294.

Yarkony, G.M., et al. 1984. Pressure sore management: Efficacy of a moisture reactive occlusive dressing. *Arch. Phys. Med. Rehabil.* 65:597–600.

Yarkony, G.M., et al. 1990. Classification of pressure ulcers. *Arch. Dermatol.* 126:1218–1219.

Chapter 9

Surgical Management of Pressure Ulcers

Victor L. Lewis, Jr.

HISTORY

The operative therapy of sores about the pelvis caused by the compression of denervated soft tissue between bone and a firm underlying surface began during and after World War II. Before this period, the length and quality of survival after spinal cord injury seldom afforded the possibility of operative reconstruction. Since World War II, the number and ingenuity of procedures to close primary and recurrent pressure sores have expanded enormously.

Historically, of course, the presence of draining, often rotting or putrescent wounds has been unavoidably recognized for millennia. Wound care was limited in most cases to débridement, topical applications, and dressings. Some factors, such as the possible role of loss of protective sensation in ulcer occurrence and the role of certain infections in wound enlargement, were recognized, but the observations did not lead to the development of effective therapy.

The fact that ulcer care has not traditionally been placed among the most desirable of surgical responsibilities has probably slowed the rate at which reconstructive managements have been developed. The current applications of interesting, successful flap reconstruction with meaningful postinjury and postoperative rehabilitation have made the aggressive treatment of pressure sores acceptable to the surgical community.

CONSULTATION

The purpose of surgical consultation for the patient with pressure sores is to determine whether the wound requires débridement and whether the wound and the patient are candidates for operative reconstruction after adequate preparation.

There are four groups of patients examined for pressure sores: patients after spinal cord injury with early or late soft tissue breakdown, myelomeningocele patients, patients with soft tissue ulceration associated with an acute illness, and those with a pressure sore in association with a chronic illness.

In requesting surgical consultation, it is useful to remember that the wounds of the acute illness group require débridement and heal by contraction and epithelialization without operative reconstruction over a period of weeks as the patient convalesces. Pressure sores in myelomeningocele patients may occur in areas of sensitivity, may cause pain, and may be associated with paralytic scoliosis and pelvic tilt that the patient cannot prevent. The chronically ill may not be candidates to undergo a major operation and significant blood loss, or, with steroid-dependent disease, the risk of failure of repair may dictate conservatism in the face of an otherwise reconstructable ulcer. In the absence of intercurrent factors, the frequency of failures of primary healing after reconstruction increases with the interval from spinal cord injury to flap repair, although no neurally mediated wound healing factor has yet been identified.

THE WOUND

At initial examination, the wounds requiring débridement contain soft tissue in various stages of decomposition. The tissues involved are skin, subcutaneous fat, and ligaments or fasciae. In the postures in which pressure sores in humans are incurred, the bony prominences of the ischiel tuberosity, sacrum, and femoral trochanter are not covered by muscle. One predisposition to breakdown in these areas is the lack of muscle padding over the bony prominence in the seated position. Therefore, muscle necrosis results, usually from extension of the wound by infection, usually of mixed colonic aerobic and anaerobic organisms; when subjected to pressure, however, muscle is less resistant to ischemia than the other tissues.

The greatest tissue ischemia and resulting necrosis are adjacent to the bone. Often the skin dies slowly as its sustaining perforating vessels are lost, leaving the eschar, a dry, black, leathery covering over the wound. The eschar may appear to expand as it demarcates from ischemia, causing the misapprehension of a growing wound. Removal of the eschar and the underlying devitalized soft tissue to bleeding may, on reinspection of the wound, result in the finding of more devitalized tissue. In this case, the bleeding may have been nonnutritive and the débridement inadequate, or the margins may have necrosed from desiccation or infection. The most serious infections in these cases are synergistic gangrenes, clostridial or nonclostridial, in which the combined aerobic and anaerobic coliform flora rapidly and progressively destroy large volumes of tissue. These constitute true surgical emergencies (Lewis et al. 1978).

The other groups of wounds seen initially are clean with granulating margins and the bony prominence at their base. These wounds usually are ready for reconstruction without débridement.

Wound Preparation

Complete débridement of a pressure sore of all devitalized soft tissue and, occasionally, bone is carried out in the operating room. Exceptionally, for the elderly, unwell patient for whose wounds the only goal is toilette, débridement is carried out at the bedside in the hospital or nursing home. Topical enzyme applications do not substitute in rate or thoroughness of tissue removal for sharp débridement. They are, however, effective, and are used in the nursing home and home settings.

Evaluation of the Patient and Preparation for Operation

Patients are prepared for operation if they are judged capable of undergoing a 2- to 3-hour operation in the prone position, blood loss of 250 to 1,500 mL, and a minimum 2-week convalescence at complete bed rest. They must not have diarrhea. Serum albumin should be at least 3.0 mg/dL. The patient should not be receiving anticoagulants or have current thromboembolic disease.

Patient prioritization for operation is based upon etiology of the pressure sore, such that self-destructive behavior was not an important factor; infrequency of previous soft tissue break-

downs; motivation for recovery and rehabilitation; and acceptance by the patient of responsibility for soft tissue integrity. The patient with a normal sensorium who accepts no responsibility for present soft tissue breakdown will certainly return with other pressure sores in the future.

Before operation, serum protein levels are optimized by adequate nutrition. Hemoglobin levels are normalized with transfusions or recombinant erythropoietin. Contractures are relieved by physical therapy or operative tendon sectioning. No perioperative enemas are administered to avoid diarrhea in the operative and postoperative periods.

Wound Dressings

After débridement, the wound is dressed with full-strength Dakin's solution until debris is gone. Dakin's solution is used even though it is known that it is toxic to fibroblasts and epithelial cells (Kozol et al. 1988); its use is discontinued when there is no more dead tissue. Normal saline is then used until reconstruction with timing between dressings such that the wound does not desiccate at the end of the interval. Organic iodides and other solutions are expensive and do not accelerate granulation. Iodoform kills the wound margins, which may never granulate while it is used, and is therefore not employed. In dressing large wounds, roller gauze such as 3-inch Kling is used rather than loose sponges, which can be lost in the wound. An elastic mesh such as Xspan is used to secure the dressing because repeated applications of adhesive tape blister and irritate the skin.

Antibiotics

Preoperative prophylactic antibiotics are not given. Topical antimicrobials (e.g., mafenide acetate or silver sulfadiazine) are indicated rarely for invasive wound infections. Both antibiotics have broad spectra and penetrate tissue well. Oral and parenteral antibiotics given for wound sepsis may not reach the devitalized wound interface and may delay reconstruction by causing diarrhea. In determining antibiotic administration, swab cultures are inadequate. Swabs will grow mixed flora of coliforms that are not contributory to the infection. Biopsy cultures of the wound margin are the best guide to therapy. Systemic antibiotics are necessary for the rare cases of rapidly spreading synergistic gangrenes usually caused by *Bacteroides* and *Proteus* organisms.

Contractures

Contractures of the joints around the sore require release before operation. The contractures are released by physical therapy in conjunction with hydrotherapy for the wound or by bedside passive range of motion. Unresponsive contractures are released operatively by the orthopedic service before reconstruction. Operative release should be judicious because it subjects the patient to an additional operation and the possibility of other open wounds.

Spasticity

In conjunction with the treatment of contractures, spasticity should be treated. Frequently the open wound itself is the trigger for the spasticity, and the spasticity is not controlled until after the reconstruction has healed.

NUTRITION

Most patients presented for reconstruction are hypoproteinemic and anemic. Their depletion is evaluated with albumin, transferrin, and total leukocyte counts and occasionally with 24-hour urinary nitrogen determinations. A plan is then developed with the dietitian for an appropriate diet and supplementation to restore nitrogen balance before operation. Antigen skin tests are applied, and anergy to these may be predictive of increased susceptibility to infection or sepsis. Recombinant erythropoietin has been used to treat the anemia of chronic disease without transfusion (Pincus et al. 1990; Watson et al. 1990).

URINARY TRACT

The urinary drainage regimen is followed until operation. During operation and afterward, until patients can sit and care for themselves, an indwelling Foley catheter is placed. The catheter is irrigated with genitourinary irrigant by protocol. Symptomatic infections are treated by culture and sensitivity. Calculi are removed when possible before operation. Postoperative symptomatic lower urinary tract infections are frequent and treated with culture-appropriate antibiotics.

PULMONARY

The patients are told that the carbon monoxide and nicotinic acid in cigarette smoke are harmful to the flaps they require (Rees et al. 1984). Most smokers will not stop and are not refused reconstruction. In quadriplegics and others with limited lung capacities, incentive spirometry is used postoperatively. Quadriplegics may not be able to breathe in the prone position and require general anesthesia and ventilatory support during operation. If in question, this should be evaluated by placing the patient in the prone position before the operation.

THROMBOEMBOLISM

Intermittent compression of the legs is employed the entire time the patient is at bed rest.

INTERCURRENT ILLNESS AND THERAPY

Anticoagulants are discontinued, and normal coagulation is confirmed before reconstruction. Steroid therapy is stabilized, and preoperative vitamin A is given if permissible. Diabetic control is optimized.

EVALUATION OF THE BONE

The treatment of the bony prominence at the base of the wound depends in part on the preoperative assessment for osteomyelitis. This assessment is best made by combining the WBC, the sedimentation rate, and the plain film appearance (Lewis et al. 1988). A WBC greater than $15,000/mm^3$, a sedimentation rate greater than 120 mm/h, and a plain film of the pelvis interpreted as positive for osteomyelitis at the site of the sore together are a good guide to the presence of active infection. Confirmation may be gained by Jamshidi needle biopsy of the bone for culture and histology. The diagnosis of osteomyelitis can most reliably be made by biopsy. Bone scan and computerized tomography have not reliably predicted the status of the bone in a prospective sequential series. One specific plain film view, the magnified view of the hip joint, in the evaluation of the trochanteric pressure sore is important to determine whether the sore extends into the joint space. If the joint has been eroded and contaminated, Girdlestone arthroplasty is required before flap reconstruction.

PSYCHOLOGICAL STATUS

Pressure sores are recognized symptoms of self-destructive behavior, depression, and possible drug and/or alcohol abuse. Preoperative psychiatric consultation and treatment of these problems is important for patient compliance in the hospital and possible prevention of further sores.

BED THERAPY

All patients are placed on an air-fluidized bed (e.g., Clinitron) the night before the operation to accustom them to the flotation therapy (Dolezal et al. 1985). Patients who are weak or febrile or who require frequent turning for wound care begin Clinitron therapy on admission. All patients remain on Clinitron therapy for the initial 2 weeks after operation to minimize flap injury from pressure and to optimize nursing care.

FLAP CHOICE

For each major pressure sore site, there is a preferred musculocutaneous flap reconstruction. Each flap is selected to preserve several reconstructive options for recurrence or flap failure. Musculocutaneous flaps, large muscle-skin units that can be repositioned on a predictable major vascular pedicle, are selected because their bulk ensures a durable soft tissue reconstruction, the high tissue oxygen levels in the muscle may help infected bone heal, muscle adheres to the bone better than subcutaneous tissue, and muscle can support skin damaged by previous scarring, which would not survive if transferred as a random skin-subcutaneous tissue unit (Fisher & Wood 1987; Mathes et al. 1982). Random flaps as used traditionally, random flaps with turnover of muscle, and axial flaps with identifiable vascular pedicles in their bases remain excellent secondary reconstructive choices and are included in the treatment cascade. It is seldom possible to achieve a durable closure with direct suture of the ulcer margins due to tension or a skin graft, due to a lack of soft tissue padding of the bone directly beneath the graft.

TREATMENT CASCADE FOR SACRAL PRESSURE SORES

The treatment of choice is gluteus maximus musculocutaneous advancement of rotation flap (Ramirez et al. 1984). Each flap contains most of the gluteus maximus muscle; it can be unilateral or bilateral and can be based upon either the su-

perior or the inferior gluteal artery, or both can be included in the flap. In the ambulatory patient, the muscle cannot be sacrificed without interference with gait. Only part of the muscle is used in the innervated patient, or, if the whole muscle is elevated and advanced, the origins are reattached to the opposite muscle to preserve hip stability.

Secondary choices include the following: (1) use of the opposite gluteus maximus flap or reutilization of the previous unilateral or bilateral flaps; (2) for the upper sacrum, the transverse lumbar or total back flap (Hill et al. 1978; Xyas et al. 1980); (3) for the upper sacrum–lumbar spine, the combined gluteus-latissimus flap or extended latissimus flap (Figure 9–1); (4) for the lower sacrum and coccyx, the tensor fascia lata (Lewis et al. 1981) and gluteal-thigh flaps (Hurwitz et al. 1981); and (5) Limberg (1966) and random flaps for small or lateral buttock defects.

TREATMENT CASCADE FOR ISCHIAL PRESSURE SORES (Figure 9–2)

The treatment of choice is the inferior gluteus maximus island musculocutaneous flap (Figure 9–3) (Scheflan et al. 1981). The body of the gluteus maximus muscle is divided in

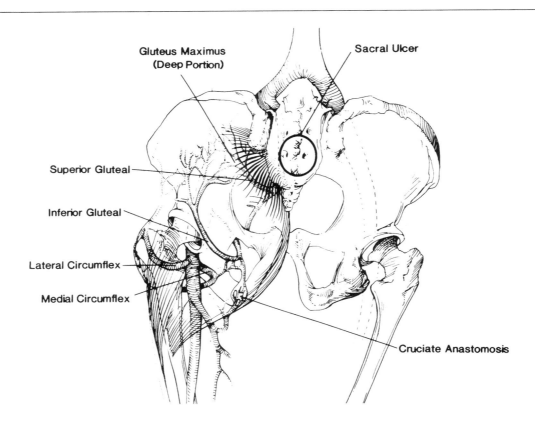

Figure 9–1 The postsacral or sacroccygeal pressure sore and the adjacent anatomy of the gluteus maximus musculocutaneous flap. *Source:* Reprinted from *Medical Management of Long-Term Disability* by D. Green (Ed.), p. 78, with permission of Aspen Publishers, Inc., © 1990.

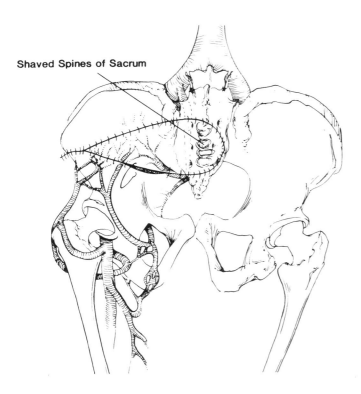

Figure 9–2 To reconstruct a postsacral pressure sore, the gluteus maximus origin is freed, sparing the vascular pedicles; the muscle is divided superiorly and inferiorly, and the muscle and overlying tissue are advanced from one or both sides partially. *Source:* Reprinted from *Medical Management of Long-Term Disability* by D. Green (Ed.), p. 79, with permission of Aspen Publishers, Inc., © 1990.

the lateral thigh, leaving the lateral muscle intact to pad the femur. The proximal body of the muscle, with a triangular wedge of overlying skin and subcutaneous tissue, is rotated medially to close the defect. This flap design leaves the entire hamstring area of the thigh free for secondary reconstructive use.

Secondary choices are as follows: (1) the gluteal thigh flap, axially designed over the descending branch of the inferior gluteal artery, which is excellent for the ambulatory patient whose gluteus maximus cannot be divided (Figure 9–4); (2) the medially based posterior thigh flap (Griffith 1975), with turnover of either or both heads of the biceps femoris, which is the traditional workhorse reconstruction; (3) the hamstring V–Y advancement (Hurteau et al. 1981), which gives good bulk and is reliable, but the medial closure is difficult and prone to dehiscence, and there is usually considerable blood loss with the dissection; (4) the medial, hockey stick myocutaneous flap for small medial ulcers (Bailey et al. 1987); (5) the tensor fascia lata myocutaneous flap, the thin tip of which reaches the area well but does not provide bulk in the atrophied limb of the chronically denervated patient; and (6)

the gracilis musculocutaneous flap (Wingate & Friedland 1978), which reaches the area well and has good bulk in the recently denervated limb. In chronic denervation, the gracilis can be thin and unreliable support for the skin island. The vastus lateralis muscle reaches the lateral ischial area well but is better reserved for secondary reconstruction of the trochanteric area or for filling the defect of a Girdlestone arthroplasty.

TREATMENT CASCADE FOR TROCHANTERIC PRESSURE SORES

The treatment of choice is the tensor fascia lata musculocutaneous flap (Nahai et al. 1978; Paletta et al. 1989), used in either a V–Y or a rotation technique (Figure 9–5). The V–Y flap places the proximal volume of the flap in the defect and has no bulky rotation point, and the donor site usually can be closed directly without skin graft. The muscle is expendable in all individuals and has a reliable single blood supply from the lateral circumflex branch of the deep femoral artery, and the flap can be rerotated easily (Figure 9–6).

Secondary choices include the following: (1) the vastus lateralis muscle flap with skin graft (Douden & McCraw 1980); (2) the gluteus medius–tensor fascia lata flap (Little & Lyons 1983), a more difficult way to move tissue into the trochanteric defect; (3) the bipedicle skin flap, a flap of limited mobility that can be tight on closure of its midpoint (Conway & Griffith 1956); and (4) the rectus femoris muscle, which will reach the area but without bulk to fill a large defect.

TREATMENT OF LESS COMMON SITES

Midline Back

The latissimus dorsi musculocutaneous flap (Casas & Lewis 1989), used as an advancement, rotation, or extended rotation flap, will cover all levels of the thoracolumbar spine. The anatomy of the muscle can be distorted by paralytic kyphoscoliosis. In each case of sacrifice of the latissimus for reconstruction, consideration needs to be given to the effect on the neurologically impaired patient's limited muscle supply.

Knee

The V–Y fasciocutaneous flap (Lewis et al. 1990) covers the knee well medially or laterally. The gastrocnemius medial belly muscle flap (Feldrian et al. 1978) will cover the medial knee, usually with its origins freed for mobility. The volume of the tip of the muscle can be quite small in chronic denervation. The vastus lateralis muscle may be turned down to cover the knee. This flap is supported by a minor pedicle to the muscle and may be unreliable.

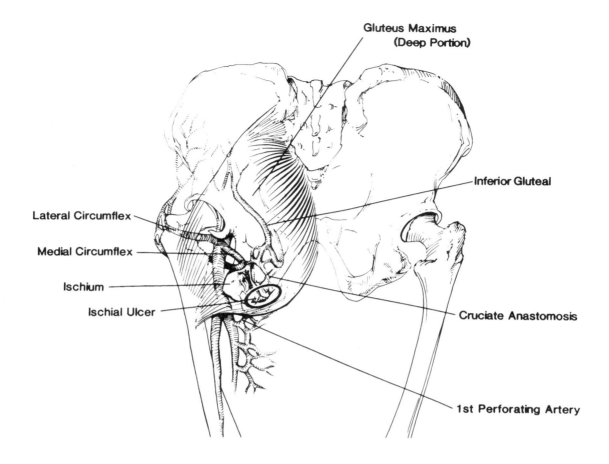

Figure 9–3 The ischial pressure ulcer underlies the ischial tuberosity. The gluteus maximus muscle does not underlie the tuberosity in the seated position. However, the gluteus maximus is adjacent and available for reconstruction. *Source:* Reprinted from *Medical Management of Long-Term Disability* by D. Green (Ed.), p. 80, with permission of Aspen Publishers, Inc., © 1990.

Malleolus

Skin grafts are tempting in this area but do not do well. Local muscle flaps are the abductor hallucis medially and the abductor digiti minimi laterally (Mathes & Nahai 1982). A local fasciocutaneous flap with skin graft of the donor site closes the area reliably (Grabb & Argenta 1981).

Heel

Whenever possible, the reversed dermal graft works well (Hynes 1954). When necessary, the lateral calcaneal flap is reliable but difficult to dissect, and it leaves an unstable donor site. The flexor digitorum brevis muscle flap is easy to dissect but can be quite thin in chronic denervation, and it does not reach the Achilles area.

OTHER OPERATIVE CONSIDERATIONS

Bone

When preoperative evaluation indicates osteomyelitis, complete ostectomy of the ischium and trochanterectomy of the femur are performed. In the postsacral area coccygectomy is performed, and the sacral spines are removed. In the absence of signs of osteomyelitis for ischial sores, the ischial tuberosity is removed; in the sacral area, the spines underlying the wound are excised. Complete trochanterectomy is performed routinely to remove the lateral pressure point. Others treating pressure sores routinely perform coccygectomy in sacral sores and ischiectomy in ischial sores, believing that the incidence of local recurrences is thereby decreased.

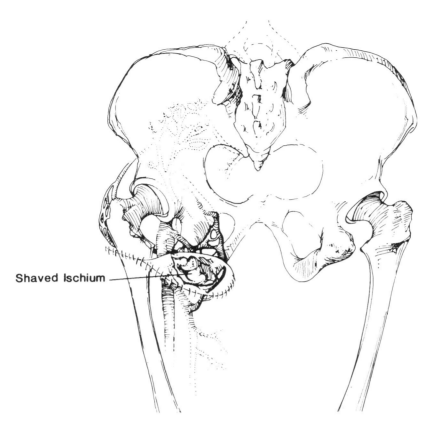

Shaved Ischium

Figure 9–4 The gluteus maximus musculocutaneous flap slides medially to cover the shaved ischial tuberosity. Clinically, the closed donor site defect does not overlie the femur. *Source:* Reprinted from *Medical Management of Long-Term Disability* by D. Green (Ed.), p. 81, with permission of Aspen Publishers, Inc., © 1990.

The excised bone is submitted for microscopic examination, and wherever infection is suspected needle biopsy specimens are submitted for culture. Documented infections are treated aggressively with antibiotics.

Anesthesia

All patients are monitored by a nurse anesthetist. General anesthesia is used when the patient has sensation in the involved area or cannot ventilate in the position in which the operation must be performed.

Antibiotics

Perioperative antibiotics are given prophylactically, usually cephalosporins. Their benefit has not been demonstrated, however.

Blood

Major pressure sore reconstructions are associated with blood loss of 250 to 1,500 mL (Wingate et al. 1992). Patients with anemia and contracted blood volumes are transfused preoperatively. Intraoperative transfusion is anticipated with cross-match of 2 to 4 units. Thrombin is used topically intraoperatively for bone and soft tissue oozing, with the application of Avitene (lyophilized bovine collagen) to the bone surface occasionally being required. Desmopressin has been shown to reduce operative blood loss in large flap reconstructions and is given routinely at the beginning of flap reconstructions.

Drains

Multiple large suction drains are placed between the layers of the closure and are kept at high suction for 14 days or until occluded. They are brought through the skin at sites away from pressure points and the sites of secondary reconstructive options.

Dressings

Bulky dressings held in place with elastic mesh are used for 24 hours after operation. Thereafter, the flap is treated open

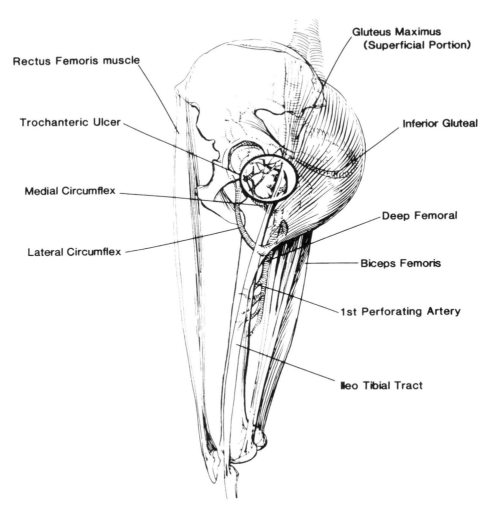

Rectus Femoris muscle

Trochanteric Ulcer

Medial Circumflex

Lateral Circumflex

Gluteus Maximus (Superficial Portion)

Inferior Gluteal

Deep Femoral

Biceps Femoris

1st Perforating Artery

Ileo Tibial Tract

Figure 9–5 The tensor fascia lata muscle belly is short and proximal, lying between the gluteus maximus and rectus femoris origins. It is adjacent to the trochanteric pressure sore, always lateral to the greater trochanter of the femur. *Source:* Reprinted from *Medical Management of Long-Term Disability* by D. Green (Ed.), p. 82, with permission of Aspen Publishers, Inc., © 1990.

when Clinitron therapy is utilized. Skin grafts require frequent moist dressings, or they will desiccate from the warm dry air flowing through the bed of the Clinitron.

Urinary

Foley catheter drainage is established before operation and is maintained until the patient can sit and resume self-care.

Operative Care

The operating table is routinely equipped with a warming blanket, and patient temperature is monitored. Bony prominences are padded with adhesive-backed foam rubber. The bean-bag mattress may be used to stabilize the patient and to avoid taping the skin.

Postoperative Care

The patient is kept on an air-fluidized bed for 2 weeks after the operation. At other centers, this period may be extended to 3 to 6 weeks. A program of sitting is then begun with the physical medicine and rehabilitation service. The patient is evaluated for orthostatic hypotension, and the range of motion at the joints proximal to the reconstruction is evaluated. The patient is then allowed to sit for 30 minutes, and the flap is evaluated for ischemia. When the flap tolerates sitting, a program of progressive sitting is begun outside the acute care setting.

The bowel program is begun at 3 days after operation and is performed by the staff, not the patient. Because dressings are omitted after operation, the staff can clean the patient easily: Feces do not soil the dressing and remain near the suture line.

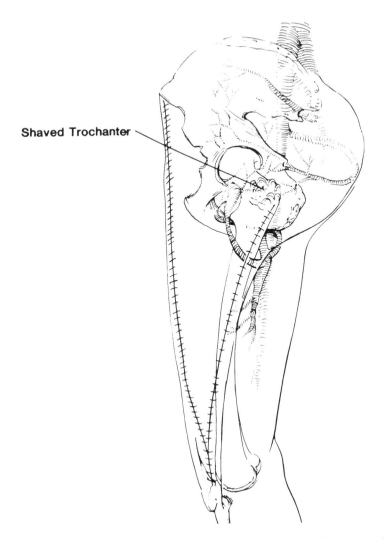

Shaved Trochanter

Figure 9–6 The tensor fascia lata musculocutaneous unit is retropositioned into the defect prepared by excision of the pseudobursa of the ulcer and complete removal of the greater trochanter. *Source:* Reprinted from *Medical Management of Long-Term Disability* by D. Green (Ed.), p. 83, with permission of Aspen Publishers, Inc. © 1990.

Sutures are left in place until a week after the patient is remobilized to prevent minor suture line dehiscences.

Complications

Early complications include wound dehiscence, hematoma, infection, and loss of flap or graft. The most frequent late complication is recurrence of a pressure sore at the same site or development of a pressure sore at another site. A rare complication of pressure sore is malignant degeneration.

Wound dehiscence may be due to the patient sitting too soon after the operation, tension on the suture line, poor flap design or lack of tissue, poor nutrition, and delayed wound healing. The treatment is reclosure of the wound without tension and immobilization until healing has occurred. Hematomas may present within hours or days to weeks after operation; some become infected and present as wound abscesses. The problem in preventing hematomas is that the large raw surface of denervated subcutaneous tissue and muscle oozes for days after the operation. It is difficult to drain every corner of the wound and to keep drains open. The treatment of acute postoperative hematomas is reoperation and hemostasis. Rare hematomas are evacuated, dressed until clean, and secondarily closed.

Wound infection is the least common of the perioperative complications; even though all the wounds reconstructed are open and contaminated, many are based on infected bone, and many are contaminated by stool after operation. The infections, when they occur, can be mixed aerobic and anaerobic coliforms and require early therapy. Tetanus immune status should be known. The treatment is adequate drainage and secondary wound closure. There seems to be a higher frequency of wound infection in patients with diarrhea before operation. Diarrhea should be controlled before flap reconstruction.

Flap loss can be due to errors of design, intraoperative damage to blood supply, tension, smoking, and arteriosclerosis. Arteriosclerosis of the pelvic and femoral vessels may suggest a preoperative arteriogram to confirm the status of the pedicle vessels. When partial flap loss occurs, débridement and closure with skin graft or a secondary flap are required.

Recurrence of additional pressure sores can be due to patient self-neglect; equipment failure of chair, cushion, or bed; falls and wounds; or loss of the home support system. All parameters need evaluation, and those that can be corrected must be dealt with. In dealing with self-neglect, patients with a second recurrence of multiple sites of pressure sores are not offered further attempts at reconstruction.

Pressure Sore Carcinoma

Squamous cell carcinoma is an uncommon complication of chronic pressure sores. It occurs in wounds of the sacral or ischial area that are present for many years, frequently 20 years or more. It can be suspected by the cauliflowerlike excrescences that grow at the wound margin, necrosis, and odor. Diagnosis is confirmed by biopsy at the time of débridement. Treatment is wide local excision, which may leave an extensive defect for reconstruction. The mortality rate is high (Berkwits et al. 1986; Grotting et al. 1987).

REFERENCES

Bailey, M.H., et al. 1987. Improved surgical management of the ischial pressure sore. *Plast. Surg. Forum* 10:86–88.

Berkwits, L., et al. 1986. Marjolin's ulcer complicating a pressure ulcer: Case report and literature review. *Arch. Phys. Med. Rehabil.* 67:831–833.

Casas, L.A., and V.L. Lewis, Jr. 1989. A reliable approach to the closure of large acquired midline defects of the back. *Plast. Reconstr. Surg.* 84:632–641.

Conway, H., and B.M. Griffith. 1956. Plastic surgical closure of decubitus ulcers in patients with paraplegia: Based on experience with 1,000 cases. *Am. J. Surg.* 91:946–954.

Dolezal, R., et al. 1985. The use of Clinitron therapy unit in the immediate post-operative care of pressure ulcers. *Am. Plast. Surg.* 17:33–36.

Douden, R.V., and J.B. McCraw. 1980. The vastus lateralis muscle flap: Technique and applications. *Am. Plast. Surg.* 4:396–404.

Feldrian, J.J., et al. 1978. The medial gastrocnemius musculocutaneous flap. *Plast. Reconstr. Surg.* 61:531–539.

Fisher, J., and M.B. Wood. 1987. Experimental comparison of bone revascularization by musculocutaneous and cutaneous flaps. *Plast. Reconstr. Surg.* 79:81–90.

Grabb, W.C., and L.C. Argenta. 1981. The lateral calcaneal artery skin flap (the lateral calcaneal artery, lesser saphenous vein and serial nerve skin flap). *Plast. Reconstr. Surg.* 68:723–730.

Griffith, B.H. 1975. "Flaps for closure of pressure sores." In *Skin flaps,* ed. W.C. Grabb and M.B. Myers, 461–469. Boston, Mass.: Little, Brown.

Grotting, J.C., et al. 1987. Pressure sore carcinoma. *Am. Plast. Surg.* 18:527–532.

Hill, H.L., et al. 1978. The transverse lumbosacral back flap. *Plast. Reconstr. Surg.* 62:177–184.

Hurteau, J.E., et al. 1981. V–Y advancement of harvesting musculocutaneous flap for coverage of ischial pressure sores. *Plast. Surg.* 68:539–542.

Hurwitz, D.J., et al. 1981. The gluteal thigh flap, a reliable, sensate flap for the closure of buttock and perineal wounds. *Plast. Reconstr. Surg.* 68:521–530.

Hynes, W. 1954. Skin-dermis graft as alternative to direct or tubed flap. *Br. J. Plast. Surg.* 7:97–101.

Kozol, R.A., et al. 1988. Effects of sodium hypochlorite (Dakin's solution) on cells of the wound module. *Arch. Surg.* 123:420–423.

Lewis, V.L., Jr., et al. 1978. Early diagnosis of crepitant nonclostridial gangrene caused by *Bacteroides melaninogenicus. Plast. Reconst. Surg.* 62:276–278.

Lewis, V.L., Jr., et al. 1981. The tensor fascia lata X–Y retroposition flap. *Am. Plast. Surg.* 6:34–37.

Lewis, V.L., Jr., et al. 1988. The diagnosis of osteomyelitis in patients with pressure sores. *Plast. Reconstr. Surg.* 81:229–232.

Lewis, V.L., Jr., et al. 1990. The fasciocutaneous flap: A conservative approach to the exposed knee joint. *Plast. Reconstr. Surg.* 85:252–257.

Limberg, A.A. 1966. "Design of local flaps." In *Modern trends in plastic surgery,* ed. T. Gibson, 2d ed. London, England: Butterworth.

Little, J.W., and J.R. Lyons. 1983. The gluteus-medius–tensor fascia lata flap. *Plast. Reconstr. Surg.* 71:366–370.

Mathes, S.J., and F. Nahai. 1982. "Clinical applications for muscle and musculocutaneous flaps." In *Foot reconstruction,* eds. S.J. Mathes and F. Nahai. St. Louis, MO: Mosby.

Mathes, S.J., et al. 1982. Use of the muscle flap in chronic osteomyelitis: Experimental and clinical correlation. *Plast. Reconstr. Surg.* 69:815–828.

Nahai, F., et al. 1978. The tensor fascia lata myocutaneous flap. *Am. Plast. Surg.* 1:372–378.

Paletta, C.E., et al. 1989. The V–Y tensor fascia lata musculocutaneous flap. *Plast. Reconstr. Surg.* 83:852–857.

Pincus, T., et al. 1990. Multicenter study of recombinant human erythropoietin in correction of anemia in rheumatoid arthritis. *Am. J. Med.* 89:161–168.

Ramirez, O.M., et al. 1984. The sliding gluteus maximus myocutaneous flap: Its relevance in ambulatory patients. *Plast. Reconstr. Surg.* 74:68–75.

Rees, T.D., et al. 1984. The effect of cigarette smoking on skin-flap survival in the face lift patient. *Plast. Reconstr. Surg.* 73:911–915.

Scheflan, M., et al. 1981. Gluteus maximus island musculocutaneous flap closure of sacral and ischial ulcers. *Plast. Reconstr. Surg.* 68:533–538.

Watson, A.J., et al. 1990. Treatment of the anemia of chronic renal failure with subcutaneous recombinant human erythropoietin. *Am. J. Med.* 89:432–435.

Wingate, G., and J.A. Friedland. 1978. Repair of ischial pressure ulcers with gracilis myocutaneous island flaps. *Plast. Reconstr. Surg.* 62:245–248.

Wingate, G., et al. 1992. Desmopressin decreases operative blood loss in spinal cord injury patients having flap reconstruction of pelvic pressure sores. *Plast. Reconstr. Surg.* 89:279–282.

Xyas, C., et al. 1980. Thoracolumbar-sacral flaps in the treatment of sacral pressure sores. *Plast. Reconstr. Surg.* 65:159–163.

Chapter 10

Management of Spastic Hypertonia after Spinal Cord Injury

Richard T. Katz

Spasticity is a nearly universal complication of spinal cord injury. Therapeutically, it is one of the most important impairments for individuals with CNS disease. This chapter focuses primarily on management of spastic hypertonia after spinal cord injury. Readers are referred to recent reviews for a complete discussion of pathophysiology and quantification of spastic hypertonia (Katz & Rymer 1989, in press).

Diagnostically, spasticity is a hallmark of an upper motor neuron disorder, and therapeutically it represents one of the most important impairments for individuals who care for patients with CNS disease; before treatment is initiated, however, the physician needs to address several important questions. Is there a functional impairment due to the spastic hypertonia? Is there a disturbance of gait? Do flexor spasms force patients from their chair or interfere with transfers? Does the pain that can be associated with spasms disturb patients' sleep? Is the lower extremity extensor tone useful to patients in supporting themselves during their gait patterns? A stereotyped therapeutic approach has been proposed (Merritt 1981), but, as in many aspects of rehabilitation, treatment is best individualized to a particular patient (Katz 1988).

BASIC PATIENT MANAGEMENT TO REDUCE SPASTICITY

Good nursing care can reduce nociceptive and exteroceptive stimuli that may be exacerbating the patient's hypertonia (Exhibit 10–1). The avoidance of noxious stimuli is therefore an important initial management step. This includes prompt treatment of urinary tract complications (infections or stones), prevention of pressure sores and contractures, releasing of tightly wrapped leg bags and clothes, proper bowel and bladder management to prevent fecal impaction and bladder distension, and deep venous thrombosis prophylaxis. Heterotopic bone has been suggested as an exacerbant, but the prevention of this complication can be difficult.

Proper bed positioning early after spinal cord injury has been suggested as an important step in the long-term reduction of spastic hypertonia (Guttmann 1976); this assertion has never been systematically evaluated, however. A daily stretching program is an integral component of any management program for spastic hypertonia. A common bedside observation is that the resistance perceived as one continuously ranges a limb progressively diminishes as one repeats the motion.

Regular ranging of a patient's limbs helps prevent contractures and can reduce the severity of spastic tone for several hours. The reasons for the carryover of ranging for several hours are not completely clear, but they could be related to mechanical changes in the musculotendinous unit as well as to plastic changes that occur within the CNS. These plastic events may correlate with short- and long-term modulation of synaptic efficacy associated with neurotransmitter changes on a cellular level. Habituation of reflex activity has been studied in the marine snail *Aplysia californica,* which has a simple nervous system. The snail has a reflex for withdrawing its respiratory organ and siphon, which is similar to the leg

Exhibit 10–1 Initial Considerations in the Management of Spastic
         Hypertonia

Preliminary considerations

Functional impairment from hypertonia?
Causes gait disturbance?
Hypertonicity needed for standing?
Flexor spasms?
Painful spasms?

Basic management

Proper bed and wheelchair positioning
Avoid noxious stimuli
Daily stretching programs

Physical measures

Therapeutic facilitation
Topical cold/anesthesia
Casting/splinting

flexion-withdrawal reflex in humans. Repetitive activation results in a decrease in synaptic transmission; this is partly due to an inactivation of calcium channels in the presynaptic terminal. The decrease in calcium influx diminishes the release of neurotransmitter, probably as a result of the calcium-dependent exocytosis of neurotransmitter vesicles (Castellucci & Kandel 1974; Castellucci et al. 1978).

SHORT-TERM STRATEGIES

Certain interventions may be valuable as temporizing strategies when a specific goal is in mind. Several schools of therapeutic exercise have suggested that reflex-inhibiting postures may temporarily decrease spastic hypertonia so that underlying movements may be unmasked (Bobath 1970; Brunnstrom 1970; Levine et al. 1954). Utilizing these strategies, therapists are able to help hemiplegic and cerebral palsy patients produce voluntary movements.

Topical cold has been reported to decrease tendon reflex excitability, reduce clonus, increase range of motion of the joint, and improve power in the antagonistic muscle group. These effects can be used to facilitate improved motor function for hours (Hartviksen 1962; Knutsson 1970; Lightfoot et al. 1975; Mecomber & Herman 1971; Miglietta 1962, 1964, 1973). Tone may be decreased shortly after the application of ice, probably as a result of decreased sensitivity in cutaneous receptors and slowing of nerve conduction. Central factors and changes in CNS excitability may take longer to occur. Thus a therapist might apply a cold pack for 20 minutes or more to obtain maximum effect (Chan 1986). Topical anesthesia may have similar effects (Mills & Pozos 1985; Sabbahi et al. 1981).

Serial casting and splinting techniques performed by occupational and physical therapists can improve the range of motion in a joint as a result of hypertonic contracture, and positioning the limb in a tonic stretch has been observed to decrease reflex tone (Booth et al. 1983; Cherry & Weigand 1981; Collins et al. 1985; Kaplan 1962; King 1982; McPherson et al. 1985; Snook 1979; Te Groen & Dommisse 1964). In one study, long-term but not short-term casting resulted in a significant decrease in both dynamic and static reflex sensitivity. Elongation of the series' elastic component of the musculotendinous unit and an increase in the number of sarcomeres within muscle fibers may each have contributed to the decrease in tone (Otis et al. 1985). Biofeedback techniques also have been observed to modulate spastic hypertonia, but they have not demonstrated much widespread usefulness (Basmajian 1981; Wolf & Binder-MacLeod 1983a, 1983b).

PHARMACOLOGICAL INTERVENTION

No medication has been uniformly useful in the treatment of spastic hypertonia. Considering the variety of problems associated with spasticity—flexor spasms in the spinal patient, dystonic posturing in the hemiplegic patient, and spastic diplegia in the cerebral palsy child—it is unlikely that one agent will be beneficial to all parties. More important, all drugs have potentially serious side effects, and these negative features should be carefully weighed when one is beginning a patient on any drug. Continued use of a drug should be contingent upon a clearly beneficial effect (Table 10–1; Davidoff 1985; Katz 1988; Young & Delwaide 1981).

Baclofen (Lioresal) is an analog of γ-aminobutyric acid (GABA), a neurotransmitter involved in presynaptic inhibition. Baclofen does not bind to the classic GABA A receptor but to a recently discovered and less well-characterized B receptor. Agonism at this site inhibits calcium influx into presynaptic terminals and suppresses the release of excitatory neurotransmitters (Davidoff 1985). Baclofen inhibits both monosynaptic and polysynaptic reflexes and also reduces activity of the γ efferent (Van Hemert 1980). Although therapeutic effects have been shown to occur when plasma levels exceed 400 ng/mL (McLellan 1977), optimal responses have been obtained at different plasma and cerebrospinal fluid levels (Knutsson et al. 1974). Baclofen is completely absorbed after oral administration and is eliminated predominantly by the renal route. The half life is approximately 3.5 hours. Baclofen readily crosses the blood-brain barrier, in contrast to GABA (Faigle et al. 1980; Koella 1980).

Baclofen is probably the drug of choice in spinal forms of spasticity. It has been demonstrated to be effective in reducing flexor spasms, increasing range of motion, and decreasing spastic hypertonia (Duncan et al. 1976; Sachais et al. 1977). Baclofen is equivalent to diazepam in efficacy but has less sedative effect (Hattab 1980). The role of baclofen in the treat-

Table 10–1 Pharmacologic Management of Spastic Hypertonia

Agent	Daily Dosage	Half-Life (hours)	Mechanism of Action
Baclofen	10–80⁺ mg	3.5	Presynaptic inhibitor by activation of γ-aminobutyric acid (GABA) B receptor
Diazepam	4–60⁺ mg	27–37*	Facilitates postsynaptic effects of GABA, resulting in increased presynaptic inhibition
Dantrolene	24–400 mg	8.7	Reduces calcium release, interfering with excitation-contraction coupling in skeletal muscle

*Half-life of the active primary metabolite is significantly longer.

ment of cerebral forms of spasticity remains unsettled (Hattab 1980; Knutsson et al. 1972; Van Hemert 1980); it may interfere with attention and memory in brain-injured patients (Sandy & Gillman 1985). Baclofen may improve bladder control by decreasing hyperreflexive contraction of the external urethral sphincter (Khanna 1979). It has been shown to be safe and effective in long-term use (Roussan et al. 1985).

Dosage begins at approximately 5 mg orally two or three times a day and may be slowly titrated upward toward a recommended maximum dosage of 80 mg/day; this recommended maximum dosage may not necessarily be the most effective dose for the patient, however, and higher doses may be well tolerated as well as additionally therapeutic (Bianchine 1985; Kirkland 1984). There is a low incidence of side effects, which may include hallucinations, confusion, sedation, hypotonia, and ataxia (Hattab 1980; Roy & Wakefield 1986). Sudden withdrawal of the drug may lead to seizures and hallucinations (Terrence & Fromm 1981). Stereospecific L-baclofen has been shown to more effective than the presently used racemic form in treatment of pain (Fromm & Terrence 1987; Sawynok & Dickson 1985). L-Baclofen deserves evaluation for treatment of spastic hypertonia.

Diazepam (Valium) facilitates postsynaptic effects of GABA, resulting in an increase in presynaptic inhibition (Costa & Guidotti 1979). It has no direct GABA-mimetic effect but exerts indirect mimetic effect only when GABA transmission is functional (Young & Delwaide 1981). In addition to its known effects on the brain (Study & Barker 1982), diazepam has been shown to have effect in patients with demonstrated spinal cord division (Cook & Nathan 1967); its effect in complete spinal lesions was not confirmed by one report, however (Verrier et al. 1977).

Diazepam has been a successful treatment for spastic hypertonia in spinal cord injury and is generally well tolerated ex-

cept for its sedative effect. Diazepam is generally unsuitable in patients with brain injury because of deleterious effects on attention and memory (Glenn 1986b). Other side effects include intellectual impairment and reduced motor coordination. Evidence of abuse and addiction is rare, but true psychological addiction may occur. Withdrawal symptoms may appear if diazepam is tapered too rapidly. There is some synergistic depression of the CNS when the drug is administered with alcohol. Although the potential for overdose exists, the benzodiazepines have an extremely large index of safety (Greenblatt et al. 1983). Dosage begins at approximately 2 mg orally twice a day and may be slowly titrated up to 15 to 20 mg or more per day in divided dosages. Although dosages as high as 60 mg/day have been used, it is our practice to use dosages less than 15 to 20 mg/day to avoid oversedation and to limit abuse potential.

Dantrolene sodium (Dantrium) reduces muscle action potential–induced release of calcium into the sarcoplasmic reticulum, decreasing the force produced by excitation-contraction coupling (Van Winkle 1976). Thus dantrolene is the only drug that intervenes in spastic hypertonia at a muscular rather than a segmental reflex level. It reduces the activity of phasic more than tonic stretch reflexes (Pinder et al. 1977). Dantrolene affects fast more than slow muscle fibers and for unknown reasons seems to have little effect on smooth and cardiac muscle tissues. It is metabolized largely in the liver and is eliminated in urine and bile. The half-life is 8.7 hours (Pinder et al. 1977).

Dantrolene is preferred for cerebral forms of spasticity such as hemiplegia or cerebral palsy (Ketel & Kolb 1984) but may be a useful adjunct to the treatment of spinal forms of spasticity. It is less likely to cause lethargy or cognitive disturbances than baclofen or diazepam (Glenn 1986). Although dantrolene theoretically weakens muscles, the effects on spastic hypertonia are generally without impairment of motor performance. Its most pronounced effect may be a reduction in clonus and muscle spasms resulting from innocuous stimuli (Joynt 1976).

Dantrolene is mild to moderately sedative and may cause malaise, nausea and vomiting, dizziness, and diarrhea. It has been suggested that the drug may exacerbate seizures in cerebral palsy patients. The most commonly considered side effect is hepatotoxicity, which may occur in about 1% of patients. Generally, liver function tests are monitored periodically, and the drug can be tapered or discontinued if enzyme elevations are noted. Fatal hepatitis has been reported in 0.1% to 0.2% of patients treated for longer than 60 days (Bianchine 1985); one expert in the use of dantrolene, however, feels that its hepatotoxic effects may have been overstated (Basmajian 1987). Dosage begins at 25 mg/day and may increase slowly up to 400 mg/day (Pinder et al. 1977); clinical results are not clearly related to dose, however, and may plateau at a dosage of 100 mg/day (Meyler et al. 1981). Because liver functions must be followed regularly, dantrolene is used only when the patient is willing to have regular blood tests and can be reliable in outpatient follow-up.

Tizanidine, an imidazoline derivative, has an agonistic action at central α_2 adrenergic receptor sites. It may facilitate the action of glycine, an inhibitory neurotransmitter (Hennies 1981), and it prevents the release of excitatory amino acids (i.e., L-glutamate and L-aspartate) from the presynaptic terminal of spinal interneurons (Davies & Quinlan 1985). It reduces tonic stretch reflexes and enhances presynaptic inhibition in animals. It enhances vibratory inhibition of the H-reflex and reduces abnormal cocontraction (Young & Shahani 1986). Tizanidine has the unusual effect of increasing the torque of spastic muscle by increasing the amplitude of the agonist electromyographic signal (Knutsson et al. 1982). It has been shown to be equivalent to baclofen as an antispastic agent (but may be better tolerated) in both cerebral and spinal forms of spasticity in divided dosages up to 36 mg/day (Hennies 1981; Hoogstraten et al. 1988; Medici et al. 1989; Smolenski et al. 1981). It has similarly been shown to be equally efficacious as and better tolerated than diazepam in patients with chronic hemiplegia (Bes et al. 1988). Multiple sclerosis patients have shown significant benefit in several large double-blind studies (Bass et al. 1988; Eyssette et al. 1988; Hoogstraten et al. 1988; Lapierre et al. 1987). Common side effects include mild hypotension, sleepiness, weakness, and dry mouth (Stien et al. 1987). Both tizanidine and baclofen are more effective in extensor than flexor musculature (Hassan & McLellan 1980). Tizanidine is not available for use in the United States.

Ketazolam, a benzodiazepine, has been shown to be equally effective as and less sedating than diazepam in spinal forms of spasticity; it may have a similar pharmacologic action. An additional benefit is that ketazolam may be administered in a single dosage of 30 to 60 mg/day (Basmajian et al. 1986; Basmajian & Yucel 1984). It is not presently approved for use in the United States. Clorazepate, a benzodiazepine analog, is transformed into desmethyldiazepam, the major metabolite of diazepam, and was shown in one study to be effective in normalizing phasic but not tonic stretch reflexes (Lossius et al. 1985).

Chlorpromazine has been applied to the treatment of hypertonia because of its α-adrenergic–blocking effect. Clinical and electrophysiological studies in humans before and after administration of α- and β-blocking agents suggest that descending adrenergic and noradrenergic pathways may have important modulatory effects on spastic hypertonia (Mai 1981); the depression of motor function by phenothiazines, however, is thought to be due largely to their effects upon the brain stem reticular formation. A small double-blind study of chlorpromazine with phenytoin suggested that a combination of these drugs may be beneficial in the treatment of spastic hypertonia. Neither drug alone was as efficacious as the combination of the two, although chlorpromazine alone was nearly as effective. Phenytoin serum levels did not correlate with therapeutic effect as long as this concentration was above 7 mg/mL. The addition of phenytoin lowered the needed optimally therapeutic dose of chlorpromazine, decreasing its sedative effect (Cohan et al. 1980).

Clonidine, an α_2-adrenergic agonist, has been used with fair success in patients with spinal cord injury (Maynard 1986; Nance et al. 1985). Syncope, hypotension, and nausea and vomiting are the most common side effects. One study cited an average dosage of 0.39 mg/day (Maynard 1986). In a second study, most of the patients who benefitted from the drug noted acceptable relief with a dosage of 0.1 mg twice a day or less (Donovan et al. 1988). Clonidine is now available in an adhesive patch for weeklong transdermal delivery.

Progabide, a systemically active GABA agonist at both A and B receptors, and tetrahydroisoxazolopyridin, a second GABA agonist, have been proposed as possible antispasticity drugs (Davidoff 1985; Mondrup & Pedersen 1983). Electrophysiological studies suggest that progabide's likely site of action is spinal interneurons (Mondrup & Pedersen 1984a). A median dose of 24.3 mg/kg (1,800 mg/day) resulted in satisfactory reduction in spastic hypertonia, tendon reflexes, and flexor spasms without a significant improvement in voluntary strength (Mondrup & Pedersen 1984b). The beneficial effects of progabide in higher dosages seem to be limited by serious side effects such as fever, weakness, and elevated liver enzymes (Rudick et al. 1987).

Glycine, a neurotransmitter involved in reciprocal inhibition, has not been thoroughly investigated in the treatment of spastic hypertonia. Glycine passes the blood-brain barrier in amounts sufficient to affect reflex activity and has decreased spasticity in small groups of patients (Barbeau 1974). Glycine is rapidly depleted in the spinal cord ventral gray matter after spinal cord transection, and the depletion correlates with the spasticity onset in a canine model (Hall et al. 1976). Similarly, threonine, a glycine precursor, has shown potential efficacy in a preliminary investigation (Barbeau et al. 1982). Cannabis, although not approved for use as an agent in the treatment of spastic hypertonia, occasionally has been noted to decrease hypertonia (Malec et al. 1982). Although various other medications such as cyclobenzaprine and carisoprodol have been forwarded in the treatment of this disorder, there is no consistent evidence to recommend their use.

INTRATHECAL MEDICATIONS

Intrathecal administration of baclofen has been successfully attempted in the treatment of spastic hypertonia. A pump may be planted subcutaneously in the abdomen wall, and a catheter can be surgically placed into the subarachnoid space. In this manner, higher dosages of these medications can be placed near the spinal cord structures of desired action, largely avoiding the CNS side effects of increased oral intake. The pump is refilled on a monthly basis by transcutaneous injection.

Baclofen has been administered in a dosage of 12 to 650 mg/day in this manner; promising preliminary results (Dralle et al. 1985; Hankey et al. 1986; Muller et al. 1987; Penn & Kroin 1985, 1987) have been confirmed in long-term follow-up evaluation (Ochs et al. 1989; Parke et al. 1989; Penn et al. 1989). In addition to beneficial effects on limb spasticity, intrathecal baclofen may have a beneficial effect on bladder management (Frost et al. 1989). Baclofen will increase bladder capacity and decrease external sphincter spasticity but will not result in normal voiding patterns. Caution concerning inadvertent overdose should be exercised because reversible coma due to baclofen toxicity has been reported (Penn & Kroin 1987; Romijn et al. 1986); patients with respiratory depression due to accidental intrathecal bolus injection, however, were treated with 2 mg physostigmine administered intravenously (Ochs et al. 1989). The half-life of intrathecal baclofen is approximately 5 hours (Penn & Kroin 1987).

One to two milligrams of intrathecal morphine has similarly caused a dramatic reduction in spasticity and pain in spinal cord patients (Erickson et al. 1985). Patients do not seem to develop drug tolerance or to lose the beneficial effect of the morphine in long-term follow-up (Erickson et al. 1989).

ELECTRICAL STIMULATION

The concept of using electrical stimulation to improve patient function, or functional electrical stimulation, has received wide medical and mainstream press. Electrical stimulation of peripheral nerves has been a potential adjunct to traditional rehabilitation therapeutics for paraplegic patients during standing (Cybulski & Jaeger 1986; Cybulski et al. 1984), walking, and exercise training (Phillips et al. 1984). Cyclical use of electrical stimulation has been shown to decrease upper extremity contractures (Baker et al. 1979), to improve motor activity in agonist muscles, and to reduce tone in antagonistic muscle groups of the hemiplegic and quadriplegic patient (Alfieri 1982; Bajd et al. 1985; Baker et al. 1979; Franek et al. 1988; Gracanin 1984; Levine et al. 1952; Robinson et al. 1988; Vodovnik et al. 1984a, 1984b). In a carefully performed study, stimulation of the sural nerve, a flexor reflex afferent, resulted in decreased extensor tonus and increased strength of ankle dorsiflexion (Petajan 1987). The therapeutic effect may last for an hour or more after stimulation has been discontinued (Vodovnik et al. 1982; Walker 1982; Waters 1984), perhaps as a result of neurotransmitter modulation within the segmental reflex. Peroneal nerve stimulation may suppress ankle clonus in ambulatory hemiplegic patients via reciprocal inhibition (Dimitrijevic & Sherwood 1980). Electrical stimulation has limited but defined applications as a dorsiflexor assist during hemiplegic gait and as a hand-opening educational device in the plegic upper extremity (Albert & Andre 1984; Waters et al. 1985).

Spinal cord stimulation, also known as dorsal column stimulation, was initially embraced enthusiastically in the treatment of spinal hypertonia (Dimitrijevic & Sherwood 1980; Illis et al. 1976; Richardson et al. 1979; Siegfried 1980). A short chain of stimulating electrodes is threaded into the epidural space, resting in the vicinity of the spinal cord dorsal columns. Maximal improvement depends upon finding the ideal combination of electrode placement, stimulation intensity, and stimulation frequency. A critical analysis of the beneficial effects of dorsal column stimulation has questioned its efficacy in improving motor and bladder functions (Illis et al. 1983; Tallis et al. 1983). In a carefully performed study where examiners were blinded as to whether stimulation was on or off, measures of joint compliance and standardized neurological examination were no better than chance in determining whether spinal cord stimulation was being received (Gottlieb et al. 1985).

PHENOL INJECTIONS

Nerve and motor point blocks with injectable phenol offer the physician a somewhat effective method of reducing spastic tone on a temporary basis. Two to six percent aqueous phenol solutions produce chemical neurolysis when applied to a nerve trunk or its terminal nerve fibers (motor point block; Dimitrijevic & Sherwood 1980; Easton et al. 1979; Garland et al. 1984; Halpern & Meelhuysen 1966; Khalili 1984; Khalili & Betts 1967; Khalili et al. 1964; Meelhuysen et al. 1968; Petrillo et al. 1980; Wainapel et al. 1984; Wood 1978). Concentrations of phenol greater than 5% cause protein coagulation and necrosis. Neurolysis of motor points is generally ineffective by itself, perhaps because of the multiplicity of motor points within a muscle (McComas et al. 1984). Nerve blocks may be quite effective and may last 3 to 6 months or more (Easton et al. 1979; Garland et al. 1982; Halpern & Meelhuysen 1966; Khalili & Betts 1967).

Musculocutaneous nerve block can be helpful in the hemiplegic with severe elbow flexion contracture or the C-5 quadriplegic with flexor contractures due to loss of triceps function (Garland et al. 1982; Wainapel et al. 1984). Elbow flexion is preserved through the action of the brachioradialis muscle, which, unlike other elbow flexors, is innervated by the radial nerve. Median nerve blocks help relax tightly contracted hemiplegic wrist and fingers. An obturator block decreases lower extremity scissoring during gait and facilitates hip abduction to ease personal hygiene. Hip flexor spasticity may be diminished by paravertebral lumbar spinal nerve block (Petajan 1987). Tibial nerve block can reduce severe equinovarus ankle posturing (Khalili 1984; Petrillo et al. 1980). A preliminary diagnostic block with local anesthetic is often useful to predict the effect of a longer-acting phenol procedure. Implantable reservoirs can be used to inject long-acting anesthetic agents repeatedly onto the brachial plexus in hemiplegics with severely spastic upper extremities (Keenan 1987).

Nerve blocks may be associated with dysesthesias and causalgia in approximately 10% of patients; patients should be advised of this before the block is administered (Wood 1978). Severe persistent dysesthesias may be treated with oral steroids or repetition of the phenol block (Glenn 1986a). Open phenol nerve blocks may be more successful by selectively blocking fibers destined for muscle groups while leaving sensory fibers unharmed. Presumably, the incidence of dysesthesias should also be lower using this method (Garland et al. 1982). Venous thromboses may complicate phenol injection for chemical neurolysis (Medical News 1983).

SPINAL BLOCKS

Intrathecal chemical neurolysis is another method of decreasing spastic hypertonia. Spinal root neurolysis may be carried out via spinal administration of 5% to 7% phenol in water or absolute alcohol, but control over affected fibers is rather imprecise (Ivan 1982). The effects of alcohol are more permanent than those of phenol (Merritt 1981). Patients must be carefully immobilized to allow precise layering of the neurolytic material. Complications of this procedure include urinary and fecal incontinence, paresis, paresthesias, and even death. Complication rates have varied from 1% to 10% in various series of patients (Wood 1978).

ORTHOPEDIC PROCEDURES

Tenotomy, the release of a tendon to a severely hypertonic muscle, is a more advanced treatment that may provide benefit in selected patients. The indications for hip abductor tenotomy are similar to those for obturator nerve block. Hamstring tenotomies may benefit those patients with severe knee flexion deformities who do not display potential for useful motor function. Care must be exercised subsequently not to extend the knee too rapidly, which will put the integrity of the neurovascular bundle at risk. Selective quadriceps release may help those patients who have a stiff-legged gait. Out-of-phase firing of the rectus femoris and vastus intermedius is the most common cause of such a gait deviation (Smith & Leventhal 1987). Achilles tenotomies are a valuable asset in many patients with plantarflexion contractures that interfere with functional goals. Although various methods of lengthening the heel cord exist, it is generally conceded that an open procedure is desirable for precision. Toe flexor tenotomies may be beneficial in the hemiplegic patient when hypertonicity of the foot intrinsics results in claw-foot type deformities (Treanor 1981). Iliopsoas myotomy has been advocated for hip flexion contractures and to decrease flexor spasms (Merritt 1981), but flexor spasms can usually be managed by less invasive procedures.

Tendon transfer in various upper extremity muscle groups has been suggested for the augmentation of motor function in hemiplegic individuals (Pinzur 1985). Transfer of the flexor digitorum sublimis to the profundus, brachioradialis transfer to the long finger extensors (Pinzur et al. 1988), and fractional lengthening of the long flexors have been advocated in stroke patients (Waters 1978), but it is not universally accepted that these procedures improve the patient's functional activities. Overlengthening of the finger flexors can result in a loss of grip strength (Keenan et al. 1987). Adequate sensory function must be present before any type of upper extremity surgery is contemplated. V–Y lengthening of the triceps muscle has been advocated in the occasional hemiplegic in whom severe triceps tone limits function (Pinzur et al. 1987). The marked complexity of upper extremity function limits the use of transfer surgery in the limb because patients tend to perform activities of daily living with the remaining functional extremity.

Lower extremity tendon transfer undoubtedly is the most successful and useful type of rehabilitative surgery in the hemiplegic patient and is used for the remediation of equinovarus posturing. The split anterior tibial transfer (SPLATT) is a procedure to help reduce excessive supination at the subtalar joint. The tibialis anterior tendon is split along its length, and the distal end of the lateral half is tunneled into the third cuneiform and cuboid bones. This creates an eversion force that is slightly greater than the varus pull of the remaining medial portion. It is generally performed in combination with an Achilles tendon lengthening (Waters et al. 1978). The SPLATT procedure is one of the most useful types of hemiplegic rehabilitative procedures and may substantially improve affected gait (Waters et al. 1982).

NEUROSURGICAL PROCEDURES

The neurosurgical options in the treatment of spastic hypertonia have been reviewed (Ivan 1982; Sindou et al. 1985a). Surgical neurectomies of the musculocutaneous, obturator, or tibial nerves can be performed rather simply to create a more permanent disturbance of nerve function than phenol for indications mentioned above.

Rhizotomies, the lesioning of spinal roots, may also be performed for the remediation of spasticity in severe cases. Rhizotomies may be categorized as open (requiring laminectomy) or closed, complete or selective, and anterior or posterior. Open rhizotomies generally are reserved as quite advanced treatment choices (Gildenberg 1982). Anterior rhizotomies are associated with severe denervation type atrophy of all innervated muscles and may place the patient at increased risk for skin breakdown. Selective rhizotomies involve cutting approximately four fifths of the posterior rootlet and may utilize electrical mapping of the rootlets to determine the role of those nerve fibers in hypertonic reflexes (Benedetti & Colombo 1981; Benedetti et al. 1982; Fraioli & Guidetti 1977; Gildenberg 1982; Peacock & Arens 1982; Privat et al.

1976; Sindou et al. 1985a, 1985b). Selective rhizotomies have been employed successfully in spastic forms of cerebral palsy with recurrence of spastic hypertonia in only 5% of cases (Fasano et al. 1978). Although selective rhizotomy is most often carried out in the lumbosacral roots, success has also been reported for treatment of spasticity and pain in the hemiplegic upper extremity (Sindou et al. 1986).

Closed rhizotomies are performed under fluoroscopic control utilizing a radiofrequency needle to destroy nerve tissue. Although percutaneous rhizotomies are not permanent, they are highly effective in reducing spastic hypertonia in the lower extremities with minimal morbidity (Herz et al. 1983; Kasdon & Lathi 1984; Kennemore 1983). Sindou and Jeanmonod (1989) utilized microsurgical dorsal root entry zone selective destruction for the treatment of spasticity and pain in the lower limbs; it is not clear what advantage this procedure offers over selective posterior rhizotomy, however.

Myelotomy, the severing of tracts in the spinal cord, has been advocated as a treatment modality in the most severe cases of spastic hypertonia. Bischoff introduced a myelotomy to interrupt the reflex arc in which the cord was approached through the lateral funiculus on one side and extended through the middle of the cord to traverse the gray matter on the other side. Only segmental analgesia resulted from the procedure, and all long tracts except the pyramidal tract remained intact. A modification of this procedure was the posterior longitudinal myelotomy, which similarly cut through the gray matter on each side using a T-shaped myelotome via a median sulcus approach. This improvement preserved lateral funiculus white matter tracts bilaterally (Laitinen & Singounas 1971). Loss of bowel and bladder function must be considered possible complications of myelotomy (Benedetti & Colombo 1981). Sectioning or excision of portions of the cord (cordotomy or cordectomy) causes severe muscle wasting, frequent voiding difficulties, and loss of erectile function and is rarely practiced (Ivan 1982; Kasdon 1986).

CONCLUSION

The functional impairment due to spasticity must be carefully assessed before any treatment is considered. Therapeutic intervention is best individualized to a particular patient (Exhibit 10–2). Basic principles of treatment to ameliorate spastic hypertonia are to avoid noxious stimuli and to provide frequent range of motion. Therapeutic exercise, cold, or topical anesthesia may decrease reflex activity for short periods of time to facilitate minimal motor function. Casting and splinting techniques are extremely valuable to extend joint range diminished by hypertonicity.

Baclofen, diazepam, and dantrolene remain the three most commonly used pharmacologic agents in the treatment of spastic hypertonia. Clonidine is being used more often because of its limited potential for abuse. Baclofen is generally the drug of choice for spinal cord types of spasticity; sodium

Exhibit 10–2 Further Options in the Management of Spastic Hypertonia

Electrical stimulation
- Peripheral nerve
- Dorsal column

Chemical neurolysis
- Peripheral
- Intrathecal

Orthopedic procedures
- Tenotomy
- Tendon transfers

Neurosurgical procedures
- Neurectomy
- Rhizotomy
  1. Anterior
  2. Posterior
  3. Open
  4. Closed
- Myelotomy

dantrolene is the only agent that acts directly on muscle tissue. Phenytoin with chlorpromazine may be potentially useful if sedation does not limit their use. Tizanidine and ketazolam, neither of which is available in the United States, may be significant additions to the pharmacological armamentarium. Intrathecal administration of antispastic medications allows high concentrations of drug near the site of action, which limits side effects. This form of treatment is the most exciting recent development in the treatment of spastic hypertonia.

Peripheral electrical stimulation may have limited use in diminishing tone and facilitating paretic muscles. Dorsal column stimulation via electrodes within the spinal column initially was hailed as a therapeutic advance but has subsequently been shown to be minimally effective. Phenol injections provide a valuable transition between short-term and long-term treatments and offer remediation of hypertonia in selected muscle groups.

Tenotomies and tendon transfers offer significant benefit in carefully chosen patients. The SPLATT procedure, transfer of the lateral portion of the tibialis anterior tendon to the lateral part of the foot, is one of the most successful rehabilitative surgeries. Hamstring tenotomies, Achilles tendon lengthening, and release of long toe flexors may all benefit selected patients with spastic hypertonia.

Surgical neurectomies can release spastic muscles in selected patient groups. Obturator neurectomies can substantially improve scissoring of gait in cerebral palsy patients. Lesions of spinal roots can decrease hypertonic reflexes; selective rhizotomies are the most invasive of these procedures but offer the most precise control of neural destruction. Closed radiofrequency rhizotomies are performed under fluoroscopic guidance but may only have temporary effect.

REFERENCES

Albert, A., and J.M. Andre. 1984. State of the art of functional electrical stimulation in France. *Int. Rehabil. Med.* 6:13–18.

Alfieri, V. 1982. Electrical treatment of spasticity: Reflex tonic activity in hemiplegic patients and selected specific electrostimulation. *Scand. J. Rehabil. Med.* 14:177–182.

Bajd, T., et al. 1985. Electrical stimulation in treating spasticity resulting from spinal cord injury. *Arch. Phys. Med. Rehabil.* 66:515–517.

Baker, L.L., et al. 1979. Electrical stimulation for wrist and fingers for hemiplegic patients. *Phys. Ther.* 59:1495–1499.

Barbeau, A. 1974. Preliminary study of glycine administration in patients with spasticity. *Neurology* 24:392 (abstract).

Barbeau, A., et al. 1982. Pilot study of threonine supplementation in human spasticity. *Can. J. Neurol. Sci.* 9:141–145.

Basmajian, J.V. 1981. Biofeedback in rehabilitation: A review of principles and practices. *Arch. Phys. Med. Rehabil.* 62:469–475.

Basmajian, J.V. 1987. Muscle relaxants in multiple sclerosis. *Int. J. Disabil. Stud.* 9:90–91.

Basmajian, J.V., and Yucel, V. 1984. Ketazolam treatment for spasticity: Double-blind study of a new drug. *Arch. Phys. Med. Rehabil.* 65:698–701.

Basmajian, J.V., et al. 1986. Ketazolam once daily for spasticity: Double-blind cross-over study. *Arch. Phys. Med. Rehabil.* 67:556–557.

Bass, B., et al. 1988. Tizanidine versus baclofen in the treatment of spasticity in patients with multiple sclerosis. *Can. J. Neurol. Sci.* 15:15–19.

Benedetti, A., and F. Colombo. 1981. Spinal surgery for spasticity (46 cases). *Neurochirurgia* 24:195–198.

Benedetti, A., et al. 1982. Posterior rhizotomies for spasticity in children affected by cerebral palsy. *J. Neurol. Sci.* 26:179–184.

Bes, A., et al. 1988. A multi-centre, double-blind trial of tizanidine, a new antispastic agent, in spasticity associated with hemiplegia. *Curr. Med. Res. Opin.* 10:709–718.

Bianchine, J.R. 1985. "Drugs for Parkinson's disease, spasticity, and acute muscle spasms." In *The pharmacological basis of therapeutics,* ed. A.G. Gilman et al., 7th ed., New York, N.Y.: Macmillan.

Bobath, B. 1970. *Adult hemiplegia: Evaluation and treatment.* London, England: Heinemann Medical.

Booth, B.J., et al. 1983. Serial casting for the management of spasticity in the head-injured adult. *Phys. Ther.* 63:1960–1966.

Brunnstrom, S. 1970. *Movement therapy in hemiplegia.* New York, N.Y.: Harper & Row.

Castellucci, V.F., and E.R. Kandel. 1974. A quantal analysis of the synaptic depression underlying habituation of the gill-withdrawal reflex in *Aplysia. Proc. Natl. Acad. Sci. U.S.A.* 71:5004–5008.

Castellucci, V.F., et al. 1978. Cellular analysis of long-term habituation of the gill-withdrawal reflex of *Aplysia californica. Science* 202:1306–1308.

Chan, C.W.Y. 1986. Some techniques for the relief of spasticity and their physiological basis. *Physiother. Can.* 38:85–89.

Cherry, D.B., and G.M. Weigand. 1981. Plaster drop-out casts as a dynamic means to reduce muscle contracture. *Phys. Ther.* 61:1601–1603.

Cohan, S.L., et al. 1980. Phenytoin and chlorpromazine in the treatment of spasticity. *Arch. Neurol.* 37:360–364.

Collins, K., et al. 1985. Customized adjustable orthoses: Their use in spasticity. *Arch. Phys. Med. Rehabil.* 66:397–398.

Cook, J.B., and P.W. Nathan. 1967. On the site of action of diazepam in spasticity in man. *J. Neurol. Sci.* 5:33–37.

Costa, E., and A. Guidotti. 1979. Molecular mechanisms in the receptor action of benzodiazepines. *Ann. Rev. Pharmacol. Toxicol.* 19:531–545.

Cybulski, G.R., and R.J. Jaeger. 1986. Standing performance of persons with paraplegia. *Arch. Phys. Med. Rehabil.* 67:103–108.

Cybulski, G.R., et al. 1984. Lower extremity functional neuromuscular stimulation in cases of spinal cord injury. *Neurosurgery* 15:132–146.

Davidoff, R.A. 1985. Antispasticity drugs: Mechanisms of action. *Ann. Neurol.* 17:107–116.

Davies, J., and J.E. Quinlan. 1985. Selective inhibition of feline dorsal horn neurons to noxious cutaneous stimuli by tizanidine and noradrenaline: Involvement of α_2 adrenoceptors. *Neuroscience* 16:673–682.

Dimitrijevic, M.R., and A.M. Sherwood. 1980. Spasticity: Medical and surgical management. *Neurology* 30:19–27.

Donovan, W.H., et al. 1988. Clonidine effect on spasticity: A clinical trial. *Arch. Phys. Med. Rehabil.* 69:193–194.

Dralle, D., et al. 1985. Intrathecal baclofen for spasticity. *Lancet* 2:1003 (letter).

Duncan, G.W., et al. 1976. An evaluation of baclofen treatment for certain symptoms in patients with spinal cord lesions. *Neurology* 26:441–446.

Easton, J.K.M., et al. 1979. Intramuscular neurolysis for spasticity in children. *Arch. Phys. Med. Rehabil.* 60:155–158.

Erickson, D.L., et al. 1985. Control of spasticity by implantable continuous flow morphine pump. *Neurology* 16:215–217.

Erickson, D.L., et al. 1989. Control of intractable spasticity with intrathecal morphine sulfate. *Neurosurgery* 24:236–238.

Eyssette, M., et al. 1988. Multi-centre, double-blind trial of a novel antiseptic agent, tizanidine, in spasticity associated with multiple sclerosis. *Curr. Med. Res. Opin.* 10:699–708.

Faigle, J.W., et al. 1980. "Chemistry and pharmacokinetics of baclofen." In *Spasticity: Disordered motor control,* ed. R.G. Feldman et al. Chicago, Ill.: Year Book Medical.

Fasano, V.A., et al. 1978. Surgical treatment of spasticity in cerebral palsy. *Child's Brain* 4:289–305.

Fraioli, B., and B. Guidetti. 1977. Posterior partial rootlet section in the treatment of spasticity. *J. Neurosurg.* 46:619–626.

Franek, A., et al. 1988. Treatment of spinal spasticity by electrical stimulation. *J. Biomed. Eng.* 10:266–270.

Fromm, G.H., and C.F. Terrence. 1987. Comparison of L-baclofen and racemic baclofen in trigeminal neuralgia. *Neurology* 37:1725–1728.

Frost, F., et al. 1989. Intrathecal baclofen infusion: Effect on bladder management programs in patients with myelopathy. *Am. J. Phys. Med. Rehabil.* 68:112–115.

Garland, D.E., et al. 1982. Current uses of open phenol nerve block for adult acquired spasticity. *Clin. Orthop. Relat. Res.* 165:217–222.

Garland, D.E., et al. 1984. Percutaneous phenol blocks to motor points of spastic forearm muscles in head-injured adults. *Arch. Phys. Med. Rehabil.* 65:243–245.

Gildenberg, P.L. 1982. "Functional neurosurgery." In *Operative neurosurgical techniques: Indications, methods and results,* ed. H.H. Schmidek and W.H. Sweet. New York, N.Y.: Grune & Stratton.

Glenn, M.B. 1986a. Antispasticity medications in the patient with traumatic brain injury. *J. Head Trauma Rehabil.* 1:71–72.

Glenn, M.B. 1986b. Update on pharmacology. *J. Head Trauma Rehabil.* 1:72–74.

Gottlieb, G.L., et al. 1985. Evaluation of cervical stimulation for chronic treatment of spasticity. *Neurology* 35:699–704.

Gracanin, F. 1984. Functional electrical stimulation in external motor control of motor activity and movements of paralysed extremities. *Int. Rehabil. Med.* 6:25–30.

Greenblatt, D.J., et al. 1983. Current status of benzodiazepines. *N. Engl. J. Med.* 309:354–358, 410–416.

Guttmann, L. 1976. *Spinal cord injury—Comprehensive management and research.* Oxford, England: Blackwell Scientific.

Hall, P.V., et al. 1976. Neurochemical correlates of spasticity. *Life Sci.* 18:1467–1472.

Halpern, D., and F.E. Meelhuysen. 1966. Phenol motor point block in the management of muscular hypertonia. *Arch. Phys. Med. Rehabil.* 45:513–519.

Hankey, G.J., et al. 1986. Intrathecal baclofen for severe spasticity. *Med. J. Aust.* 145:465–466.

Hartviksen, K. 1962. Ice therapy in spasticity. *Acta Neurol. Scand.* 38:79–84.

Hassan, N., and D.L. McLellan. 1980. Double-blind comparison of single doses of DS 103-282, baclofen, and placebo for suppression of spasticity. *J. Neurol. Neurosurg. Psychiatry* 43:1132–1136.

Hattab, J.R. 1980. "Review of European clinical trials with baclofen." In *Spasticity: Disordered motor control,* ed. R.G. Feldman et al. Chicago, Ill.: Year Book Medical.

Hennies, O.L. 1981. A new skeletal muscle relaxant (DS 103-282) compared to diazepam in the treatment of muscle spasm of local origin. *J. Int. Med. Res.* 9:62–68.

Herz, D.A., et al. 1983. Percutaneous radiofrequency foraminal rhizotomies. *Spine* 8:729–732.

Hoogstraten, M.C., et al. 1988. Tizanidine versus baclofen in the treatment of spasticity in multiple sclerosis patients. *Acta Neurol. Scand.* 77:224–230.

Illis, L.S., et al. 1976. Dorsal column stimulation in the rehabilitation of patients with multiple sclerosis. *Lancet* 1:1383–1386.

Illis, L.S., et al. 1983. Spinal cord stimulation in the United Kingdom. *J. Neurol. Neurosurg. Psychiatry* 43:299–304.

Ivan, L.P. 1982. "Longitudinal (Bischoff's) myelotomy." In *Operative neurosurgical techniques: Indications, methods and results,* ed. H.H. Schmidek and W.H. Sweet. New York, N.Y.: Grune & Stratton.

Joynt, R.L. 1976. Dantrolene sodium: Long-term effects in patients with muscle spasticity. *Arch. Phys. Med. Rehabil.* 57:212–217.

Kaplan, N. 1962. Effect of splinting on reflex inhibition and sensorimotor stimulation in treatment of spasticity. *Arch. Phys. Med. Rehabil.* 43:565–569.

Kasdon, D.L. 1986. Controversies in the surgical management of spasticity. *Clin. Neurosurg.* 33:523–529.

Kasdon, D.L., and E. Lathi. 1984. A prospective study of radiofrequency rhizotomy in the treatment of post-traumatic spasticity. *Neurosurgery* 15:526–529.

Katz, R. 1988. Management of spasticity. *Am. J. Phys. Med. Rehabil.* 67:108–116.

Katz, R., and W.Z. Rymer. 1989. Spastic hypertonia: Mechanisms and measurement. *Arch. Phys. Med. Rehabil.* 70:144–155.

Katz, R., and W.Z. Rymer. (In Press). Pathophysiology and quantification of spastic hypertonia. *J. Head Trauma Rehabil.*

Keenan, M.A.E. 1987. The orthopedic management of spasticity. *J. Head Trauma Rehabil.* 2:62–71.

Keenan, M.A.E., et al. 1987. Results of fractional lengthening of the finger flexors in adults with upper extremity spasticity. *J. Hand Surg.* 12A:575–581.

Kennemore, D. 1983. Radiofrequency neurotomy for peripheral pain and spasticity syndromes. *Contemp. Neurosurg.* 5:1–6.

Ketel, W.B., and M.E. Kolb. 1984. Long-term treatment with dantrolene sodium of stroke patients with spasticity limiting the return of function. *Curr. Med. Res. Opin.* 9:161–169.

Khalili, A.A. 1984. "Physiatric management of spasticity by phenol nerve and motor point block." In *Current therapy in physiatry,* ed. A.P. Ruskin. Philadelphia, Pa.: Saunders.

Khalili, A.A., and H.B.B. Betts. 1967. Peripheral nerve block with phenol in the management of spasticity. *J.A.M.A.* 200:1155–1157.

Khalili, A.A., et al. 1964. Management of spasticity by selective peripheral nerve block with dilute phenol solutions in clinical rehabilitation. *Arch. Phys. Med. Rehabil.* 45:513–519.

Khanna, O.P. 1979. "Nonsurgical therapeutic modalities." In *Clinical neurology,* ed. R.J. Krane and M.B. Siroky. Boston, Mass.: Little, Brown.

King, T. 1982. Plaster splinting to reduce elbow flexor spasticity. *Am. J. Occup. Ther.* 36:671–673.

Kirkland, L.R. 1984. Baclofen dosage: A suggestion. *Arch. Phys. Med. Rehabil.* 65:214 (letter).

Knutsson, E. 1970. On effects of local cooling upon motor functions in spastic paresis. *Prog. Phys. Ther.* 1:124–131.

Knutsson, E., et al. 1972. Lioresal and spasticity. *Acta Neurol. Scand.* 48(suppl. 51):449–450.

Knutsson, E., et al. 1974. Plasma and cerebrospinal fluid levels of baclofen (Lioresal) at optimal therapeutic responses in spastic paresis. *J. Neurol. Sci.* 23:473–484.

Knutsson, E., et al. 1982. Antipyretic and anti-spastic effects induced by tizanidine in patients with spastic paresis. *J. Neurol Sci.* 53:187–204.

Koella, W.P. 1980. "Baclofen: Its general pharmacology and neuropharmacology." In *Spasticity: Disordered motor control,* ed. R.G. Feldman et al. Chicago, Ill.: Year Book Medical.

Laitinen, L., and E. Singounas. 1971. Longitudinal myelotomy in the treatment of spasticity of the legs. *J. Neurosurg.* 35:536–540.

Lapierre, Y., et al. 1987. Treatment of spasticity with tizanidine in multiple sclerosis. *Can. J. Neurol. Sci.* 14:513–517.

Levine, M.G., et al. 1952. Relaxation of spasticity by electrical stimulation of antagonistic muscles. *Arch. Phys. Med. Rehabil.* 11:668–673.

Levine, M.G., et al. 1954. Relaxation of spasticity by physiological technics. *Arch. Phys. Med. Rehabil.* 35:214–223.

Lightfoot, E., et al. 1975. Neurophysiological effects of prolonged cooling of the calf in patients with complete spinal transection. *Phys. Ther.* 55:251–258.

Lossius, R., et al. 1985. Effect of clorazepate in spasticity and rigidity: A quantitative study of reflexes and plasma concentrations. *Acta Neurol. Scand.* 71:190–194.

Mai, J. 1981. Adrenergic influences on spasticity. *Acta Neurol. Scand.* 63(suppl.):1–143.

Malec, J., et al. 1982. Cannabis effect on spasticity in spinal cord injury. *Arch. Phys. Med. Rehabil.* 63:116–118.

Maynard, F.M. 1986. Early clinical experience with clonidine in spinal spasticity. *Paraplegia* 24:175–182.

McComas, A.J., et al. 1984. Multiple innervation of human muscle fibers. *J. Neurol. Sci.* 64:55–64.

McLellan, D.L. 1977. Co-contraction and stretch reflexes in spasticity during treatment with baclofen. *J. Neurol. Neurosurg. Psychiatry* 40:30–38.

McPherson, J.J., et al. 1985. Dynamic splint to reduce the passive component of hypertonicity. *Arch. Phys. Med. Rehabil.* 66:249–252.

Mecomber, S.A., and R.M. Herman. 1971. Effects of local hypothermia on reflex with voluntary activity. *Phys. Ther.* 51:271–282.

Medical News. 1983. *J.A.M.A.* 249:1807.

Medici, M., et al. 1989. A double-blind, long-term study of tizanidine in spasticity due to cerebrovascular lesions. *Curr. Med. Res. Opin.* 11:398–407.

Meelhuysen, F.E., et al. 1968. Treatment of flexor spasticity of hip by paravertebral lumbar spinal nerve block. *Arch. Phys. Med. Rehabil.* 49:717–722.

Merritt, J. 1981. Management of spasticity in spinal cord injury. *Mayo Clin. Proc.* 56:614–622.

Meyler, W.J., et al. 1981. The effect of dantrolene sodium in relation to blood levels in spastic patients after prolonged administration. *J. Neurol. Neurosurg. Psychiatry* 44:334–339.

Miglietta, O. 1962. Evaluation of cold in spasticity. *Am. J. Phys. Med.* 41:148–151.

Miglietta, O. 1964. Electromyographic characteristics of clonus and influence of cold. *Arch. Phys. Med. Rehabil.* 45:508–512.

Miglietta, O. 1973. Action of cold on spasticity. *Am. J. Phys. Med.* 52:198–205.

Mills, W.J., and R.S. Pozos. 1985. Decrease in clonus amplitude by topical anesthesia. *Electroencephalogr. Clin. Neurophysiol.* 61:509–518.

Mondrup, K., and E. Pedersen. 1983. "The acute effect of THIP in human spasticity—A pilot study." In *Actual problems in multiple sclerosis research,* ed. E. Pedersen et al. Copenhagen, Denmark: FADL's Forlag.

Mondrup, K., and E. Pedersen. 1984a. The effect of the GABA-agonist, progabide, on stretch and flexor reflexes and on voluntary power in spastic patients. *Acta Neurol. Scand.* 69:191–199.

Mondrup, K., and E. Pedersen. 1984b. The clinical effect of the GABA-agonist, progabide, on spasticity. *Acta Neurol. Scand.* 69:200–206.

Muller, H., et al. 1987. The effect of intrathecal baclofen on electrical muscle activity in spasticity. *J. Neurosurg.* 234:348–352.

Nance, P.W., et al. 1985. Clonidine in spinal cord injury. *Can. Med. Assoc. J.* 133:41–42.

Ochs, G., et al. 1989. Intrathecal baclofen for long-term treatment of spasticity: A multi-centre study. *J. Neurol. Neurosurg. Psychiatry* 52:933–939.

Otis, J.C., et al. 1985. Measurement of plantar flexor spasticity during treatment with tone-reducing casts. *J. Pediatr. Orthop.* 5:682–686.

Parke, B., et al. 1989. Functional outcome after delivery of intrathecal baclofen. *Arch. Phys. Med. Rehabil.* 70:30–32.

Peacock, W.J., and L.J. Arens. 1982. Selective posterior rhizotomy for the relief of spasticity in cerebral palsy. *Sa Med. Tydskr. Deel* 62:119–124.

Penn, R.D., and J.S. Kroin. 1985. Continuous intrathecal baclofen for severe spasticity. *Lancet* 2:125–127.

Penn, R.D., and J.S. Kroin. 1987. Long-term intrathecal baclofen infusion for treatment of spasticity. *J. Neurosurg.* 66:181–185.

Penn, R.D., et al. 1989. Intrathecal baclofen for severe spinal spasticity. *N. Engl. J. Med.* 320:1517–1521.

Petajan, J.H. 1987. Sural nerve stimulation and motor control of tibialis anterior muscle in spastic paresis. *Neurology* 37:47–52.

Petrillo, C.R., et al. 1980. Phenol block of the tibial nerve in the hemiplegic patient. *Orthopedics* 3:871–874.

Phillips, C.A., et al. 1984. Functional electrode exercise: A comprehensive approach for physical conditioning of the spinal cord injured patient. *Orthopedics* 7:1112–1123.

Pinder, R.M., et al. 1977. Dantrolene sodium: A review of its pharmacological properties and therapeutic efficacy in spasticity. *Drugs* 13:3–23.

Pinzur, M.S. 1985. Surgery to achieve dynamic motor balance in adult acquired spastic hemiplegia. *J. Hand Surg.* 10A:547–553.

Pinzur, M.S., et al. 1987. Triceps spasticity in traumatic hemiplegia: Diagnosis and treatment. *Arch. Phys. Med. Rehabil.* 68:446–449.

Pinzur, M.S., et al. 1988. Brachioradialis to finger extensor tendon transfer to achieve hand opening in acquired spasticity. *J. Hand Surg.* 13A:549–552.

Privat, J.M., et al. 1976. Sectorial posterior rhizotomy, a new technique of surgical treatment for spasticity. *Acta Neurochir.* 35:181–195.

Richardson, R.R., et al. 1979. Percutaneous epidural neurostimulation in modulation of paraplegic spasticity. *Acta Neurochir.* 49:235–243.

Robinson, C.J., et al. 1988. Spasticity in spinal cord injured patients: 1. Short-term effects of surface electrical stimulation. *Arch. Phys. Med. Rehabil.* 69:598–604.

Romijn, J.A., et al. 1986. Reversible metabolic coma due to intrathecal baclofen. *Lancet* 2:696.

Roussan, M., et al. 1985. Baclofen versus diazepam for the treatment of spasticity and long-term follow-up of baclofen therapy. *Pharmatherapeutica* 4:278–284.

Roy, C.W., and I.R. Wakefield. 1986. Baclofen pseudopsychosis: Case report. *Paraplegia* 24:318–321.

Rudick, R.A., et al. 1987. The GABA-agonist progabide for spasticity in multiple sclerosis. *Arch. Neurol.* 44:1033–1036.

Sabbahi, M.A., et al. 1981. Topical anesthesia: A possible treatment for spasticity. *Arch. Phys. Med. Rehabil.* 62:310–314.

Sachais, B.A., et al. 1977. Baclofen, a new antispastic drug. *Arch. Neurol.* 34:422–428.

Sandy, K.R., and M.H. Gillman. 1985. Baclofen-induced memory impairment. *Clin. Neuropharm.* 8:294–295.

Sawynok, J., and C. Dickson. 1985. D-Baclofen is an antagonist at baclofen receptors mediating anti-nociception in the spinal cord. *Pharmacology* 31:248–259.

Siegfried, J. 1980. Treatment of spasticity by dorsal cord stimulation. *Int. Rehabil. Med.* 9:31–34.

Sindou, M., and D. Jeanmonod. 1989. Microsurgical DREZ-otomy for the treatment of spasticity and pain in the lower limbs. *Neurosurgery* 24:655–670.

Sindou, M., et al. 1985a. "Surgical selective lesions of nerve fibers and myelotomies for modifying muscle hypertonia." In *Recent achievements in restorative neurology: Upper motor neuron function and dysfunction,* ed. J. Eccles and M.R. Dimitrijevic. Basel, Switzerland: Karger.

Sindou, M., et al. 1985b. Microsurgical selective procedures in peripheral nerves and the posterior root-spinal cord junction for spasticity. *Appl. Neurophysiol.* 48:97–104.

Sindou, M., et al. 1986. Selective posterior rhizotomy in the dorsal root entry zone for treatment of hyperspasticity and pain in the hemiplegic upper limb. *Neurosurgery* 18:587–595.

Smith, C.W., and L. Leventhal. 1987. Surgical treatment of lower extremity deformities in adult head-injured patients. *J. Head Trauma Rehabil.* 2:53–57.

Smolenski, C., et al. 1981. A double-blind comparative trial of a new muscle relaxant, tizanidine (DS 103-282) and baclofen in the treatment of chronic spasticity in multiple sclerosis. *Curr. Med. Res. Opin.* 7:374–383.

Snook, J. 1979. Spasticity reduction splint. *Am. J. Occup. Ther.* 33:648–651.

Stien, R., et al. 1987. Treatment of spasticity in multiple sclerosis: A double-blind clinical trial of a new anti-spastic drug tizanidine compared with baclofen. *Acta Neurol. Scand.* 75:190–194.

Study, R.E., and J.L. Barker. 1982. Cellular mechanisms of benzodiazepine action. *J.A.M.A.* 247:2147–2151.

Tallis, R.C., et al. 1983. The quantitative assessment of the influence of spinal cord stimulation on motor function in patients with multiple sclerosis. *Int. Rehabil. Med.* 5:10–16.

Te Groen, J.A., and G.F. Dommisse. 1964. Plaster casts in the conservative treatment of cerebral palsy. *S. Afr. Med. J.* 18:502–505.

Terrence, D.V., and G.H. Fromm. 1981. Complications of baclofen withdrawal. *Arch. Neurol.* 38:588–589.

Treanor, W.J. 1981. Improvement of function in hemiplegia after orthopaedic surgery. *Scand. J. Rehabil. Med.* 13:123–135.

Van Hemert, J.C.J. 1980. "A double-blind comparison of baclofen and placebo in patients with spasticity of cerebral origin." In *Spasticity: Disordered motor control,* ed. R.G. Feldman et al. Chicago, Ill.: Year Book Medical.

Van Winkle, W.B. 1976. Calcium release from skeletal muscle sarcoplasmic reticulum: Site of action of dantrolene sodium? *Science* 193:1130–1131.

Verrier, M., et al. 1977. Diazepam effect on reflex activity in patients with complete spinal lesions and in those with other causes of spasticity. *Arch. Phys. Med. Rehabil.* 58:148–153.

Vodovnik, L., et al. 1982. Functional improvement of pathological neuromuscular systems by means of electrical stimulation. In *Proceedings of the Rehabilitation Engineering International Seminar,* Tokyo.

Vodovnik, L., et al. 1984a. Effect of electrical stimulation on spasticity in hemiparetic patients. *Int. Rehabil. Med.* 6:153–156.

Vodovnik, L., et al. 1984b. Effects of electrical stimulation on spinal spasticity. *Scand. J. Rehabil. Med.* 16:29–34.

Wainapel, S.F., et al. 1984. Spastic hemiplegia in a quadriplegic patient: Treatment with phenol nerve block. *Arch. Phys. Med. Rehabil.* 65:786–787.

Walker, B.J. 1982. Modulation of spasticity: Prolonged suppression of a spinal reflex by electrical stimulation. *Science* 216:203–204.

Waters, R.L. 1978. Upper extremity surgery in stroke patients. *Clin. Orthop. Relat. Res.* 131:30–37.

Waters, R.L. 1984. The enigma of "carry over." *Int. Rehabil. Med.* 6:9–12.

Waters, R.L., et al. 1978. Surgical correction of gait abnormalities following stroke. *Clin. Orthop. Relat. Res.* 131:54–63.

Waters, R.L., et al. 1982. Electromyographic gait analysis before and after operative treatment for hemiplegic equinus and equinovarus deformity. *J. Bone Joint Surg. Am.* 64:284–288.

Waters, R.L., et al. 1985. Functional electrical stimulation of the peroneal nerve for hemiplegia. *J. Bone Joint Surg. Am.* 67:792–793.

Wolf, S.L., and S.A. Binder-MacLeod. 1983a. Electromyographic biofeedback applications to the hemiplegic patient: Changes in upper extremity neuromuscular and functional status. *Phys. Ther.* 63:1393–1403.

Wolf, S.L., and S.A. Binder-MacLeod. 1983b. Electromyographic biofeedback applications to the hemiplegic patient: Changes in lower extremity neuromuscular and functional status. *Phys. Ther.* 63:1404–1413.

Wood, K.M. 1978. The use of phenol as a neurolytic agent. *Pain* 5:205–229.

Young, R.R., and P.J. Delwaide. 1981. Drug therapy: Spasticity. *N. Engl. J. Med.* 304:28–33, 96–99.

Young, R.R., and B.T. Shahani. 1986. "Spasticity in spinal cord injured patients." In *Management of spinal cord injuries,* ed. R.F. Bloch and M. Basbaum. Baltimore, Md.: Williams & Wilkins.

Chapter 11

Posttraumatic Syringomyelia

Richard B. Lazar

Since its original description in the 16th century by Etienne (1546), no discrete clinicopathologic entity has been associated with a more diverse group of neuroanatomic disorders than syringomyelia. Whether syringomyelia is a primary or secondary disease of the CNS has not been determined. The literature is replete with examples of both. Syringomyelia has been associated with developmental anomalies at the foramen magnum and in the posterior fossa, acquired abnormalities at the base of the brain, posterior fossa tumors and cysts, spinal arachnoiditis, and spinal cord tumors. Finally, there are instances where none of the known etiopathogenic factors is identified; these cases are categorized as idiopathic syringomyelia (Barnett 1973). The most unifying and operational concept of syringomyelia is a pathologic one, referring to that clinical syndrome that results from cystic cavitation and gliosis of the spinal cord.

One rare but nevertheless important form of syringomyelia occurs in association with spinal cord injury (Barnett & Jousse 1973). Its pathogenesis, clinical and pathologic features, diagnosis, and treatment are the focus of this chapter.

INCIDENCE

One of the largest and most thoroughly described groups of patients with posttraumatic syringomyelia was described by Barnett and Jousse (1973). Progressive cystic cavitation of the spinal cord occurred in 1.8% of 864 paraplegic patients and in 0.2% of 523 quadriplegic patients. Other clinical series reported to date generally corroborate an incidence of between 1% and 2% in paraplegics and less than 1% in quadriplegics (Scher 1976; Vernon et al. 1982).

The age of patients at the time of injury who develop syringomyelia has been reported to range from 8.0 to 59.5 years. The interval from the date of injury to the development of the syrinx has varied in the literature from less than 2 months to more than 30 years as newer, improved diagnostic modalities have evolved (Barnett & Jousse 1973; Barnett et al. 1966). There appears to be no clear relationship between the development of the syrinx and the mechanisms of injury, type of early treatment, or completeness or incompleteness of the lesion; most major series of patients with posttraumatic syringomyelia, however, report a relative preponderance in association with thoracolumbar over cervical injuries (Barnett & Jousse 1973; Vernon et al. 1982).

PATHOLOGY

Syringomyelia is one neuropathologic entity where an understanding of the gross and cellular morphologic changes as well as the clinically relevant neuroanatomy leads directly to a clear understanding of the clinical manifestations. Upon gross inspection, the spinal cord is enlarged along at least several segments in its transverse axis and has a hollow, tubular appearance. The swelling or dilatation of the cord may be symmetric or asymmetric with enlargement of the coronal, axial, or horizontal plane. The leptomeninges appear normal.

The cavity itself may extend from the uppermost cervical segments of the spinal cord and even the medulla (syringobulbia) to the filum terminale. Fusiform widening of the cord may be noted, and on close inspection the cord may appear to be fluctuant at the site of cavitation.

On cross-section of the cord, the cavity may be either symmetric or asymmetric and usually contains clear or xanthochromic fluid originating dorsal to the central spinal canal. The size of the cavities is highly variable. The shape of the cavity may be cylindric or multiloculated with glial septae. Communication of the cavity with the central spinal canal can be demonstrated in some instances with clear preservation of the integrity of the ependymal cell lining. In other instances multiple cavities may be demonstrated, some with and some without clear communication with the central canal.

How the late sequelae of spinal cord cavitation relate to the early acute formation of a microhemorrhagic response to injury in the central gray matter is a matter of conjecture (Waggener & Beggs 1979). Furthermore, in the subacute gross pathologic response to spinal injury, myelomalacic cores of material have been noted that may be a pathologic precursor to syrinx formation (Barnett et al. 1966; Holmes 1915).

Microscopic examination of the spinal cord is marked by cystic cavitation and sparsely cellular gliosis of the cord. Thickly matted glial fibers can be noted in a circumferential array. There is a distortion of the normal architecture of the spinal cord with secondary myelin and neuronal changes. The cavity may occupy almost the entire cross-sectional area of the cord, compressing the posterior columns and the dorsolateral funiculi. The spinothalamic tracts are involved early, usually at the decussation ventral to the central spinal canal, as is the central gray matter.

CLINICAL MANIFESTATIONS

The clinical features of syringomyelia are protean, chiefly dependent on the longitudinal extent and cross-sectional nature of the lesion. Signs and symptoms may be unilateral or bilateral, symmetric or asymmetric. Under most circumstances, the nature of the presentation can be directly predicted and derived from a knowledge of the clinically relevant anatomy.

Pain may be the presenting symptom and is described as tingling or burning in nature. It may be exacerbated by straining, coughing, or sneezing. The insidious onset of lower motor neuron dysfunction, including weakness, atrophy, and a loss of the muscle stretch reflexes appropriate to the lesion, are customary. Scoliosis is common, because of early involvement of the dorsomedian and ventromedian nuclei with denervation of the paraspinous muscles. In most instances, a dissociated sensory loss (loss of pain with preservation of tactile sensation) can be demonstrated as a result of early encroachment of the cystic cavity upon the decussating spinothalamic tracts. Sparing of position, vibration, and light touch sensation is the rule because of the relatively late involvement of the posterior columns. The presence of Horner's syndrome usually indicates extension of the lesion to the interomediolateral cell column with involvement of the sympathetic nervous system. Trophic disturbances and neurogenic arthropathy may supervene (Rhoades et al. 1983). Progressive involvement of the corticospinal tracts occurs in the more advanced stage of the disease but may be difficult to find in cases of posttraumatic syrinx. In some cases of incomplete spinal cord injury, progression of lower limb weakness occurs. Abnormal patterns of sweating and orthostatic hypotension may occur.

Few patients have been described with brain stem involvement (syringobulbia) from posttraumatic syrinx (Klawans 1968). Dysphagia, facial numbness, and tongue weakness and atrophy may occur (Barnett et al. 1966). The development and progression of any or all of these clinical signs or symptoms superimposed upon a fixed traumatic neurologic deficit at any time after spinal cord injury should suggest the possibility of syringomyelia, syringobulbia, or both.

PATHOGENESIS

The etiopathogenesis of posttraumatic syringomyelia has been a matter of great interest and uncertainty. No theory or hypothesis to date can be invoked to explain even a majority of the diverse forms of congenital and acquired syringomyelia or that associated with traumatic myelopathy.

Under some circumstances, it appears that the syrinx develops as a secondary softening and resorption of previously injured neural tissue. A secondary cavitation may result from hematomyelia that occurs at the time of injury. In others, alteration of the normal spinal fluid hemodynamics by spinal cord injury occurs and may become symptomatic after normal closure of the central spinal canal during the second and third decades of life. This obviously would not explain the onset of posttraumatic syrinx in a significant group of older individuals.

A vascular etiology has been suggested by some to account for the cavitation within the spinal cord (Feigin et al. 1971; Klawans 1968). An experimental animal model devised to test this hypothesis has been developed (Tauber & Langworthy 1935).

Gardner's (1965) theory of the etiopathogenesis of syringomyelia has achieved great notoriety but probably has little relevance to posttraumatic syrinx. He postulated that syringomyelia is secondary to occlusion of the foramina of the fourth ventricle, leading to transmission of spinal fluid pressure downward into the central spinal canal and producing hydrocephalus. Although this mechanism cannot explain all types of syringomyelia, it may be operative in some cases of posttraumatic syrinx where traumatic occlusion of the fourth ventricular outlet occurs. In some clinical reports, the patency of these outlets has been demonstrated to be preserved (Cahan & Bentson 1982). Nevertheless, hemodynamically significant pressures may be transmitted without fourth ventricular outlet obstruction. Furthermore, experimental models of chronic communicating hydrocephalus in dogs and primates failed to produce significant morphologic or histologic changes in the cervical spinal canal (James et al. 1978).

Williams (1969) proposed that, rather than hydrodynamic pressure directed into the central spinal canal from fourth ventricular outlet obstruction, intermittent fluctuations in venous pressure may occur from below a partial obstruction at the foramen magnum, leading to dilation of the central spinal canal. He emphasized the dissociation of craniospinal pressures in the development of the syrinx, with hydrodynamic pressure being delivered from below the foramen magnum rather than above.

Syringomyelia is much less common in paraplegics of nontraumatic origin, a fact that supports the importance of trauma to the cord in its etiopathogenesis. In some instances, the central spinal cord may undergo traumatic expansion with a funicular presentation of the syrinx related to injury. Hyperextension of the neck may result in inspissation of the cerebellar tonsils sufficient to cause enlargement of the syrinx. Greenfield (1984) has suggested that extension of the syrinx occurs as a consequence of secondary cord trauma with tension and torsion directed to the cervical cord and medulla from compensatory dependence on vigorous upper extremity, head, neck, and trunk activity.

DIAGNOSIS

In spite of recent major advances in neuroradiologic investigation, posttraumatic syringomyelia remains a clinical diagnosis. When a previously stable patient develops the insidious onset of weakness above or below a fixed neurologic deficit in association with a dissociated sensory loss, syringomyelia must be suspected until proven otherwise. Trophic disturbances, Charcot's joints, atrophy and fasciculations, scoliosis, and Horner's syndrome are useful in establishing a clinical diagnosis.

Routine spine radiographs are usually normal at onset but later reveal progressive kyphoscoliosis. Conventional electromyographic examination may indicate positive sharp waves and fibrillation potentials in the affected myotomes with a decreased number of motor units. F-wave latency may be prolonged. Single fiber electromyography may suggest increased fiber density, reflecting the pattern of muscle involvement (Schwartz et al. 1980). The usefulness of somatosensory evoked potentials in detecting syringomyelia is at this point open to question.

Myelography with either lipid- or water-soluble contrast material may demonstrate fusiform enlargement of the spinal cord or complete subarachnoid block at the site of the syrinx. The sagittal diameter of the spinal canal may also be increased (Conway 1961; Heinz et al. 1966). In general, spinal cord dimensions are unreliable because of the high degree of variability in techniques. Under most circumstances, the ratio of the coronal dimension of the spinal cord on frontal view to the total width of the subarachnoid space should not exceed 80%. Occasionally in the first year from the onset of symptoms, myelography may be normal or equivocal (Barnett et al. 1966). In rare instances, myelography defines a cause for the patient's symptoms other than syringomyelia. Cerebrospinal fluid analysis is nearly always normal. In the case of partial or complete subarachnoid block, the protein may be elevated or even xanthochromic.

High-resolution computed tomography (CT) of the spine with the intrathecal injection of water-soluble contrast material has added a new dimension in the diagnosis of syringomyelia. Water-soluble contrast myelography followed by a CT scan after a delay of 2 to 6 hours may show concentration of the contrast medium in the cavity. Cross-sectional views of the spinal cord in relation to the subarachnoid space are now readily available. Occasionally, magnification views of the spinal cord by CT under contrast enhancement will reveal one or more cysts. Even modern techniques of CT scanning have limitations in certain areas of the neuraxis, particularly near bone, such as in the temporal lobe, posterior fossa, and spinal cord.

In these areas, magnetic resonance imaging (MRI) has been particularly useful. Recently MRI has become the procedure of choice for diagnosing syringomyelia for several reasons. First, it is noninvasive. Second, standard pulse sequences with both T1- and T2-weighted images can, in most instances, discriminate between a syrinx and myelomalacia. In syringomyelia, the cord typically appears enlarged with a clear, low-signal cavity with characteristics similar to those of cerebrospinal fluid; if normal tissue contiguous with the syrinx is included in the slide thickness, however, it can alter the low signal of the syrinx, making radiologic definition of the cavity difficult.

CLINICAL COURSE

Untreated, posttraumatic syringomyelia has a variable course, sometimes characterized by improvement, plateau, or relentless progression. There is no way of predicting, based on the nature and extent of the lesion, what clinical pattern the syrinx will follow (McIlroy & Richardson 1965). Complications of thermoanesthesia may supervene early, leading to burns, decubitus ulceration, and contractures. Neurogenic arthropathies develop in a significant number of patients, chiefly involving the elbow and shoulder joints. Complete joint destruction or ankylosis, neurogenic bladder and bowel, and respiratory failure may occur.

TREATMENT

The benchmark of sound rehabilitative treatment is prevention of the sequelae of progressive immobilization by judicious skin care and rigorous range of motion exercise. The effects of surgical treatment, in view of the variable clinical course of syringomyelia, are extremely difficult to determine. Nevertheless, myelotomy and syringostomy have been time-honored surgical treatments of choice (Abbe & Coley 1892; McIlroy & Richardson 1965). When subarachnoid block is present, surgical decompression of the syrinx by placement of a stent tube from the cavity to the subarachnoid space appears to lead to improvement rapidly in many patients. In others, surgical intervention is palliative at best.

Recently, microlaser myelotomy combined with syringostomy has been employed to reduce morbidity by more acute separation of tissue planes. Nevertheless, complication rates are between 5% and 10%, usually related to shunt malfunction. Current indications for surgery appear to be rapid progression of a neurologic deficit with a clinically appropriate cystic lesion 1 cm in diameter or greater, intractable pain, and cerebrospinal fluid block. Although the effect of surgery in arresting neurologic deterioration has been strongly advocated, others experienced in the care of spinal cord injury advocate a conservative approach with vigorous attention to prevention of complications and physical restoration (Adelstein 1938; Griffiths & McCormick 1981).

REFERENCES

Abbe, R., and W.B. Coley. 1892. Syringomyelia: Operation, exploration of cord, withdrawal of fluid, exhibition of patient. *J. Nerv. Ment. Dis.* 19:512.

Adelstein, L.J. 1938. The surgical treatment of syringomyelia. *Am. J. Surg.* 40:384.

Barnett, H.J.M. 1973. "Epilogue." In *Syringomyelia*, ed. H.J.M. Barnett et al. Philadelphia, Pa.: Saunders.

Barnett, H.J.M., and A.T. Jousse. 1973. "Syringomyelia as a late sequel to traumatic paraplegia and quadriplegia." In *Syringomyelia*, ed. H.J.M. Barnett et al. Philadelphia, Pa.: Saunders.

Barnett, H.J.M., et al. 1966. Progressive myelopathy as a sequel to traumatic paraplegia. *Brain* 89:159–178.

Cahan, L.D., and J.R. Bentson. 1982. Considerations in the diagnosis and treatment of syringomyelia and the Chiari malformation. *J. Neurosurg.* 57:24–31.

Conway, L.W. 1961. Radiographic studies of syringomyelia. *Trans. Am. Neurol. Assoc.* 86:205.

Etienne, C. 1546. *Dissection du corps humain.* Paris, France: Simon de Colines.

Feigin, I., et al. 1971. Syringomyelia: The role of edema in its pathogenesis. *J. Neuropathol. Exp. Neurol.* 30:216–232.

Gardner, W.J. 1965. Hydrodynamic mechanism of syringomyelia: Its relationship to myelocele. *J. Neurol. Neurosurg. Psychiatry* 28:247–259.

Greenfield, J.G. 1984. *Neuropathology.* New York, N.Y.: Wiley.

Griffiths, E.R., and C.C. McCormick. 1981. Post-traumatic syringomyelia (cystic myelopathy). *Paraplegia* 19:81–88.

Heinz, E.R., et al. 1966. Radiologic signs of hydromyelia. *Radiology* 86:311–318.

Holmes, G. 1915. Spinal injuries of warfare. *Br. Med. J.* 2:769–774.

James, A.E., Jr., et al. 1978. Evaluation of the central canal of the spinal cord in experimentally produced hydrocephalus. *J. Neurosurg.* 48:970–974.

Klawans, H.L. 1968. Delayed traumatic syringomyelia. *Dis. Nerv. Syst.* 29:525.

McIlroy, W.J., and J.C. Richardson. 1965. Syringomyelia: A clinical review of 75 cases. *Can. Med. Assoc. J.* 93:731–734.

Rhoades, C.E., et al. 1983. Diagnosis of post-traumatic syringomyelia presenting as neuropathic joints: Report of two cases and a review of the literature. *Clin. Orthop.* 180:182–187.

Scher, A.T. 1976. Syringomyelia secondary to paraplegia due to fractures of the thoracic spine. *S. Afr. Med. J.* 50:1406–1408.

Schwartz, M.S., et al. 1980. Pattern of segmental motor involvement in syringomyelia: A single fiber EMG study. *J. Neurol. Neurosurg. Psychiatry* 43:150–155.

Tauber, E.J., and O.R. Langworthy. 1935. A study of syringomyelia and the formation of cavities within the spinal cord. *J. Nerv. Ment. Dis.* 81:245.

Vernon, J.D., et al. 1982. Post-traumatic syringomyelia. *Paraplegia* 20:339–364.

Waggener, J.D., and J.L. Beggs. 1979. The acute microvascular response to spinal cord injury. *Adv. Neurol.* 22:179–189.

Williams, B. 1969. Hypothesis: The distending force in the production of communicating syringomyelia. *Lancet* 2:189–193.

Chapter 12

Cognitive Dysfunction in Spinal Cord Injury

Jeri Morris and Elliot J. Roth

Cognitive dysfunction is a frequent and serious comorbid condition in patients with spinal cord injury (SCI) and has important implications for assessment and rehabilitation management. Depending on the definition and method of study of cognitive dysfunction, between 10% and 60% (Davidoff et al. 1985b; Richards et al. 1988; Roth et al. 1989; Wilmot et al. 1985) of patients with acute SCI may have various types of cognitive impairments. These include difficulty with attention, concentration, memory, problem solving, and abstract reasoning. Assessment of cognitive abilities is important because rehabilitation after SCI involves an intensive program of learning new knowledge and skills and of adapting to a new life style. Careful and comprehensive evaluation of neuropsychologic function provides the opportunity for more focused treatment.

A variety of factors may contribute to the frequency with which neuropsychological deficits occur in patients with SCI: concomitant acute closed head injury (CHI) at the time of SCI, premorbid history of CHI before SCI, cerebral effects of chronic alcohol and substance abuse, medication effects, depression and anxiety, motivational problems, preinjury learning disability, poor educational background, and others.

Although clearly not the only factor contributing to the concomitance of cognitive dysfunction and SCI, associated CHI is the most extensively investigated comorbidity. Indeed, when the group at the Rehabilitation Institute of Chicago (RIC) first explored this important issue on both a clinical and a research level, attention was directed specifically toward the coexistence of head injury and SCI and its implications. Experience over time, however, demonstrated that concomitant CHI could not explain all the cognitive deficits detected in this group; other potentially contributing factors appeared to be important. The other factors were considered at that time and continue to be evaluated at present. The current focus is cognitive dysfunction from any cause and how it is reflected in daily behavior, mental status examination, and formal neuropsychological tests. This is the important issue for inquiry in both patient care and research.

The present chapter follows a similar course of consideration of the literature. First, the incidence and pattern of CHI associated with SCI are reviewed, followed by a discussion of the frequency and nature of cognitive dysfunction in these patients regardless of the cause. Finally, implications for rehabilitation management are considered.

CHI IN SCI

Craniocerebral injury and cognitive deficits resulting from it are frequent concomitants of traumatic SCI (Davidoff et al. 1985a, 1985b, 1988a, 1988b; Dubo & Delaney 1984; Guttmann 1963, 1973; Harris 1965, 1968; Maynard et al. 1979; Meinecke 1968; Richards et al. 1988; Rimel 1981; Roth et al. 1989; Schneider & McGillicuddy 1976; Schueneman & Morris 1982; Silver et al. 1980; Wagner et al. 1983; Wilmot et al. 1985; Young et al. 1982). In some types of trauma, an impact that is sufficiently severe and extensive in nature to injure the spine and spinal cord may also cause other associated injuries, including those to the head. Indeed, a number of investigators (Davidoff et al. 1985a, 1985b, 1988a, 1988b; Dubo & Delaney 1984; Guttmann 1963, 1973; Harris 1965, 1968; Maynard et al. 1979; Meinecke 1968; Richards et al. 1988; Rimel 1981; Roth et al. 1989; Schneider & McGillicuddy 1976; Schueneman & Morris 1982; Silver et al. 1980; Wagner et al. 1983; Wilmot et al. 1985; Young et al. 1982) have demonstrated that many patients with SCI sustain a concomitant craniocerebral injury at the time of trauma.

The nature and severity of craniocerebral injury may vary among patients. Although these associated injuries may include severe traumatic brain injuries, skull fractures, or intracranial hematomas, it is more common to see concussion, contusion, and diffuse brain injury resulting from global shearing forces in the deep white matter among these patients.

Direct brain injury, as evidenced by any period of loss of consciousness (LOC) or posttraumatic amnesia (PTA), may cause significant disturbances in cognitive (Brooks 1972; Denny-Brown 1945; Gronwall & Wrightson 1974; Mandelberg 1975; Mandelberg & Brooks 1975; Rimel et al. 1981; Russell, W.R. 1932, 1971; Russell & Nathan 1946; Russell & Smith 1961; Steadman & Graham 1970) and emotional (Dikmen & Reitan 1977; Fordyce et al. 1983; Levin & Grossman 1978; Lishman 1968, 1973) functioning, regardless of the cause. Deficits in attention, concentration, memory, and judgment (Brooks 1972; Denny-Brown 1945; Gronwall & Wrightson 1974; Mandelberg 1975; Mandelberg & Brooks 1975; Rimel et al. 1981; Russell, W.R. 1932, 1971; Russell & Nathan 1946; Russell & Smith 1961; Steadman & Graham 1970) and in coping skills caused by associated head trauma may place the patient with SCI at risk for unsuccessful rehabilitation programs and unfavorable outcomes. Unfortunately, even today many of these problems often remain unrecognized by health care professionals (Davidoff et al. 1985a).

Early Studies of Associated Injuries in SCI

Sir Ludwig Guttmann (1963, 1973) emphasized the importance of recognition and management of associated injuries in patients with spinal trauma. He observed cerebral concussion to be associated frequently with SCI and noted that brain injuries could occur in patients with spinal injuries at virtually any segmental level. He also noted some deaths from associated head injury in his series of patients with SCI.

In 1968, Meinecke noted that one out of every four patients with traumatic SCI in his series sustained concomitant head injuries, the majority of which were concussion or contusion. Some of these injuries were fractures of the skull. He noted that, although head injuries were most likely to occur in patients whose SCIs were caused by sporting accidents, other causes such as bicycle accidents, motor vehicle accidents, and falls also contributed to these associated injuries.

In 1965 and again in 1968, Harris found an incidence of coexistent head and spinal injury similar to that of Meinecke,

with a range between 27% and 33% depending on the level of injury. He reported that head injuries were more common but not necessarily more serious in patients with cervical SCI. He observed that most (two thirds) of the associated head injuries could be classified as mild, which was defined as unconsciousness for only a few minutes and PTA for less than 12 hours.

An excellent systematic study of associated injuries in 100 consecutive patients with SCI admitted to the Stoke-Mandeville National Spinal Center in England was reported by Silver et al. in 1980. In that study, head injury was the most frequent concomitant injury. Exactly half the patients had an associated head injury, 84% of which were classified as minor, defined as occurring with brief periods of LOC. In this study, patients with cervical injuries sustained fewer and less severe head injuries than patients with thoracic or lumbar injuries. No associations were made between head injuries and etiology of SCI.

SCI Database Reports

Several databases exist in the U.S. spinal injury care centers that record the frequency and nature of associated injuries occurring at the time of the SCI. The results of many of these have been published recently, some of the reports include documentation of the coincidence of head trauma and SCI.

In the California Regional Spinal Cord Injury Care System, a 3-year summary reported that 10% of all patients with traumatic quadriplegia sustained head injuries impairing consciousness for more than 72 hours (Maynard et al. 1979). In that report, no mention was made of milder head injuries or of patients with paraplegia. The investigators did note that performance of a thorough neurologic examination and establishment of an accurate diagnosis were difficult in the SCI patient with coexistent cognitive dysfunction; all patients who apparently had complete SCIs 72 hours after injury and who later recovered motor function to useful or normal levels (Frankel grades D and E) were also later found to have sustained concomitant head injuries that impaired cognition and compromised the reliability of the initial diagnosis.

The neurotrauma database in Virginia reported that 47% of patients with SCI had concomitant craniocerebral injuries (Rimel 1981). In Texas, the coincidence frequency was found to be only 25%, but this included only patients with brain injury (Wagner et al. 1983). Most injuries in the Texas study were considered mild. As with the findings in some of the previous studies, the frequencies of associated traumatic brain injury were similar between patients with quadriplegia and those with paraplegia. Although level of spinal injury appears to have little effect on the likelihood of associated head injury, it is likely that etiology does affect the coincidence of head injury: patients whose SCIs were caused by motor vehicle accidents appear to be the most likely to sustain associated cerebral trauma. One study found the frequency of head injury in patients with SCI caused by motor vehicle accident to be 58% (Dubo & Delaney 1984).

Finally, the original summary of information obtained by the National Database of the National Institute of Disability and Rehabilitation Research–supported Regional Spinal Cord Injury Care Systems reported that 13% of patients with traumatic SCI sustained concomitant brain injury, three fourths of which were classified as mild (Young et al. 1982). In that report, concussion was the third most common associated injury in patients with quadriplegia. Major brain injury was also seen in about 3% to 4% of patients.

RIC Studies of Mild CHI in SCI

Because of the high prevalence, unique nature, special diagnostic considerations, and particular therapeutic implications of problems associated with mild CHI in patients with SCI, a preliminary study was undertaken at the RIC. Schueneman and Morris (1982) determined that more than half of 35 consecutively admitted patients with SCI sustained LOC, PTA, or both at the time of trauma. These investigators were the first to describe potential short-term and long-term sequelae and their implications for patients with SCI; they noted that such a silent CHI may be accompanied by the development of postconcussion syndrome with symptoms of headache, fatigue, vertigo, irritability, attentional deficits, lack of concentration, loss of memory, and impaired judgment. Clearly, these problems may complicate rehabilitation and compromise outcome.

To explore further the incidence and clinical features of CHI in patients with SCI, Davidoff et al. (1985a) retrospectively reviewed 101 complete medical records of patients admitted to the Midwest Regional Spinal Cord Injury Care System with acute traumatic SCI. In this study, 42 patients (42%) had evidence of an acute CHI as evidenced by a period of LOC, PTA, or both at the time of the SCI. There was no association between the presence of CHI and the level of injury, but etiology appeared to have affected CHI incidence. As expected, patients whose SCIs were caused by gunshot wounds rarely sustained concomitant concussions, whereas 40% of patients who sustained their injuries by motor vehicle accidents, falls, sporting accidents, or other causes appeared to have cerebral damage.

An additional finding of that study was the larger than expected frequency of unrecognized and undocumented concomitant CHI. Although LOC was assessed frequently in the emergency department by acute care physicians, this assessment was performed with only moderate consistency (67%) in the rehabilitation center by rehabilitation physicians. PTA was assessed infrequently (14% to 22% of cases) in both settings. This is important because PTA has been found to be a highly reliable and probably the most sensitive indicator of the occur-

rence and severity of CHI (Davidoff et al. 1988a; Russell, W.R. 1971; Russell & Nathan 1946; Russell & Smith 1961; Smith 1971; Steadman & Graham 1970; VonWowern 1966).

The observation that few patients were assessed for PTA together with the wide range of figures quoted for the incidence of associated CHI casts doubt on the reliability of the incidence figures reported in this and other studies on the frequency of CHI in patients with SCI. It is likely that estimates of the incidence of CHI in those studies are lower than the true incidence because assessment of PTA was performed so infrequently. Patients who denied LOC in those studies may have sustained intervals of PTA that were not assessed by the examining physicians, were forgotten by the patients, or were never known about by the patients. The likelihood of this is supported by the finding in the study by Davidoff et al. (1985a) that half the patients who admitted PTA denied LOC.

More Recent, Detailed Studies of Head Injury in SCI

Because of the importance of determining the occurrence of PTA in the establishment of a diagnosis of CHI, and because of the inconsistency with which PTA is documented in patients with SCI, a study was conducted to evaluate the utility of an objective measure of PTA in these patients (Davidoff et al. 1988a). This instrument, the Galveston Orientation and Amnesia Test (GOAT; Levin et al. 1979), was administered serially for 3 to 5 days to 34 patients with acute SCI. Based on medical history alone, the reported incidence of PTA was only 20%. The observed incidence of PTA increased significantly to 44% when the GOAT was used. Using the GOAT appeared to increase the sensitivity of the assessment of PTA in these patients.

Finally, in 1988 a prospective study was conducted to evaluate carefully and systematically 82 consecutively admitted patients with SCI for the incidence and factors associated with the presence of acute concomitant CHI (Davidoff et al. 1988b). The incidence of CHI, as defined by the presence of PTA, was 49%, with a significantly increased risk of CHI occurring in patients whose SCI resulted from motor vehicle accidents. There was no increased risk of head injury associated with any particular level of spinal injury. The investigators suggested that all patients with SCI, regardless of level of injury sustained, should undergo an evaluation for associated CHI.

Overall Findings of CHI in SCI

Although accurate coincidence figures for the occurrence of concomitant head injury and SCI depend on the use of appropriate selection criteria, consistent definitions, and meticulous assessment methodologies, published reports suggest that approximately half of all patients with SCI may have sustained an acute CHI at the time of the SCI, with a range between 13%

and 58%. Studying only brain injury (rather than cranial trauma or any blow to the head) and using sensitive criteria and specific definitions for cerebral injury (as demonstrated by careful and systematic evaluation of LOC and PTA) greatly enhance the sensitivity of the evaluation process. Patients whose SCI results from motor vehicle accidents are at the greatest risk for associated CHI, but they are not the only group at risk. Level of SCI is unrelated to the presence of a concomitant CHI. When an acute CHI is present, initial assessment of the functional level and extent of the SCI may be compromised. In addition, the patients may be at risk for a variety of neuropsychologic deficits, including impairments of concentration, memory, general intelligence, sequencing, organizational skills, spatial relations, problem solving, and abstract reasoning. Studies of associated head injury in patients with SCI are important in that they illustrate the extent to which associated problems may affect the patient's future course and outcome. These findings underscore the necessity of performing comprehensive initial and ongoing assessments of patients with SCI.

COGNITIVE DYSFUNCTION IN SCI

After acute head injury, symptoms of easy fatigability, irritability, impaired concentration, and memory deficits may occur (Brooks 1972; Denny-Brown 1945; Gronwall & Wrightson 1974; Mandelberg 1975; Mandelberg & Brooks 1975; Rimel et al. 1981; Russell, W.R. 1932, 1971; Russell & Nathan 1946; Russell & Smith 1961; Steadman & Graham 1970). Subtle cognitive and emotional deficits may persist for months after onset of head injury, paralleling the time interval during which maximum participation in a rehabilitation program occurs; it is important to note, however, that these problems, and others, may also be the long-term sequelae of older CHIs that predated the SCI. Other possible factors that may compromise cognition include chronic alcohol or substance abuse, psychotropic medication use, and other contributing factors. A few studies have examined the frequency, magnitude, nature, and pattern of specific cognitive deficits regardless of cause in patients with SCI.

Early Prevalence Studies

Davidoff et al. (1985b) conducted a study that was prompted by their earlier findings that craniocerebral injury was common in patients with SCI and that it was frequently unrecognized and underreported (Davidoff et al. 1985a). The Halstead Category Test (HCT; Reitan 1979) of the Halstead-Reitan Neuropsychological Battery was administered to 30 consenting inpatients with SCI admitted to RIC for rehabilitation. The HCT evaluates deficits in attention, concentration, visual problem-solving skills, abstract reasoning (Boll 1981; Lansdell & Donnelly 1977; Lynch 1983; Pendleton & Heaton 1982), and ability to adapt to new situations (Rothke 1986).

The test has been reported to be a sensitive and strong indicator of cognitive dysfunction among patients with brain damage (DeFillipis et al. 1979; DeWolfe et al. 1971; Fitzhugh & Fitzhugh 1961; Kimura 1981; Reitan 1955; Shaw 1966) and has been reported to be nearly as sensitive an indicator of cognitive dysfunction as all the other tests of the entire Halstead-Reitan Neuropsychological Battery. Importantly, results are not influenced by hand function.

In the study, subjects underwent testing between 8 and 12 weeks after SCI to allow time for them to adapt to the new disability and to the rehabilitation environment and to avoid possible confounding effects of general anesthesia in those patients who recently underwent surgical procedures.

Based on clinical histories of impaired consciousness and PTA at the time of injury, 12 (40%) of the 30 patients were found to have sustained mild CHI concurrently with SCI. Six of the remaining 18 had a premorbid history of head injury. Twelve patients had no history of CHI at any time. On neuropsychological testing, 17 (57%) of the 30 patients with SCI scored in the impaired range on the HCT, a level defined as 51 errors or more on the 208 items on the test (Reitan 1979).

Analysis of variance did not reveal any significant differences in HCT scores among patients with concomitant CHI, those with pre-SCI CHIs, and those with no history of CHI; there was, however, a general trend toward poorer performance on the HCT among patients who sustained head injuries at any time, either before or at the time of the SCI, compared with those who had no CHI history. Premorbid factors, such as age and educational level, did not correlate with HCT scores, but patients who sustained their SCI in motor vehicle accidents had a greater frequency of CHI (with LOC or PTA) than patients with other etiologies of SCI.

In another investigation of what was called occult head injury among patients with traumatic SCI, Wilmot et al. (1985) studied 67 patients with SCI admitted to the California Regional Spinal Cord Injury Care Center who were at high risk for head trauma. Patients were not randomly selected; rather, they were chosen based on the presence of any one of four high-risk inclusion criteria: quadriplegia associated with deceleration impact, history of documented LOC, presence of neurologic indicators, or need for respiratory support.

An extensive neuropsychologic test battery of 11 tests was administered to all the patients, providing a comprehensive assessment of a wide variety of cognitive functions. The GOAT (Reitan 1979) was used to assess orientation, memory for events, and PTA. The Quick Test (Ammons & Ammons 1962) was given because it measures vocabulary and simple verbal reasoning. The three subtests of the Stroop Color/Word Tests (Golden 1978) were used to evaluate reading, perception, and ability to use information simultaneously. Serial 7s (Taylor 1981) were used to assess attention, concentration, and simple calculation. Raven Progressive Matrices (Raven 1960) tested general intellectual ability, mental organization, spatial relationship, and analogous reasoning. The two trials of the Associated Learning Subtest of the Wechsler Memory Scale (WMS; Larabee et al. 1983; Lezak 1983; Wechsler 1945) were used to test verbal learning. Finally, the Vocabulary Scale of the Shipley Hartford Test was used because it measures preinjury general vocabulary knowledge; the Abstraction Scale of the Shipley Hartford Test was used because it measures capacity for abstract conceptual thinking (Shipley 1946).

Despite the breadth of scope of the tests, the scoring and reporting were rather limited. No individual test means were reported. An overall 6-point impairment rating was used, summarizing all test results in one measure. Using this method, the investigators found that 64% of the patients were rated as mildly impaired or worse on the 6-point scale and that one third of the patients in the study sample who had pre-SCI learning disabilities had the most impaired scores. They concluded that the patients without premorbid learning disabilities but with impaired neuropsychological test scores represented the group that was most likely to have sustained a concomitant CHI at the time of the SCI.

The Raven Progressive Matrices were found to correlate best with the overall score, and the Shipley Hartford Test Vocabulary Scale correlated least. No significant relationships were found between neuropsychological impairments and spinal lesion level or degree of completeness of the spinal lesion. Surprisingly, test results appeared to have no relationship to length of stay in the rehabilitation program.

Persistence of Cognitive Deficits

To evaluate the persistence of cognitive deficits in patients with SCI, Richards et al. (1988) studied the results of serial neuropsychological testing in patients with acute SCI. A comprehensive neuropsychological test battery was administered to 150 patients shortly after injury and then again to 67 of those same patients an average of 38 weeks later.

The battery was extensive and included measures of both right and left hemisphere functioning. The Benton Visual Retention Test (L'Abate et al. 1962, 1963) was used because it tests visual memory and perception. The Benton Facial Recognition Test (Dricker et al. 1978; Hamsher et al. 1979) was used to test visuospatial and linguistic function. The HCT was used to measure abstract concept formation and attention (Boll 1981; DeFillipis et al. 1979; DeWolfe et al. 1971; Fitzhugh & Fitzhugh 1961; Kimura 1981; Lansdell & Donnelly 1977; Lynch 1983; Pendleton & Heaton 1982; Reitan 1955, 1979; Rothke 1986; Shaw 1966). The Benton Judgement of Line Orientation Test (Benton et al. 1978) was used to measure perceptual ability. The Rey Auditory Verbal Learning Test (RAVLT; Lezak 1983) was administered because it measures memory span, provides a learning curve, and reflects learning strategies and retention after distraction. The Russell Memory Test (Russell, E.W. 1975) was used as a measure of long-term retention of semantic material presented auditorily. The

Stroop Test (Dodril 1978; Golden 1978) was used to measure ability to shift perceptual sets, concentration, and reading fluency. The Wechsler Adult Intelligence Scale–Revised (WAIS-R) Verbal IQ (Larabee et al. 1983; Lezak 1983; Wechsler 1945) was employed as an overall indicator of intellectual functioning, and the WMS Memory Quotient (Larabee et al. 1983; Lezak 1983; Wechsler 1945) was used because it assesses immediate recall, new learning, attention, concentration, and orientation. The Controlled Oral Word Association Test (Benton 1968) assesses verbal fluency, and the Selective Reminding Task (Buschke & Fuld 1974) measures retention, storage, and retrieval of semantic information.

Significant improvement was noted over time for results on the HCT, Stroop Color Test, WAIS-R Information Test, WAIS-R Vocabulary Test, WAIS-R Comprehension Test, WAIS-R Verbal IQ, WMS Memory Quotient, and Verbal Fluency. The pattern of recovery was judged to be similar to that seen in mild to moderate CHI: Improvement in memory, complex reasoning, mental speed, and persistence predominated.

Comparisons and Controls

One of the limitations in the applicability of findings from many previous investigations of neuropsychological test abnormalities among patients with SCI consistently has been related to the failure of those studies to compare the frequency and severity of cognitive impairment in these patients with those of concurrent, noninjured control subjects matched for a number of sociodemographic factors. It is extremely important to consider those factors, including age, gender, education, and geographic location, because they have been found to influence neuropsychological performance (Bornstein & Matarazzo 1985; Grant et al. 1984; Hillbom & Holm 1986; Levin et al. 1987; Lezak 1983; McGlone 1978; Prigatano & Parsons 1976; Sundet 1988). To address the issue of controlling for social factors, a study was conducted in which a broad range of cognitive abilities were assessed and compared in 81 patients with acute SCI and 61 paid, noninjured volunteer control subjects (Roth et al. 1989).

A comprehensive, motor-free neuropsychologic test battery was administered an average of 72 days after injury. The HCT, Booklet Form, measured attention, concentration, visual problem-solving ability, abstract reasoning, ability to use feedback, and ability to adapt to new situations (Boll 1981; DeFillipis et al. 1979; DeWolfe et al. 1971; Fitzhugh & Fitzhugh 1961; Kimura 1981; Lansdell & Donnelly 1977; Lynch 1983; Pendleton & Heaton 1982; Reitan 1955, 1979; Rothke 1986; Shaw 1966). The WAIS-R Vocabulary Subtest (Larabee et al. 1983; Lezak 1983; Wechsler 1945) assessed verbal and general mental ability. The WMS Mental Control Subtest (Larabee et al. 1983; Lezak 1983; Wechsler 1945) tested automatic and simple conceptual tracking. Two trials each and percentage of information retained from the WMS–Russell Adaptation Logical Memory and Paired Associates subtests (Larabee et al. 1983; Lezak 1983; Wechsler 1945) were used to test immediate recall of verbal ideas, verbal retention from word pairs, and long-term verbal and nonverbal storage capacity. The RAVLT (Lezak 1983) measured immediate memory span and retention after interpolated activity and provided a learning curve. Separate scores were documented and reported for each test.

Impairment levels for each test were defined as values that exceeded two standard deviations from the mean scores of the controls on each test. With these criteria, impairment was found on all tests in 10% to 40% of all patients with SCI. Impaired test performance was noted most frequently on the 30-minute recall trial of the Paired Associates Subtest (40%), the recognition trial of the RAVLT (31%), and the WAIS-R Vocabulary Subtest (24%). Impaired test performance was noted least frequently on the interference trial of the RAVLT (10%). Significantly more patients than controls scored in the impaired range on each test. Mean scores of the patients were significantly more impaired than mean scores of the control subjects for most, but not all, of the tests.

In general, results of this study suggested diffuse or global cognitive impairments, with concentration and initial learning being particularly impaired (as reflected by the impaired performance on the Mental Control Subtest, initial trials of the Logical Memory and Paired Associates subtests, the first six trials of the RAVLT, and the recognition trial of the RAVLT); storage and retrieval of long-term verbal and non-verbal material were relatively preserved (as reflected by the percentage of information retained on the Logical Memory and the Paired Associates subtests). Ability to adapt to new situations and to shift to new mental sets also was found to be impaired (as seen on the HCT), as were word retrieval and syntax use (as measured by the WAIS-R Vocabulary Subtest).

Clearly, these cognitive impairments have the potential to affect adversely ability to achieve the goals of rehabilitation, including independence in self-care and mobility skill performance, prevention of medical complications, adjustment to the disability, and reintegration into the community. An accurate and thorough description of specific cognitive strengths and weaknesses in an individual patient provides the opportunity to modify a patient's treatment program. The observation in the study that concentration and new learning are significantly impaired but that retention of information committed to long-term memory is relatively intact suggests that repeated instruction and opportunity for repeated practice of skills might enhance storage and cognitive integration.

Relationship with Depression

The prevalence of clinically significant depression in patients with acute SCI has been found to range between 10% and 30% (Davidoff et al. 1990a; Frank et al. 1985; Fullerton et al. 1981; Judd et al. 1986; Richards 1966). Because of the possibility that depression may alter patient motivation, impair

concentration and memory, and hamper neuropsychological test performance, a study was undertaken to determine the extent, if any, to which depression ratings influence cognitive performance in patients with SCI (Davidoff et al. 1990b). Sixty-six patients with acute SCI were administered the same comprehensive, motor-free neuropsychologic test battery described above, including the HCT, Booklet Form; the WAIS-R Vocabulary Subtest, the WMS Mental Control Subtest; the WMS–Russell Adaptation Logical Memory Subtest (two trials), Paired Associates Subtest (two trials), and Visual Reproduction Subtests; and the RAVLT. All patients were also administered the Zung Self-Rating Depression Scale (Zung 1965, 1971). This instrument is a 20-item inventory of affective and somatic attributes of depression. It has been found to be a valid and reliable objective measure of depression (Blumenthal & Dielman 1975; Schaeffer et al. 1985; Zung 1965, 1971).

Results indicated minimal relationship between neuropsychological performance and depression as evaluated in several different ways. There were no significant differences in mean scores on any of the 20 neuropsychological tests between patients who scored in the depressed range on the Zung scale and those who scored in the not depressed range on the Zung scale. In addition, there were only two (with the recall trials of the Paired Associates and the Visual Reproduction subtests) significant correlations from 20 possible relationships between scores on each of the neuropsychological tests and the Zung scores. These findings suggest that the magnitude and nature of cognitive dysfunction is largely unrelated to the presence or severity of depression in patients with SCI and that these two psychological issues should be treated as separate problems.

Summary of Neuropsychological Deficits in SCI

Several special considerations are necessary for the proper assessment of cognitive functioning in patients with SCI. Factors such as absent upper extremity dexterity, skin maintenance procedures, bowel and bladder regulation programs, poor endurance, and limited sitting tolerance require that appropriate modifications be made to the design of a comprehensive neuropsychological test battery.

Many of the neuropsychological abnormalities found in patients with SCI are related to the occurrence of a concomitant acute CHI at the same time as the SCI, but some may reflect the long-term effects of chronic problems such as alcohol and substance abuse or preinjury learning disability. To the extent that the deficits may recover within the first year after injury, these may more likely reflect sequelae of the acute CHI. Recognition and evaluation of cognitive dysfunction in patients with SCI allow the opportunity for more directed and focused treatment. Alterations in the treatment regimen may include both cognitive training programs for the neuropsychological abnormalities and modifications in the physical training program for the disability resulting from the SCI. These special treatment considerations may help maximize function, facilitate adaptation, and optimize outcome after SCI.

IMPLICATIONS OF COGNITIVE DYSFUNCTION IN SCI

The Research Strategy—Driven by Clinical Needs

The initial research by Schueneman and Morris (1982), which first discussed therapeutic implications of problems associated with mild CHI in patients with SCI, grew from clinical needs. At that point, in 1980, although the coincidence of brain and spinal injuries had been reported, head injury and its effects in patients with SCI were not generally recognized in treatment settings. The investigators frequently encountered situations in which cognitive and personality sequelae of brain injury were mistaken for character traits in these patients. As a consequence, therapists often complained that the patient was not motivated to learn when in fact the patient's learning difficulties represented memory deficits or other cognitive problems associated with head trauma. A common scenario would involve a therapist expressing frustration with a patient with whom it was difficult to work; when asked whether he or she thought the patient's problems might be related to the head injury, the therapist would reply, "What head injury?" It was not unusual to receive this reply even when the patient had experienced 1 or 2 weeks of PTA.

It became clear that the treatment team, often made up of the same individuals who worked with patients whose primary diagnosis was head injury, simply was unaccustomed to considering that their patients with SCI might have had a dual injury. Once sensitized to this possibility, therapists were able to bring to the treatment situation any knowledge they already had about sequelae of head injury and were able to add to this knowledge base through additional experience and training.

The first study documented the frequency of patients' reports of PTA. The research strategy that followed, including work by Davidoff et al. (1985a) and subsequent studies (Davidoff et al. 1985b; Roth et al. 1989), grew from the clinical need to understand the phenomenon of head injury in this group. Given the fact that head injury was common in patients with SCI, those investigators and others (Richards et al. 1988; Wilmot et al. 1985) examined whether such injuries were actually in evidence in the form of cognitive deficits during rehabilitation. After it was determined that such deficits were, in fact, frequently in evidence, ongoing research has focused on the effects of head injury on the rehabilitation process itself and on the long-term adjustment to spinal injury.

Implications for the Treatment Team

Since World War II, tremendous strides have been made in the medical management and rehabilitation of patients with

SCI. We now are in a position to be more sophisticated in our treatments, taking into account the needs of the individual. Fortuitously, brain injury rehabilitation has also become more highly developed during the past decade; in working with our patients, we can now integrate such treatments into rehabilitation programs when appropriate.

It is necessary that someone, preferably a clinical neuropsychologist who has knowledge of brain functioning and who can assess the patient, be available to the spinal treatment team. At a minimum, each patient should be screened with an extended mental status examination soon after admission to the program. This needs to be done in the context of answering the question, "Who is this person?" Thus there needs to be an emphasis on evaluating the particular patient, not just making an assessment of cognitive functioning. Such an evaluation should include consideration of pretrauma capabilities, schooling, and the like as well as assessment of personality characteristics. It would be a serious error to consider either cognitive or emotional functioning outside the context of the patient's personal history.

Although statistics have varied in different studies, as cited above, as to the exact percentage of patients with SCI who have also sustained head trauma, certainly even if the lowest estimates are accurate the coincidence of head and spinal injury is of such a magnitude as to be clinically significant. Many of these injuries can be classified as mild, according to the definition of mild traumatic brain injury as developed by the American Congress of Rehabilitation Medicine (Appendix 12-A). By that definition, such injuries frequently result in a constellation of physical symptoms often labeled postconcussion syndrome, including nausea, vomiting, dizziness, headache, tinnitus, blurred vision, other sensory loss such as taste or smell, or extended periods of fatigue and lethargy. Cognitive deficits, such as deficits to attention, concentration, memory, language, or perception, can also follow as sequelae to even mild head injuries. Exploration of such sequelae at a minimum with an extended mental status examination is critical before treatments are planned for patients with SCI.

Neuropsychological Evaluation

An extended mental status examination is similar to a physician's general examination in that it is clinical (the procedures are not standardized). Furthermore, there is typically a broad outline of areas to be covered, with the opportunity to explore any given area more extensively if needed. An extended mental status examination usually involves assessment of cognitive functions such as attention, concentration, memory processes, expressive and receptive language functioning, visuospatial processing, judgment, reasoning, and problem-solving abilities (see Appendix 12–B for a sample of an extended mental status examination).

If findings are questionable or more specific information is needed as to the patient's cognitive functioning, formal evaluation might be undertaken. Such tests as the RAVLT, the HCT, portions of the WMS-Revised (WMS-R), the Wisconsin Card Sort (WCS), the Raven Progressive Matrices, portions of the WAIS-R, and the Peabody Individual Achievement Test (PIAT) are measures that are used frequently in such formal evaluations because they are well standardized and normed and also because they do not require upper extremity functioning and thus can be employed with patients of any spinal injury level. These tests are sensitive to cognitive functioning that is frequently disrupted or impaired as a consequence of head injury.

The RAVLT assesses the ability to acquire new verbal information when it is presented auditorily and evaluates the patient's ability to improve with repetition of verbal information. The HCT, WCS, and Raven Progressive Matrices are measures that assess problem solving, mental flexibility, and the ability to shift mental sets. They are primarily dependent upon visual input and evaluate the patient's ability to develop novel solutions to problems. The HCT is also considered an excellent indicator of the presence or absence of brain damage and can therefore be useful for diagnostic purposes as well. Furthermore, the HCT also assesses the patient's ability to use feedback in developing alternative hypotheses when solving problems. The WMS-R assesses orientation to place and time, screens for fund of personal and current information, and provides additional information about the patient's ability to store and retain new verbal information. Portions of the WAIS-R (particularly the verbal scales) can be useful in evaluating the patient's fund of general information. This not only provides insight into the patient's pretrauma fund of acquired information but also contributes to our understanding of his or her current ability to retrieve information from long-term storage. This ability to retrieve pretrauma acquired information is often better preserved than the ability to store new information. Other useful subtests of the WAIS-R that do not involve upper extremity functioning include those that measure echoic memory, social and practical judgment, verbal abstraction processes, vocabulary knowledge, and arithmetic skills to the seventh grade. Finally, the PIAT measures the amount of acquired information in the domains of reading, spelling, and mathematics. Because such information generally is preserved even after head injury (unless the injury is severe), these achievement measures help us understand the patient's pretrauma functioning and provide information that can help us assess whether the patient's current functioning is at levels consistent with his or her preinjury functioning.

Although a clinical neuropsychologist might conduct such an examination, it is critical that all members of the treatment team be familiar with such evaluations as well as the common sequelae of head injury, so that they can integrate the findings of the evaluation into their treatment program. Texts such as those by Levin et al. (1982) and Rosenthal et al. (1983) provide excellent information about head injury and its consequences. Furthermore, to get a sense of what is involved in an extended mental status evaluation, therapists working with patients with SCI might want to read the work of Strub and Black (1985), which provides excellent examples of assessment techniques as well as an overview of the rationale for their use.

It is also critical to appreciate that head injuries can cause emotional problems as well. Certainly irritability is among the most common emotional sequelae of head injury. Patients who once were considered easy going can become quickly annoyed, flying off the handle at the slightest provocation. This reaction is considered a primary, brain-related phenomenon, representing physiological disinhibition rather than simply a secondary, emotional response to the injury. Other common emotional responses are depression, anhedonia, and apathy as well as primary brain-related responses. In more severe injuries, it is not unusual to find paranoid thinking as a consequence of misinterpretation of the motives of others and of what is occurring; for example, a patient may believe the team is keeping him or her a prisoner against his or her will.

Results of Neuropsychological Assessment I: Cognitive Rehabilitation

Assessment of the patient's cognitive and emotional functioning in the context of pretrauma abilities, personality, and history can assist us in three major ways. When deficits are significant, the assessment can provide information that will be useful in guiding cognitive rehabilitation. Over the past 5 to 10 years, methods of cognitive rehabilitation have become increasingly sophisticated and are used routinely in programs that are focused on treating patients with brain injury (Davidoff et al. 1990a). For the most part, these treatments are aimed at improving the patient's awareness of his or her specific deficits so that he or she can learn and appropriately use compensatory strategies. The strategies generally are designed to help the patient perform, on a voluntary and intentional basis, functions that before the injury were automatic and did not require conscious awareness.

In programs where treatment is guided by this or a similar philosophy, it is clear that patients' understanding of their deficits is usually critical if they are to generalize what they have learned and employ the techniques they have been taught, not just in the rehabilitation setting but in everyday life. Therefore, identifying the specific deficits to be focused on is essential in effective treatment planning. The standardized neuropsychological evaluation can provide information regarding areas of cognitive deficits that then can be assessed in a more detailed manner at the pace of the patient in making specific treatment plans. For example, if the neuropsychological evaluation indicates that the patient shows deficits in visual memory, additional assessment can identify the specific problem that underlies the visual memory deficit. For one patient, the problem may be that he does not take the time to view the entirety of the visual image. For another, it may be that she cannot perceive which of the details of the image are essential or important and which are not. For still another patient, the deficit may be due to an inability to perceive the whole ("the forest") rather than just the parts ("the trees"). Each of these problems leads to deficits in the ability to recall visual material later but suggests the need for different treatment strategies. A program based on this type of assessment process contrasts strongly with "canned" methods (e.g., a particular group of computer programs) that are always used in rehabilitation of general deficits (e.g., visual memory problems) without regard for the underlying specific cause of the general deficit. Although the "canned" or preplanned approach may be helpful to certain patients in the long term, it is likely to be less efficient, less effective, and less generalized by the patient in nontherapy settings than individually designed programs based on rehabilitation of specific, underlying problems.

Results of Neuropsychological Assessment II: Prevention of Adverse Reactions

Assessment of cognitive and emotional functioning can help the SCI rehabilitation treatment team maintain empathy for patients whose behavior might otherwise lead us to believe they are simply being uncooperative. A patient who shows irritability, impulsiveness, poor judgment, or lack of cooperation often is labeled difficult, a problem patient, or a management problem. It is much easier for therapists to sustain a professional relationship and a positive alliance with such a patient if the patient's problems are understood as an outcome of his or her injury rather than as unattractive character traits.

Without insight into the genesis of the patient's behavior, it is difficult for the therapist to avoid feeling angry and inadequate in response. As a consequence, the therapist may react to the patient with frank dislike and hostility, avoidance, or rejection. Conversely, if the relationship is understood, team members are more likely to be able to avoid interpreting the patient's behavior as a personal affront.

Optimal treatment takes place in situations in which there is mutual respect between therapist and patient. Establishing a positive therapeutic alliance should therefore precede treatment, especially with patients with brain injury who may be learning of their deficits for the first time. Typically, increased understanding of the patient by the therapist promotes mutual respect.

Results of Neuropsychological Evaluation III: Tailoring the Rehabilitation Program

The neurological assessment can allow us to alter appropriately the standard rehabilitation program when necessary. The results of the initial assessment of these areas by the neuropsychologist should be accompanied by specific suggestions for treatment whenever possible. They should include recommendations for how best to teach the patient new skills and information as well as guidance in managing the patient's behavioral problems.

Addressing memory functioning generally is central in this process. For example, patients often have a preferred sensory modality in which they learn. As a result, some will learn best by what they see and will therefore benefit from watching a demonstration. Others will learn best by what they hear and will profit from hearing an explanation. Others profit most from what they read and still others from the tactile and kinesthetic feedback of physically going through the steps of the tasks themselves. Although most able-bodied individuals do best with a combination of these methods wherein information is taken in a redundant manner using more than one sensory modality, after head trauma many patients are poor at storing new information received in one or more modality. This is a matter of degree and may be a mild problem in one individual and a severe problem in another. One common phenomenon after head trauma is the inability to remember what has been said. A patient with this problem may seem otherwise cognitively intact, and team members working with the patient might easily mistake the patient's ability to learn as normal and fail to adjust the teaching format accordingly. Team members often feel frustrated later when their expectations of what the patient will remember do not meet the reality of the patient's ability to learn.

The neuropsychologist should provide guidance about memory in a manner that will facilitate appropriate alterations of teaching methods. Information about how the patient takes in new information is essential in making these alterations. In the case of a patient who has difficulty remembering what he or she has heard, the team might be told that the patient does profit from repetition of verbal information (not all patients do) and that repetitions should be incorporated into teaching sessions. Alternatively, they might be told that the patient takes in little information at any given time and that giving more overtaxes the patient, putting him or her on overload and preventing him or her from remembering any of what he or she has heard. With this information, team members would know to keep their instructions brief for any given session. The team might be told that the patient will retain verbal information if he or she takes it in accurately but that he or she frequently becomes confused when the material is initially presented and often does not accurately take in the details or the sense of what is said. With this information, team members can alter their teaching by having the patient repeat what he or she has heard and correct any patient misperception. Through this method, the chances of the patient later recalling the material correctly would be increased. For other patients, difficulty in processing information because of slowed mentation can also affect the ability to store and retain new material. With this insight about the patient, the team can slow their presentations to a speed that is manageable for that individual.

There are also some types of memory problems that are not amenable to direct compensatory techniques. For example, some patients have a profound deficit to the ability to encode new verbal information into long-term storage, not because it is presented too rapidly or in too great a quantity or anything that would lend itself to a shift in teaching technique, but as a consequence of a physiologically based inability to engage in that encoding process. This problem is occasionally seen in severely injured patients long after their injury. More commonly, it is encountered in the early stages after injury when the patient is experiencing PTA. During this period, no new memories are being stored. Engaging in any of the techniques mentioned above, such as repetition or slowed presentations, will do little but frustrate the therapist. Under those circumstances, some amount of teaching might still be attempted. Teaching based on appropriate expectations on the part of the therapist, however, is likely to leave both the patient and the therapist feeling less frustrated and inadequate. For the team to have appropriate expectations, it is clear that the patient's deficits need to have been evaluated.

Although deficits are important to understand, it is also of the utmost importance that the patient's strengths be known as well. Teaching can be geared toward using the patient's better preserved modalities. No individual likes to experience failure, and the degree to which teaching can be centered on the patient's strengths and therefore can provide him or her with success experiences is important in preserving the patient's self-esteem and maintaining his or her motivation to continue in treatment. When one is teaching any patient, but particularly under the kinds of frustrating and depressing conditions experienced by patients who have both spinal and head injuries, praise and encouragement are critical components of the experience.

Communication with the Patient

The team should be sensitive in communicating the results of such assessments. Certainly, no recently spinal-injured patient wants to learn that there is also a component of brain injury. Nevertheless, many patients need reassurance of the likelihood of recovery in the case of mild injuries. When the head trauma is more severe, the patient is apt to need to understand the specific repercussions of that injury so that he or she may best engage in head injury rehabilitation with cooperation. Furthermore, such findings are frequently important to share with family members who might be confused about why the patient is responding as he or she is and what they might expect in the future.

CONCLUSION

In this chapter and much of the research in this field, heavy emphasis is placed on the problem of concomitant head injury in the population with spinal injury. It is widely accepted, however, that there are a number of other causes of cognitive dysfunction that frequently affect this population. These include the effects of chronic alcohol and other recreational drug use and the existence of learning disabilities before the spinal injury that may have an impact on the patient's adaptive abilities in general and on the acquisition of new skills and information during rehabilitation in particular. These are important areas for further research to improve our ever evolving treatment methods. It is clear that we are no longer satisfied with one standard rehabilitation program for spinal injury. The better we understand the effects of neuropsychological dysfunction on the patient's overall functioning, the easier it will be for us to tailor our treatments to the specific needs of the individual patient.

REFERENCES

Ammons, R.B., and C.H. Ammons. 1962. Quick Test (QT): Provisional manual. *Psychol. Rep.* 11(Monograph Suppl. I-VII):111–161.

Benton, A.L. 1968. Differential behavioral effects in frontal lobe disease. *Neuropsychologia* 6:53–60.

Benton, A.L., et al. 1978. Visuospatial judgment: A clinical test. *Arch. Neurol.* 35:364–367.

Blumenthal, M.D., and T.E. Dielman. 1975. Depression symptomatology and role function in a general population. *Arch. Gen. Psychiatry* 32:985–991.

Boll, T.J. 1981. "The Halstead-Reitan Neuropsychology Battery." In *Handbook of clinical neuropsychology*, ed. S.B. Filskov and R.J. Boll. New York, N.Y.: Wiley Interscience.

Bornstein, R.A., and J.D. Matarazzo. 1985. Wechsler VIQ versus PIQ differences in cerebral dysfunction: A literature review with emphasis on sex differences. *J. Clin. Neuropsychol.* 4:319–334.

Brooks, D.N. 1972. Memory and head injury. *J. Nerv. Ment. Dis.* 155:350–355.

Buschke, H., and P.A. Fuld. 1974. Evaluating storage, retention and retrieval in disordered memory and learning. *Neurology* 11:1019–1025.

Davidoff, G., et al. 1985a. Closed head injury in spinal cord injured patients: Retrospective study of loss of consciousness and post-traumatic amnesia. *Arch. Phys. Med. Rehabil.* 66:41–43.

Davidoff, G., et al. 1985b. Cognitive dysfunction and mild closed head injury in traumatic spinal cord injury. *Arch. Phys. Med. Rehabil.* 66:489–491.

Davidoff, G., et al. 1988a. Galveston Orientation and Amnesia Test: Its utility in the determination of closed head injury patients. *Arch. Phys. Med. Rehabil.* 69:432–434.

Davidoff, G., et al. 1988b. Closed head injury in traumatic spinal cord injury: Incidence and risk factors. *Arch. Phys. Med. Rehabil.* 69:869–872.

Davidoff, G., et al. 1990a. Depression among acute spinal cord injury patients: A study utilizing the Zung Self-Rating Depression Scale. *Rehabil. Psychol.* 35:171–180.

Davidoff, G., et al. 1990b. Depression and neuropsychological test performance in acute spinal cord injury patients: Lack of correlation. *Arch. Clin. Neuropsychol.* 5:77–88.

DeFillipis, N.A., et al. 1979. Development of a booklet form of the Category Test: Normative and validity data. *J. Clin. Neuropsychol.* 1:339–342.

Denny-Brown, D. 1945. Disability arising from closed head injury. *J.A.M.A.* 127:429–436.

DeWolfe, A.S., et al. 1971. Intellectual deficit in chronic schizophrenia and brain damage. *J. Consult. Clin. Psychol.* 36:197–204.

Dikmen, S., and R.M. Reitan. 1977. Emotional sequelae of head injury. *Ann. Neurol.* 2:492–494.

Dodril, C.B. 1978. A neuropsychological battery for epilepsy. *Epilepsia* 19:611–623.

Dricker, J., et al. 1978. The recognition and encoding of faces by alcoholic Korsakoff and right-hemisphere patients. *Neuropsychologia* 16:683–695.

Dubo, H., and G. Delaney. 1984. 101 Spinal cord injuries due to motor vehicle accidents. In *Proceedings of the tenth annual meeting of the American Spinal Injury Association.* 10:35.

Fitzhugh, K.B., and L.C. Fitzhugh. 1961. Psychological deficits in relationship to acuteness of brain dysfunction. *J. Consult. Psychol.* 25:61–65.

Fordyce, D.J., et al. 1983. Enhanced emotional reactions in chronic head trauma patients. *J. Neurol. Neurosurg. Psychiatry* 46:620–624.

Frank, R.G., et al. 1985. Depression and adrenal function in spinal cord injury. *Am. J. Psychiatry* 142:243–252.

Fullerton, D.T., et al. 1981. Psychiatric disorders in patients with spinal cord injuries. *Arch. Gen. Psychiatry* 38:1369–1371.

Golden, C.J. 1978. *Stroop Color and Word Test: Manual for clinical and experimental uses.* Chicago, Ill.: Stoelting.

Grant, I., et al. 1984. Aging, abstinence and medical risk factors in the prediction of neuropsychologic deficit among long-term alcoholics. *Arch. Gen. Psychiatry* 41:710–718.

Gronwall, D., and P. Wrightson. 1974. Delayed recovery of intellectual function after minor head injury. *Lancet* 2:605–609.

Guttmann, L. 1963. "Surgical management: Initial treatment of traumatic paraplegia and tetraplegia." In *Spinal injuries*, ed. P. Harris. Edinburgh, Scotland: Royal College of Surgeons.

Guttmann, L. 1973. "Associated injuries." In *Spinal cord injuries: Comprehensive management and research*, ed. L. Guttmann. Oxford, England: Blackwell Scientific.

Hamsher, K., et al. 1979. Facial recognition in patients with focal brain lesions. *Arch. Neurol.* 36:837–839.

Harris, P., ed. 1965. *Proceedings of the Third International Congress of Neurological Surgeons* (Excerpta Medica International Congress Series 110). Copenhagen, Denmark: International Congress of Neurological Surgeons.

Harris, P. 1968. Associated injuries in traumatic paraplegia and tetraplegia. *Paraplegia* 5:215–220.

Hillbom, M., and L. Holm. 1986. Contribution of traumatic head injury to neuropsychological deficits in alcoholics. *J. Neurol. Neurosurg. Psychiatry* 49:1348–1353.

Judd, F.K., et al. 1986. Depression following acute spinal cord injury. *Paraplegia* 24:358–363.

Kimura, S. 1981. Card form of the Reitan modified Halstead Category Test. *J. Consult. Clin. Psychol.* 49:145–146.

L'Abate, L., et al. 1962. The diagnostic usefulness of four potential tests of brain damage. *J. Consult. Psychol.* 26:479.

L'Abate, L., et al. 1963. The diagnostic usefulness of two tests of brain damage. *J. Clin. Psychol.* 19:87–91.

Lansdell, H., and E.F. Donnelly. 1977. Factor analysis of the Wechsler Adult Intelligence Scale subtests and the Halstead-Reitan Category and Tapping tests. *J. Consult. Clin. Psychol.* 45:412–416.

Larabee, G.J., et al. 1983. Factor analysis of the WAIS and Wechsler Memory Scale. *J. Clin. Psychol.* 5:159–168.

Levin, H.S., and R.G. Grossman. 1978. Behavioral sequelae of closed head injury: A quantitative study. *Arch. Neurol.* 35:720–727.

Levin, H.S., et al. 1979. Galveston Orientation and Amnesia Test: Practical scale to assess cognition after head injury. *J. Nerv. Ment. Dis.* 167:675–684.

Levin, H.S., et al. 1982. *Neurobehavioral consequences of closed head injury.* New York, N.Y.: Oxford University Press.

Levin, H.S., et al. 1987. Neurobehavioral outcome following minor head injury: A three-center study. *J. Neurosurg.* 66:234–243.

Lezak, M.D. 1983. *Neuropsychological assessment.* New York, N.Y.: Oxford University Press.

Lishman, W.A. 1968. Brain damage in relation to psychiatric sequelae after head injury. *Br. J. Psychiatry* 114:373–410.

Lishman, W.A. 1973. The psychiatric sequelae of head injury: A review. *Psychol. Med.* 3:304–318.

Lynch, W. 1983. "Neuropsychological assessment." In *Rehabilitation of the head injured adult*, ed. M. Rosenthal et al. Philadelphia, Pa.: Davis.

Mandelberg, I.A. 1975. Cognitive recovery after severe head injury. I. Verbal and performance IQs as a function of post-traumatic amnesia: Duration and time from injury. *J. Neurol. Neurosurg. Psychiatry* 38:1001–1006.

Mandelberg, I.A., and D.N. Brooks. 1975. Cognitive recovery after severe head injury. III. Serial testing on the Wechsler Adult Intelligence Scale. *J. Neurol. Neurosurg. Psychiatry* 38:1121–1126.

Maynard, F.M., et al. 1979. Neurological prognosis after traumatic quadriplegia. *J. Neurosurg.* 50:611–616.

McGlone, J. 1978. Sex differences in functional brain asymmetry. *Cortex* 14:122–128.

Meinecke, F.W. 1968. Frequency and distribution of associated injuries in traumatic paraplegia and tetraplegia. *Paraplegia* 5:196–211.

Pendleton, M.G., and R.K. Heaton. 1982. A comparison of the Wisconsin Card Sorting Test and the Halstead Test. *J. Clin. Psychol.* 38:392–396.

Prigatano, G.P., and O.A. Parsons. 1976. Relationship of age and education to Halstead test performance in different patient populations. *J. Consult. Clin. Psychol.* 44:527–533.

Raven, J.C. 1960. *Guide to standard progressive matrices.* London, England: Lewis.

Reitan, R.M. 1955. Investigation of the validity of Halstead's measure of biological intelligence. *Arch. Neurol. Psychiatry* 73:28–35.

Reitan, R.M. 1979. *Manual for administration of neuropsychological test batteries for adults and children.* Tucson, Ariz.: R.M. Reitan.

Richards, J.S. 1966. Psychological adjustment to spinal cord injury during the first post-discharge year. *Arch. Phys. Med. Rehabil.* 67:362–365.

Richards, J.S., et al. 1988. Spinal cord injury and concomitant traumatic brain injury: Results of a longitudinal investigation. *Am. J. Phys. Med. Rehabil.* 67:211–216.

Rimel, R.W. 1981. A prospective study of patients with central nervous system trauma. *J. Neurosurg. Nurs.* 13:132–141.

Rimel, R.W., et al. 1981. Disability caused by minor head injury. *Neurosurgery* 9:221–228.

Rosenthal, M., et al., eds. 1983. *Rehabilitation of the head injured adult.* Philadelphia, Pa.: Davis.

Roth, E., et al. 1989. A controlled study of neuropsychological deficits in acute spinal cord injury patients. *Paraplegia* 27:480–489.

Rothke, S.E. 1986. The role of set shifting cues on the Wisconsin Card Sorting Test and Halstead Category Test. *Int. J. Clin. Neuropsychol.* 8:11–14.

Russell, E.W. 1975. A multiple scoring method for the assessment of complex memory functions. *J. Consult. Clin. Psychol.* 43:800–809.

Russell, W.R. 1932. Cerebral involvement in head injury. *Brain* 55:549–603.

Russell, W.R. 1971. *The traumatic amnesias.* London, England: Oxford University Press.

Russell, W.R., and P.Q. Nathan. 1946. Traumatic amnesia. *Brain* 69:280–300.

Russell, W.R., and A. Smith. 1961. Post-traumatic amnesia in closed head injury. *Arch. Neurol.* 5:4–17.

Schaeffer, A., et al. 1985. Comparison of the validities of the Beck, Zung and MMPI depression scales. *J. Consult. Clin. Psychiatr.* 53:415–418.

Schneider, R.C., and J.E. McGillicuddy. 1976. "Concomitant craniocerebral and spinal trauma with special reference to the cervico-medullary region." In *Handbook of clinical neurology*, ed. P.J. Vinken and G.W. Bruyn. Vol. 24, part 2. New York, N.Y.: Elsevier.

Schueneman, A.L., and J. Morris. 1982. Neuropsychological deficits associated with spinal cord injury. *Spinal Cord Inj. Digest* 4:35–36, 64.

Shaw, D.J. 1966. The reliability and validity of the Halstead Category Test. *J. Clin. Psychol.* 22:176–179.

Shipley, W.C. 1946. *Shipley-Institute of Living Scale for measuring Intellectual Impairment, manual of directions and scoring key.* Los Angeles, Calif.: Western Psychological Services.

Silver, J.R., et al. 1980. Associated injuries in patients with spinal injury. *Injury* 12:219–224.

Smith, A. 1971. Duration of impaired consciousness as an index of severity in closed head injury: A review. *Dis. Nerv. Syst.* 22:69–74.

Steadman, J.H., and J.G. Graham. 1970. Head injuries: An analysis and follow-up study. *Proc. R. Soc. Med.* 63:23–28.

Strub, R.L., and F.W. Black. 1985. *The mental status examination in neurology.* Philadelphia, Pa.: Davis.

Sundet, K. 1988. Sex differences in cognition impairment following unilateral brain damage. *J. Clin. Exp. Neuropsychol.* 8:51–61.

Taylor, M.A. 1981. *Neuropsychiatric mental status examination.* New York, N.Y.: SP Medical & Scientific.

VonWowern, F. 1966. Post-traumatic amnesia and confusion as an index of severity in head injury. *Acta Neurol. Scand.* 42:373–378.

Wagner, K.A., et al. 1983. Head and spinal cord injury patients: Impact of combined sequelae. *Arch. Phys. Med. Rehabil.* 64:519.

Wechsler, D. 1945. Standardized memory scale for clinical use. *J. Psychol.* 19:87–95.

Wilmot, C.B., et al. 1985. Occult head injury: Its incidence in spinal cord injury. *Arch. Phys. Med. Rehabil.* 66:227–231.

Young, J.S., et al. 1982. *Spinal cord injury statistics: Experience of the Regional Spinal Cord Injury Systems.* Tucson, Ariz.: Good Samaritan Medical Center.

Zung, W.W.K. 1965. A self-rating depression scale. *Arch. Gen. Psychiatry* 12:63–70.

Zung, W.W.K. 1971. Depression in the normal adult population. *Psychosomatics* 12:164–167.

Appendix 12–A

Definition of Mild Traumatic Brain Injury (Revised)[*]

DEFINITION

A patient with mild traumatic brain injury is a person who has had a traumatically induced physiological disruption of brain function as manifested by at least one of the following:

1. any period after LOC
2. any loss of memory for events immediately before or after the accident (retrograde or anterograde amnesia), even in the absence of LOC or amnesia
3. any alteration in mental state at the time of the accident (e.g., feeling dazed, disoriented, or confused)
4. focal neurological deficit that may or may not be transient

but where the severity of the injury does not exceed the following:

A. LOC of approximately 30 minutes or less
B. after 30 minutes, an initial Glasgow Coma Scale score of 13 to 15
C. PTA not greater than 24 hours

COMMENTS

This definition includes trauma such as hitting the head, the head being struck, or whiplash injury but excludes stroke, anoxia, tumor, encephalitis, and the like. Computed tomography or magnetic resonance imaging studies and, in practice, routine neurological evaluations may be read as normal. Because of the lack of medical emergency or the realities of certain medical systems, some patients may not have the above factors medically documented in the acute stage. In such cases, it is appropriate to consider symptomatology that, when linked to a traumatic head injury, can suggest the existence of a mild traumatic brain injury.

SYMPTOMATOLOGY

The above criteria define the event of a mild traumatic brain injury. Symptoms of brain injury may or may not persist for variable lengths of time after such a neurological event. It should be recognized that patients with mild traumatic brain injury can exhibit persistent emotional, cognitive, and behavioral symptoms, alone or in combination, that may produce a functional disability even when the initial signs of injury are no longer present. Other patients may not become aware of, or admit, the extent of their symptoms until they attempt to return to normal functioning. In such cases, the evidence for mild traumatic brain injury only emerges with time, and the existence of the acute criteria must be reconstructed. Mild traumatic brain injury may also be overlooked in the face of more dramatic physical injury (e.g., orthopedic or spinal cord injury). The constellation of problems has been referred to as minor head injury, postconcussive syndrome, traumatic head syndrome, traumatic cephalalgia, post–brain injury syndrome, and posttraumatic syndrome.

---

[*]Developed by the Head Injury Interdisciplinary Special Interest Group of the American Congress of Rehabilitation Medicine.

Appendix 12–B

Sample Extended Mental Status Examination

I.   LOC (coma, stupor, lethargy, alert).

II. Behavioral observations (patient's appearance, motor movements such as gait, grooming).

III. Attention and concentration
   A. State days of the week backward.
   B. State days of the month backward.
   C. When I say the letter "A," I want you to say, "Stop":
      LRPTANCTARPRUTAALPNCTRGPQMALM.

IV. Repeating digits forward

7–2–8	5–4–6
3–9–8–2	5–1–4–7
5–9–7–1–8	6–4–9–5–3
2–4–9–3–7–5	9–7–3–2–6–4
7–9–1–3–6–2–8	3–7–8–2–5–6–9

V.   Repeating digits backward

9–4	6–8
3–2–7	1–6–3
9–6–8–2	5–3–6–7
2–5–7–3–6	6–3–5–9–2
7–1–2–5–4–6	8–2–5–3–6–4

VI. Following commands
   A. Point to the door.
   B. Show me the pencil.
   C. Point to my watch.

VII. Commands requiring motor movements
   A. Show me how you would brush your teeth.
   B. Show me how you would cut with a knife.
   C. Show me how you would cut with scissors.
   D. Show me how you would throw a ball.

VIII. Repetitions
   A. Ball.
   B. Help.
   C. Airplane.
   D. Hospital.
   E. Mississippi River.
   F. The little boy went home.
   G. No ifs, ands, or buts.
   H. We all went home together.
   I. Let's go to the store for sugar.
   J. The short fat boy dropped the china vase.
   K. Each fight readied the boxer for the championship bout.

IX. Naming

   Colors, body parts, clothing, room objects, parts of a watch, or other objects.

X.   Verbal fluency

   In 1 minute, name all the animals you can think of.
   In 1 minute, name all the parts of a car you can think of.

XI. Calculations

3 + 8	7 + 5	21 + 32	
9 − 4	17 − 5	21 − 9	35 − 7
3 × 4	4 × 12	21 × 5	
15 ÷ 5	40 ÷ 8	60 ÷ 12	

XII. Reading

Read the following letters of the alphabet in random order:

THE CAT IS BIG.

HE RAN TO THE GIANT TREE AND SHOOK THE LOWER BRANCHES.

XIII. Orientation

A. Self (name, age, birthday).
B. Place (name of place, address, city).
C. Time (year, month, date, day of week, time of day, season).

XIV. Remote memory

A. Personal historical information.
B. Mother's maiden name.
C. Who was president during the Vietnam War? World War II?
D. Inquire about historical events that occurred during the patient's lifetime.

XV. Memory for new information

Repeat three words (e.g., Chevrolet, zebra, purple).
Tell the patient you will ask again in 5 minutes.
Words remembered after 5 minutes.
Give prompts if necessary (e.g., car, animal, color).
Words remembered after 5 minutes with prompts.
Give three choices if necessary.
Words remembered after 5 minutes with choices.
Ask again after 10 or 15 minutes.

XVI. Story for immediate recall

Phillip Taylor, / a 26-year-old / sheetmetal worker / from Kenton County, / Nevada, / was leaving for vacation / when he began experiencing a stomach ache. / He entered Central Community Hospital / for 2 days of tests. / A harmless virus was diagnosed, / and he, his dog, / and two cats / left for their holiday trip.

Number of correct memories immediately following presentation _____ After 20 minutes _____

XVII. Visual neglect

A. Draw a daisy.
B. Draw a clock. Make the hands say 10 minutes after 11.
C. Bisect a line.

XVIII. Constructional dyspraxia

Copy a square, a cube, a Greek cross.

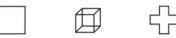

XIX. Visual memory

Show the patient designs such as those from the Wechsler Memory Scale. Have the patient reproduce the designs from memory immediately and again after a half hour. Show all three at one time.

XX. Fund of information

A. How many months are there in a year?
B. What does the bear do?
C. Where is Brussels?
D. How far is it from London to New York?
E. What is the capital of Peru?
F. What causes metal to rust?
G. Who wrote the *Odyssey*?
H. What is the Acropolis?

XXI. Interpreting idioms

What would it mean if I said he:
A. is walking on air?
B. is seeing red?
C. is thick-skinned?
D. has a chip on his shoulder?

XXII. Interpreting proverbs

A. Rome wasn't built in a day.
B. Don't cry over spilled milk.
C. A rolling stone gathers no moss.

XXIII. Similarities

In what way are the following alike?
A. Apple–pear.
B. Happy–angry.
C. Desk–bookcase.

XXIV. Right-left orientation

Show me your left hand, your right eyebrow, etc.
Touch your left elbow with your right hand, etc.
Point to my right hand.
Point to my left foot (with the examiner's legs crossed).

Chapter 13

Management of the Ventilator-Dependent Patient with Quadriplegia

Mary Elizabeth Keen

HISTORICAL PERSPECTIVE

Many of the management problems of ventilator dependence and quadriplegia have been encountered by rehabilitation and other medical practitioners during the polio epidemics of the recent past. Many technological innovations in respiratory care and rehabilitation of persons with ventilator dependence were in large part spurred by the needs of polio patients (Drinker & McKhann 1986; Goldberg et al. 1984). Mechanical means of providing ventilatory support were among these developments.

The first mechanical ventilators used negative pressure around the body to produce passive breathing. Although such a device was first described in 1832, the first known clinical trial took place in 1928. An 8-year-old girl with polio who was comatose from anoxia was placed in a tank ventilator and was successfully resuscitated. Although she died in a few days from pneumonia, news of the machine's success led to a great demand for these respirators, which became known as iron lungs (Drinker & McKhann 1986).

This life-saving device was effective only in cases of anterior polio, involving the cervical and thoracic spinal cord. Bulbar polio, which affects swallowing and oral motor control, was still fatal because of aspiration and pneumonia. During the polio epidemics of the early 1950s intubation and positive pressure ventilation were utilized to manage these complica-

tions and significantly reduced the mortality of poliomyelitis (Drinker & McKhann 1986). Intubation and positive pressure ventilation offered the additional advantages of improved access to the patient and more precise control of tidal volume and delivery of supplemental oxygen.

The iron lung is still in use by an estimated 300 individuals, most of whom are polio survivors (Drinker & McKhann 1986). Positive pressure ventilation with intubation or tracheostomy has been used more commonly than negative pressure devices in the management of spinal cord injury (SCI). Negative pressure ventilation and noninvasive means of positive pressure ventilatory support have some distinct advantages, however, and can be equally effective in the management of individuals with SCI (Bach 1991; Bach & Alba 1990b; Hill 1986).

How is a ventilatory assist device selected? An understanding of ventilatory mechanics and the pathophysiology of ventilation in SCI is necessary for logical selection of an appropriate means of ventilatory support.

PHYSIOLOGY OF VENTILATION: THE MECHANICS OF NORMAL BREATHING

Normal breathing consists of respiration (gas exchange) and ventilation (movement of air in and out of the lungs). Normal ventilation occurs as a result of the coordinated contrac-

The author gratefully acknowledges the assistance of Dr. Alan Goldberg and Charles Kirchoff who reviewed the manuscript and made many helpful suggestions.

tion of the muscles of inspiration and expiration. The muscles of inspiration include the diaphragm (innervated by C3–5), the scalenes (C4–8), the external intercostals (T1–11), and the accessory muscles. The muscles of expiration include the abdominals and the internal intercostals, all of which are innervated by thoracic spinal segments. Contraction of these muscle groups causes pressure changes in the thoracic and abdominal cavities, resulting in inspiration and expiration (Roussos & Macklem 1982).

When the diaphragm contracts and pushes against the abdominal contents while the abdominal wall contracts isotonically, the thorax is lifted and the chest expands. This elevation and expansion of the thorax depend on the resistance of the abdominal contents and the mobility of the ribs. Expansion of the lungs displaces the abdominal contents downward and outward, thereby decreasing intrathoracic pressure and creating a vacuum effect within the chest. The diaphragm, the intercostals, and the abdominal wall contract in a coordinated fashion for maximum efficiency. Expiration follows as the muscular pump relaxes and passively contracts. Forceful expiration (e.g., coughing) requires the coordinated contraction of the abdominal and chest wall musculature.

When greater ventilatory efforts are necessary, the accessory muscles of ventilation are recruited. The accessory muscles include the muscles of the neck and upper chest, such as the sternocleidomastoids, the scalenes, and the cervical paraspinals, and the muscles of the back and abdomen.

Ventilation is affected by position. Rib cage motion is greater in the upright posture. In the supine position most breathing movements are abdominal, and there is little motion of the rib cage. Lung compliance also decreases in the horizontal position because of the lower end-expiratory reserve volume in the supine chest (Mansel & Norman 1990).

VENTILATORY DYSFUNCTION IN SCI

In uncomplicated SCI the lungs are normal, and the chest wall is intact. Ventilatory failure rather than respiratory failure is more common in acute high-level SCI. Respiratory failure and impaired gas exchange, however, can occur as well with bulbar involvement, atelectasis, pulmonary embolus, or pneumonia. After any complete SCI at the cervical levels, the coordination of the ventilatory musculature is lost.

During spinal shock, when paralyzed muscles are flaccid, the paralyzed abdominal wall moves outward rather than contracting to augment chest wall expansion. Paralyzed intercostals are drawn inward with inspiration. These paradoxical movements of the intercostals and abdominal muscles result in a significant drop in the efficiency of breathing (Mansel & Norman 1990).

When the diaphragm (injuries at C-4 or above) is also paralyzed and only the accessory muscles are available for inspiration, the abdominal wall is drawn inward with the negative pressure generated on inspiration, and the abdominal contents are both pushed and pulled upward. Therefore, the lungs cannot be inflated fully. Breathing in this manner is extremely inefficient and energy consuming and usually cannot maintain adequate ventilation for more than a brief period of time.

These changes in ventilatory mechanics are associated with changes in pulmonary function tests. Vital capacity, maximum static inspiratory pressure, maximum static expiratory pressure, inspiratory capacity, and expiratory reserve volume all drop significantly. Acute injuries at the midcervical levels can result in vital capacities less than 1500 mL and not infrequently require ventilatory assistance. Injuries at the C-4 level or above that result in bilateral diaphragmatic paralysis generally require long-term ventilatory assistance for survival (Mansel & Norman 1990).

Ventilator-dependent patients with SCI are sometimes classified as respiratory quadriplegics or pentaplegics. Respiratory quadriplegics have head and neck control and thus have some use of accessory muscles for breathing. Pentaplegics have no head or neck control or use of accessory muscles for breathing. Many of these individuals also have bulbar involvement because several cranial nerve nuclei extend down into the upper cervical spine (Stauffer & Bell 1978). With bulbar involvement there is also loss of upper airway protection, placing these individuals at high risk for aspiration of pharyngeal and gastric secretions.

TYPES OF VENTILATOR SUPPORT

Negative Pressure Ventilation

The iron lung was the first mechanical ventilator effectively used on a wide scale. The iron lung and a modified version called the Porta-lung are the most efficient of the negative pressure ventilators (Hill 1986). The body below the neck is enclosed in a tank within which negative pressure is generated. Passive inspiration is induced by the pull on the chest wall. Expiration can be augmented as well if positive pressure is applied, but more commonly expiration is allowed to occur passively.

The chest cuirass and the pneumowrap (pulmowrap) are smaller and less efficient but more portable negative pressure ventilators. The tortoise shell–shaped cuirass forms a negative pressure chamber over the thorax. It can be custom made by orthotists. The plastic pneumowrap, also known as the raincoat or poncho ventilator, forms a negative pressure chamber over the chest and abdomen.

These devices are most effective in individuals with normal lungs and normal chest compliance. Achieving a comfortable fit can be difficult especially in patients who are thin or obese or who have deformities of the spine or extremities. None of these ventilators can be used in a wheelchair (Hill 1986). They should not be used in cases of upper airway obstruction or significant bulbar weakness.

Positive Pressure Ventilation

Positive pressure ventilation offers several advantages over negative pressure ventilation. Ventilation volume, humidity, flow rates, and fraction of inspired oxygen can be accurately controlled. Positive pressure ventilators are less bulky and more portable. They allow improved access to the patient for medical and nursing care. They are also more effective in cases of lung pathology (e.g., pneumonia, abnormal chest wall compliance, or chest trauma). Positive pressure ventilators are most often used in combination with endotracheal or tracheostomy tubes. These devices offer the advantage of airway protection, especially in cases of bulbar involvement, but they may interfere with speaking and swallowing.

There are two prototypes of positive pressure ventilators: pressure regulated and volume regulated (Drinker & McKhann 1986). Pressure-regulated positive pressure ventilators deliver air for gas exchange with a stable pressure. The pressure in the system determines the tidal volume. The volume delivered changes if resistance to flow changes. For example, if there is a leak in the system, the volume delivered will be increased to maintain a stable pressure within the system. Conversely, if lung compliance decreases for some reason, the volume delivered will be decreased. Volume-regulated positive pressure ventilators deliver a specific volume of air with each cycle. These ventilators do not compensate for a leak in the system. Hence if there is a leak in the system, a lower volume of air is delivered. Variable leaks around tracheostomy tubes can be problematic and may result in hypoventilation during sleep with volume-regulated ventilators (Goldberg 1992).

Portable ventilators, which are smaller and lighter than stationary ones, and console type ventilators are available for use with wheelchairs. Internal and external batteries allow freedom of movement, including community mobility.

Volume- and pressure-regulated ventilators are usually used with intubated or tracheostomized patients, but they can be used with oral or nasal interfaces as well. Bach and Alba recently reported on 25 ventilator-dependent traumatic quadriplegic patients who were supported with noninvasive ventilatory assistance, including mouth intermittent positive pressure ventilation (IPPV). Twenty were able to have their tracheostomy sites closed (Bach 1991; Bach & Alba 1990b). Noninvasive IPPV will not be effective in cases of severe weakness of the oropharyngeal musculature or depressed mental status. It also may interfere with the use of mouth wands. Aerophagia and abdominal distension are occasionally problematic.

Diaphragmatic Assist Devices

There are two devices in use today that assist ventilation by augmenting diaphragmatic movement: the pneumobelt, also known as the intermittent abdominal pressure ventilator (IAPV), and the rocking bed (Hill 1986).

The pneumobelt consists of a motorized inflatable bladder secured over the abdomen. The bladder alternately expands and contracts as air is forced into and released from it. The abdomen is thus intermittently compressed, causing passive movement of the diaphragm upward and augmenting expiration (exhalation). Deflation of the bladder allows the diaphragm to descend passively and the rib cage to expand by elastic recoil. With the pneumobelt, inhalation is largely passive and dependent on gravity; hence the device is effective only when used in the sitting or standing position. The pneumobelt has been used successfully by patients with SCI who previously used tracheostomy-dependent means of ventilatory support (Bach 1991).

The rocking bed is a motorized bed that moves continuously in the longitudinal plane. When the head is higher than the rest of the body, the diaphragm is passively pulled down by gravity, and inhalation is assisted. When the head is lower than the rest of the body, gravity pulls the abdominal contents cephalad and passively assists expiration.

Phrenic Nerve Pacing

Phrenic nerve stimulation was first used for ventilatory insufficiency in the late 1940s. A technique of radiofrequency electrophrenic respiration was first described in 1968 (Sharkey et al. 1989). This system has since been successfully used in hundreds of patients with chronic respiratory failure, including many with ventilator-dependent SCI (Lee et al. 1989).

Phrenic pacing causes inhalation by inducing a contraction of the diaphragm through electrical stimulation of the phrenic nerve(s). A stimulating electrode is surgically placed on the phrenic nerve. Each stimulating electrode is attached to a radiofrequency receiver, which is also implanted subcutaneously. A small external transmitter supplies electrical power and stimulus through the intact skin via magnetic coupling with a loop-shaped antenna placed over the receiver. The transmitter produces a coded signal that is transmitted to the subcutaneous receiver and induces a series of electrical impulses to the phrenic nerve. Each train of impulses causes movement of the hemidiaphragm.

Diaphragmatic pacing is effective only when the lower motor neurons of the phrenic nerve are intact. Therefore, it may not be effective in cases of injury at the C3–5 levels. Function of the phrenic nerve can be verified via observation under fluoroscopy, measurement of phrenic nerve conduction and latency, and visualization of contraction of a hemidiaphragm at the costal insertion of the muscle when the phrenic nerve is stimulated.

High-intensity stimulation causes fatigue of the phrenic nerve and myopathic changes in the diaphragm. Low-frequency pulses and rates of stimulation with bilateral pacing produce larger minute volumes and improved air mixing at a lower intensity of stimulation.

Implantation of a pacing system is usually delayed until any spontaneous recovery is complete. Pacing is initiated gradually for the diaphragm to develop the endurance necessary for full-time stimulation. The pulse frequency can be lowered gradually as the strength and endurance of the diaphragm improve.

Advantages of electrophrenic respiration include improved cosmesis, less bulky and heavy equipment, and improved voicing. Families find phrenic pacers less intimidating than positive pressure ventilators (Lee et al. 1989). Problems with phrenic nerve pacing include a significant risk of system failure, risk of phrenic nerve damage during electrode implantation, and scarring and fibrosis around the electrodes (Sharkey et al. 1989). As with negative pressure devices, an adequate upper airway is necessary and should be verified by bronchoscopy.

VENTILATOR WEANING AND INTERVENTIONS TO IMPROVE VENTILATORY FUNCTION

A significant percentage of patients who initially present with ventilatory compromise due to high cervical SCI do not require long-term mechanical assistance for survival (Mansel & Norman 1990; McMichan et al. 1980; Wicks & Menter 1986). After experiencing an acute drop in vital capacity and other measures at the time of injury, many individuals with cervical SCI experience an improvement in ventilatory function over the first weeks to months after the injury. Wicks and Menter (1986) found that most of those who were weaned from ventilatory support developed a mean vital capacity of almost 2,000 mL. Those who remained ventilator dependent did not achieve an adequate vital capacity. Mechanisms of improvement in pulmonary function probably include neurologic recovery as swelling and posttraumatic inflammation within the injured spinal cord resolve; the development of spasticity and the recovery of stretch reflexes in the abdominal and intercostal segments, which help the diaphragm work more efficiently by stabilizing the rib cage; and recruitment of accessory muscles of the neck and upper chest to augment elevation of the rib cage and chest wall expansion (Mansel & Norman 1990).

Although ventilatory function initially may improve over time, some individuals develop progressive ventilatory fail-

ure, especially with advancing age, or experience recurrent pulmonary complications after weaning (Bach 1993). Others develop chronic alveolar hypoventilation from nocturnal respiratory insufficiency (Bach & Alba 1990a). Therefore, patients with ventilator-dependent SCI require close follow-up and periodic reassessment of their ventilatory and respiratory status. Also, medical management of individuals with high cervical SCI requires familiarity with means to preserve, improve, or augment ventilatory function.

Rest

When muscle mass is marginal for the daily work of breathing, periodic rest and ventilatory support may be necessary. Some individuals require support during times of illness, when the work of breathing is increased; others require intermittent rest during the day or may utilize nighttime ventilatory support (Hill 1986; Splaingard et al. 1985).

Positioning

Although vital capacity is lower in the supine than in the upright position in normal individuals, inspiratory capacity and tidal volume are improved in the supine position in persons with quadriplegia. The abdominal contents displace the diaphragm cephalad into a mechanically more efficient position of relative stretch. The diaphragm is stretched more by the pressure of the abdominal organs, but the abdominal contents provide less resistance in the supine than in the upright position and allow more diaphragmatic excursion (Mansel & Norman 1990).

Strengthening Exercises

Individuals with quadriplegia have reduced muscle mass available for the work of breathing. Therefore, they are susceptible to fatigue. The contractile force (strength) and resistance to fatigue (endurance) of muscles can improve with training, however. Gross et al. (1980) found that an exercise training program using inspiratory resistance improved ventilatory function in a group of quadriplegic patients. These findings have been confirmed in subsequent studies (Mansel & Norman 1990).

Glossopharyngeal Breathing

Accessory muscles can be used to increase inspiratory volumes dramatically via a technique known as glossopharyngeal or frog breathing. First described in the late 1940s, it has since been used effectively by hundreds of individuals with polio, SCI, and other neurologic disorders affecting ventilation. The lips, mouth, tongue, soft palate, pharynx, and larynx are used repetitively as a pump to force air into the lungs. By closure of the larynx, air is trapped within the lungs. Frog breathing can be used to help clear secretions, to augment expiration by increasing the stretch of the chest wall and thereby increasing the elastic recoil of the chest, and to provide free time off the ventilator for minutes to hours (Dail et al. 1955; Donovan & Taylor 1973). It has been used successfully in children as young as 3 years of age (Gilgoff et al. 1988).

Medication

Aminophylline may improve diaphragmatic contractility and fatigue resistance (Aubier et al. 1981). Inhaled bronchodilators have also improved pulmonary function in cervical SCI, even in patients without a history of reactive airway disease (Spungen et al. 1993). This effect may be related to unopposed parasympathetic tone causing bronchial smooth muscle constriction.

Corsets

An abdominal corset may improve vital capacity, inspiratory capacity, and tidal volume by supporting the abdominal contents and thereby elevating the diaphragm and positioning it in a mechanically advantageous position (Mahoney 1979).

Assisted Cough

Among the causes of respiratory failure in high-level SCI is the inability to cough and clear secretions. Maximum expiratory pressure, a measure of expiratory function, is greatly reduced in patients with high-level SCI (McMichan et al. 1980). Manually assisted coughing, the practice of pushing upward on the abdomen forcefully to augment expiration after a full inspiration, has been in use for decades to compensate for this difficulty. Manually assisted coughing may be more effective than tracheal suctioning for removing airway secretions (Bach et al. 1993).

A study using functional electrical stimulation (FES) of abdominal wall muscles found that FES significantly increased the maximal expiratory pressure in a group of patients with cervical SCI. Manually assisted cough was more effective, however (Linder 1993). Mechanical exsufflation devices have been used by polio patients for years. Bach et al. (1993) recently reviewed the use of manually assisted cough and mechanical insufflation-exsufflation (MIE) in postpolio ventilator-assisted individuals and measured the peak cough expiratory flows with these techniques. MIE was superior to manually assisted coughing in that it produced air flow and velocity more comparable with those in normal coughing with less abdominal and intrathoracic pressure.

Nutrition

The extremes of obesity and emaciation are not uncommon among ventilator-dependent patients with quadriplegia. Either extreme can have an adverse effect on ventilatory function. Malnutrition can cause muscle weakness and increased susceptibility to infections. Hypercalcemia, a complication encountered especially among teenage patients with SCI, can cause muscle weakness and can transiently interfere with respiratory function.

SELECTION OF APPROPRIATE VENTILATORY SUPPORT

Endotracheal intubation with subsequent tracheostomy is typically used in acute respiratory failure of any cause, including SCI, and is necessary for airway protection in cases of bulbar or oropharyngeal weakness. Hence it has been customary to use tracheostomies with phrenic pacing and/or volume-regulated ventilators among persons with SCI and ventilatory dependence. Noninvasive means of ventilatory support, however, such as negative pressure ventilation, have also been shown to be effective in individuals with chronic SCI and have been used among these patients for decades (Bach & Alba 1990b; Donovan & Taylor 1973; Splaingard et al. 1985). Advantages of non–tracheostomy-dependent means of ventilatory support include more natural voicing and elimination of the hazards of accidental disconnection from a ventilator, mucous plugging of a tracheostomy tube, and other complications of tracheostomy such as tracheomalacia or tracheal stenosis. Noninvasive means of ventilatory support may also be less expensive than electrophrenic respiration or positive pressure ventilation via tracheostomy (Bach & Alba 1990b).

A pneumobelt (IAPV) may be sufficient for an individual who requires partial ventilatory assistance. A pneumobelt may become less effective as pulmonary volumes and compliance change with age, however, and can be used only in the upright position. Positive pressure ventilation via the mouth, nose, and oral–nasal interfaces (masks, etc.) are alternatives for part-time or full-time ventilator support (Bach & Alba 1990b). Negative pressure ventilation via pneumowrap, cuirass, body ventilators, or the rocking bed is also an option, especially for individuals who require only nighttime ventilator support.

COMMUNICATION

An effective means of communication is critical for any individual with high-level SCI. Voicing can be problematic in cases in which tracheostomy or endotracheal tubes are necessary, but several management options exist. Many individuals learn to talk around a tracheostomy tube by making use of a leak around the tube and timing speech production with inspiration rather than expiration. Fenestrated tracheostomy tubes and one-way inhalation valves (Passy-Muir tracheostomy speaking valve) attached to a tracheostomy allow air to enter the lungs via the tracheostomy tube but then divert it through the vocal cords and mouth during exhalation for voicing. Augmentive communication systems or talking tracheostomy systems may be necessary for pentaplegics with bulbar involvement and impaired oral-motor control or for those who require cuffed tracheostomy tubes. Electrolarynges and intraoral voice prostheses are also available (Levine et al. 1987; Manzano et al. 1993).

DISCHARGE PLANNING AND HOME CARE

Discharge planning for patients with ventilator-dependent quadriplegia must begin early in the rehabilitation process. The medical, physical, economic, psychosocial, and community needs of these individuals are many. Home care is not an option for all patients, but there has been growing recognition of significant advantages of home care, including economic savings. Before discharge, a detailed home care plan must be designed, including alternative caregivers, respite care, community-based health care, provision of necessary supplies and equipment maintenance, and community access.

The first criterion for discharge is medical stability. Adequacy of ventilation must be verified with the equipment to be used at home. Sleep studies may be necessary to rule out nocturnal hypoventilation.

Ventilator-dependent quadriplegic patients may require full-time or nearly full-time attendant or nursing care for safety. The patient, family members responsible for care, and nurses and attendants require detailed, hands-on training for management of any potential complications and must be comfortable using all necessary equipment well before discharge. A detailed home care manual must be prepared for reference and for training of subsequent caregivers.

The community must be prepared to support the individual with SCI as well. Local power companies, fire departments, and hospital emergency departments should be notified in writing of the patient's special needs and presence in the community in advance of any emergency that may develop. Back-up emergency generators may be necessary in rural communities (Goldberg et al. 1984; Lee et al. 1989; Splaingard et al. 1983).

The potential for medical instability in these patients is high (Goldberg 1992). Alarm systems are necessary because of the risks such as accidental disconnections, equipment malfunction, and mucous plugging of tracheostomy tubes. A back-up mechanical ventilator may be necessary, especially for individuals with no free time off ventilatory support. Patients who need long-term mechanical ventilation require ongoing reassessment to ensure optimal management and to avoid complications such as nocturnal hypoventilation. Ongoing case

Exhibit 13–1 Manufacturers, Suppliers, and Other Resources

Iron lung, rocking bed, cuirass, negative pressure generator, mechanical insufflation/exsufflation device—JH Emerson Co., Cambridge, MA 02140

Porta-lung—Porta-lung, Inc., Boulder, CO

Pneumobelt—Thompson Products, Boulder, CO

Vertivoice Communication Aid—Bear Medical Systems, Inc., Riverside, CA 92507

Passy-Muir tracheostomy speaking valve—Passy & Muir, Inc., 4521 Campus Drive, Suite 273, Irvine, CA 92715

Chest shell—Life Care International, 655 Aspen Ridge Drive, Lafayette, CO 80026-9341

Additional Resources

International Ventilator Users Network Directory of Sources for Ventilator Face Masks—Gazette International Networking Institute (G.I.N.I.), 5100 Oakland Avenue, Suite 206, St. Louis, MO 63110-1406

monitoring is necessary to ensure that support services remain adequate for home care.

LONG-TERM OUTCOME

The lifespan of ventilator-dependent quadriplegic patients is reduced compared with normal. There is a high risk of system failure and unexpected early death with all forms of mechanically assisted ventilation of persons with traumatic quadriplegia (Fuhrer et al. 1987; Sharkey et al. 1989; Splaingard et al. 1983, 1985; Wicks & Menter 1986). Information about the perceived quality of life of patients with ventilator-dependent SCI is limited. Glass (1993), however, recently reported the results of a survey of 6 ventilator-dependent quadriplegic patients and their families. All patients and their families responded positively to the question, "Are you glad to be alive?" Similarly, Whiteneck et al. (1985), in a survey of 30 ventilator-dependent individuals with SCI, found that quality of life was excellent or good in the majority of cases and that self-esteem was high. There were no significant differences in self-esteem or life satisfaction between patients who were ventilator dependent and those who were not.

CONCLUSION

There are many options for ventilatory support for patients with cervical SCI (Exhibit 13–1). The long-term survival and quality of life of these individuals may be improved with careful management, including periodic reassessment and use of noninvasive means to improve ventilatory function.

REFERENCES

Aubier, M., et al. 1981. Aminophylline improves diaphragmatic contractility. *N. Engl. J. Med.* 305(5):249–252.

Bach, J.R. 1991. New approaches in the rehabilitation of the traumatic high level quadriplegic. *Am. J. Phys. Med. Rehabil.* 70:14–19.

Bach, J.R. 1993. Inappropriate weaning and late onset ventilatory failure of individuals with traumatic spinal cord injury. *Paraplegia* 31:430–438.

Bach, J.R., and A.S. Alba. 1990a. Management of chronic alveolar hypoventilation by nasal ventilation. *Chest* 97:52–57.

Bach, J.R., and A.S. Alba. 1990b. Noninvasive options for ventilatory support of the traumatic high level quadriplegic patient. *Chest* 98:613–619.

Bach, J.R., et al. 1993. Airway secretion clearance by mechanical exsufflation for post-poliomyelitis ventilator-assisted individuals. *Arch. Phys. Med. Rehabil.* 74:170–177.

Dail, C.W., et al. 1955. Clinical aspects of glossopharyngeal breathing. *JAMA* 158:445–449.

Donovan, W.H., and N. Taylor. 1973. Ventilatory assistance in quadriplegia. *Arch. Phys. Med. Rehabil.* 54:485–488.

Drinker, P.A., and C.F. McKhann. 1986. The iron lung—First practical means of respiratory support. *JAMA* 255:1476–1480.

Fuhrer, M.J., et al. 1987. Postdischarge outcomes for ventilator-dependent quadriplegics. *Arch. Phys. Med. Rehabil.* 68:353–356.

Gilgoff, I.S., et al. 1988. Neck breathing: A form of voluntary respiration for the spine injured ventilator-dependent quadriplegic child. *Pediatrics* 82:741–745.

Glass, C.A. 1993. The impact of home based ventilator dependence on family life. *Paraplegia* 31:93–101.

Goldberg, A.I. 1992. The management of long-term mechanical ventilation at home. *Chest* 101:1483–1484.

Goldberg, A.I., et al. 1984. Home care for life-supported persons: An approach to program development. *J. Pediatr.* 104:785–795.

Gross, D., et al. 1980. The effect of training on strength and endurance of the diaphragm in quadriplegia. *Am. J. Med.* 68:27–35.

Hill, N.S. 1986. Clinical applications of body ventilators. *Chest* 90:897–905.

Lee, M.Y., et al. 1989. Rehabilitation of quadriplegic patients with phrenic nerve pacers. *Arch. Phys. Med. Rehabil.* 70:549–552.

Levine, S.P., et al. 1987. Independently activated talking tracheostomy systems for quadriplegic patients. *Arch. Phys. Med. Rehabil.* 68:571–573.

Linder, S.H. 1993. Functional electrical stimulation to enhance cough in quadriplegia. *Chest* 103:166–169.

Mahoney, F.P. 1979. Pulmonary function in quadriplegia: Effects of a corset. *Arch. Phys. Med. Rehabil.* 60:261–265.

Mansel, J.K., and J.R. Norman. 1990. Respiratory complications and management of spinal cord injuries. *Chest* 97(6):1446–1452.

Manzano, J.L., et al. 1993. Verbal communication of ventilator dependent patients. *Crit. Care Med.* 21:512–517.

McMichan, J.C., et al. 1980. Pulmonary dysfunction following traumatic quadriplegia. *JAMA* 243:528–531.

Roussos, C., and P.T. Macklem. 1982. The respiratory muscles. *N. Engl. J. Med.* 30(13):786–797.

Sharkey P.C., et al. 1989. Electrophrenic respiration in patients with high quadriplegia. *Neurosurgery* 24:529–535.

Splaingard, M.L., et al. 1983. Home positive-pressure ventilation. *Chest* 84:376–382.

Splaingard, M.L., et al. 1985. Home negative pressure ventilation: Report of 20 years of experience in patients with neuromuscular disease. *Arch. Phys. Med. Rehabil.* 66:239–242.

Spungen, A.M., et al. 1993. Pulmonary obstruction in individuals with cervical spinal lesions unmasked by bronchodilator administration. *Paraplegia* 31:404–407.

Stauffer, E.S., and G.D. Bell. 1978. Traumatic respiratory quadriplegia and pentaplegia. *Orthop. Clin. North Am.* 9:1081–1089.

Whiteneck, G.G., et al. 1985. A collaborative study in quadriplegia. Englewood, Colo.: Rocky Mountain Regional SI System.

Wicks, A.B., and R.R. Menter. 1986. Longterm outlook in quadriplegic patients with initial ventilator dependency. *Chest* 90:406–410.

Chapter 14

Surgical Options after Spinal Cord Injury

Judy Hill

Rehabilitation after cervical spinal cord injury should include consideration of surgical options to restore active elbow extension, grasp, release, and pinch. Since Bunnell (1948, 1949) suggested tenodeses and tendon transfers for patients with quadriplegia, the array of procedures used has expanded significantly. As experience increased with techniques, preferred methods were described in the rehabilitation and surgical literature. Lipscomb et al. (1958) reported their results with tendon transfers to restore hand function in patients with preserved function of the extensor carpi radialis longus and brevis, brachioradialis, flexor carpi radialis, and pronator teres. House et al. (1976) reported their experience with restoration of grasp and lateral pinch in 10 limbs of 7 patients. House and Shannon (1985) later reported their experiences with more than 50 patients and a comparison of two methods of restoring thumb control. Zancolli (1975) described his experience with 76 patients over a 25-year period who received surgical reconstructive procedures to improve hand function. Moberg (1987) reported his cumulative experience with 200 reconstructions, including hand grip and elbow extension restoration. Other surgeons contributing significantly to the body of knowledge regarding these procedures include Freehafer (1969), Freehafer and Mast (1967), Freehafer et al. (1974), Lamb (1963), Lamb and Landry (1971, 1972), and Lamb and Chan (1983). These cumulative experiences offer insight not only into the surgical options but also into consideration of the following:

- a method systematically to classify upper limb function
- timing of surgery
- expected outcomes
- postsurgical management

COMMON PROCEDURES

Exhibit 14–1 represents a summary of established procedures that have evolved over the years. Although the majority of the experience is with the restoration of thumb and hand function, the significance of the option of restoring elbow extension should not be overlooked. The ability to lift the forearm and hand against gravity aids greatly in performing self-care activities requiring overhead reach and more complete forward reach to retrieve objects. Elbow extension also provides necessary stability of the elbow after brachioradialis transfer to achieve active wrist extension. Lateral pinch is preferred to two- or three-point prehension because of the increased stability it offers and the frequency of use of this pattern in functional tasks. Irreversible procedures such as arthrodeses are rarely used.

CLASSIFICATION OF UPPER LIMB FUNCTION

A classification system describing both sensory and motor function has been agreed upon by surgeons performing the procedures. The classification stresses the importance of sensation for function by first grading the extremity as functioning with ocular afference if adequate vision is present. If two-point discrimination is present at 10 mm or less in the thumb, cutaneous sensation is present and is recorded as cu. Motor

Exhibit 14–1 Frequently Cited Surgical Procedures Used To Enhance Upper Extremity Function in Quadriplegia

International Motor Classification	Procedures
0	Posterior deltoid to triceps for elbow extension (Moberg 1975, 1987) Biceps to triceps transfer for elbow extension (Zancolli 1979)

1	Above elbow extension procedures
	    Brachioradialis to extensor carpi radialis brevis (ECRB) for wrist extension
	      (Freehafer & Mast 1967; Moberg 1975; Zancolli 1979)
	    Stabilization of thumb interphalangeal joint with Kirschner wire, resection of annular ligament
	      to release flexor pollicis longus (FPL) tendon over thumb metacarpophalangeal (MCP) joint, and tenodesis of FPL
	      to volar surface of radius for lateral pinch (Moberg 1975)
	    FPL tendon looped deep to flexor tendons to ulnar side of hand then proximally through Guyon's canal to volar radius,
	      where it is tenodesed to radius for pinch (Brand procedure described by McDowell et al. 1986)
	    Thumb MCP arthrodesis; FPL, extensor pollicis longus (EPL), and abductor pollicis longus (APL) tenodesis for
	      pinch and release (Zancolli 1979)

2	Thumb carpometacarpal (CMC) joint fusion, EPL and FPL tenodesis for pinch and release (House & Shannon 1985) Thumb MCP arthrodesis; tenodesis of EPL, APL, and extensor digitorum communis (EDC) to radius for release and brachioradialis to flexor digitorum profundus (FDP) for grasp; FPL tenodesis for pinch (Zancolli 1979) Brachioradialis to FPL (Waters et al. 1985)

3	Extensor carpi radialis longus (ECRL) to FDP for grasp and brachioradialis to FPL for pinch
	    (Lamb & Landry 1972; Lamb & Chan 1983)
	 ECRL to FDP for grasp and brachioradialis opponensplasty (Freehafer et al. 1974)
	 Two-stage Zancolli (1975)
	    Extensor phase: thumb CMC fusion, brachioradialis to EDC and EPL, flexor digitorum superficialis (FDS)
	      to intrinsic function/MCP stabilization (lasso procedure)
	    Flexor phase: ECRL to FDP, ECR (supranumerary) to FPL, or ECRB to FPL side-by-side suture or FPL tenodesis

4–7	Zancolli (1975) as above, adding pronator teres to flexor carpi radialis (FCR) to augment wrist flexion (group 4)
	 Brachioradialis to FDP, pronator teres opponensplasty for grasp (Freehafer et al. 1984)
	 Thumb CMC fusion, EPL tenodesis, pronator teres to FPL for pinch (House & Shannon 1985)
	 Two-stage House:
	    Flexor phase: ECRL to FDP for finger flexion, pronator teres to FPL for pinch, and brachioradialis-FDS graft
	      for thumb adduction/opposition
	    Extensor phase: EDC, ERL, and APL tenodesis for extension; free tendon graft for intrinsic tenodesis
	 Pronator teres, FCR, and ECRL may also be used to FDP for grasp (Johnstone et al. 1988)

8, 9	FDS lasso for intrinsic balance (House & Shannon 1985; Zancolli 1975)
	 Two-stage Zancolli (1979)
	    Stage I: brachioradialis to FPL for thumb flexion, side-to-side suture of FDP of index to the others, ECRL
	      to FDS to create active indirect lasso
	    Stage II: extensor indicis around FCR tendon to EPL for thumb abduction, extensor digiti minimi to
	      flexor pollicis brevis for thumb adduction

classification is based on muscles present with a grade 4 or 5 strength (Medical Research Council grades), starting with the brachioradialis (Exhibit 14–2). Using this classification system, a patient with only ocular afferent input and brachioradialis grade 4 but no other of the specified muscles would be graded 0:1. Patients without cutaneous sensibility generally are not considered for bilateral reconstructions.

EXPECTED OUTCOMES

With restoration of elbow extension, the ability to extend the elbow in gravity-eliminated planes and against gravity is expected. Although achievement of grade 4 or 5 strength is not expected, the ability to perform activities such as pressure reliefs using the arms to balance, reaching overhead to retrieve

Exhibit 14–2 International Classification of the Upper Limb in
Quadriplegia (McDowell et al. 1986; Johnstone et al. 1988)

Motor Grouping

0, no muscle below elbow suitable for transfer
1, brachioradialis
2, extensor carpi radialis longus
3, extensor carpi radialis brevis
4, pronator teres
5, flexor carpi radialis brevis
6, finger extensors
7, thumb extensors
8, partial digital flexors
9, lacks intrinsics only
X, exceptions

Sensory Grouping

0 if two-point discrimination is greater than 10 mm in thumb
cu if two-point discrimination is less than 10 mm in thumb

---

objects, and assisting with transfers is enhanced (Lamb 1987).
Results are dependent upon a closely supervised postoperative
period because these transfers are highly subject to overstretch
if the transferred muscle is mobilized too quickly.

With restoration of hand function, grip strengths of 4.5 to
10.0 lb and pinch strengths of 2 to 5 lb can be achieved. Although these gains may seem objectively minimal, they can be
extremely useful in self-care and vocational pursuits, especially when combined with other compensatory techniques.
Patients generally are pleased with the results, even after en-
during the postoperative period, when some independence is
lost (House & Shannon 1985; Lamb 1987; Moberg 1975).

The results of these surgeries are dependent not only on the
skill of the surgeon but also on the motivation of the patient.
Spasticity interferes with optimal results and may
contraindicate reconstructive procedures. The availability of
closely supervised and well-coordinated postoperative
therapy is essential to preserve the transfers after surgery and
to maximize the functional applications. Moberg (1975) suggests that poor results can be expected if the patient must remain bedridden during the recovery period and if the patient
has not understood and accepted the permanence of disability.

TIMING OF SURGERY

The proceedings of the 1979 International Conference on
Surgical Rehabilitation of the Upper Limb in Tetraplegia indicated agreement among the attendees that surgeries should not
be performed until 1 year in most cases and in any case not
sooner than 6 months after onset (McDowell et al. 1979). Repeated examination by the surgeon of both sensibility and
muscle strength is suggested to ensure that the condition has
stabilized. Moberg (1975) reported performing reconstructive
surgeries from 6 months to many years after onset. Hentz et al.
(1983) suggested that results are less predictable if surgery is
performed later than 5 years after onset.

POSTSURGICAL MANAGEMENT

All procedures involve a period of immobilization after surgery followed by varying periods of gradual mobilization. Too
rapid mobilization can result in overstretching and compromised function. As more active motion is allowed, the patient
begins to learn how to activate the transferred muscle to
achieve a new motion through muscle reeducation. Electromyographic biofeedback can be useful in this process. Because many patients are used to compensating for the missing
motions before reconstructive surgery, it is advisable for the
therapist to set up trials with tasks that incorporate the reconstructed function. For example, a patient might need to be encouraged to try reconstructed lateral pinch for holding a pen to
compare this method with writing with the penholder he or she
was using before surgery.

Hand procedures generally require immobilization for up to
3 weeks. After that, gradual mobilization and graded active
exercise are introduced. Overstretching is carefully avoided
for the first 3 months, and night splinting is sometimes used to
maintain transfer tightness.

The recovery process with restoration of elbow extension is
more exacting. Immobilization occurs for 6 weeks. Gradual
mobilization is then introduced in increments of 10° per week
(Moberg 1975) until 90° of flexion is achieved. Once 90° of
flexion is achieved in this manner, day splinting is discontinued, but night splinting in extension is continued. Lamb
(1987) introduces extension against gravity when 60° is
achieved and resistance at 75° of flexion.

REFERENCES

Bunnell, S. 1948. *Surgery of the hand.* 2d ed. Philadelphia, Pa.: Lippincott:
388–395.

Bunnell, S. 1949. "Tendon transfers in the hand and forearm." In *Instructional
course lectures,* ed. American Academy of Orthopedic Surgeons, 106–
112. Ann Arbor, Mich.: Edwards.

Freehafer, A.A. 1969. Care of hands in spinal cord injuries. *Paraplegia*
7:118–129.

Freehafer, A.A., and W.A. Mast. 1967. Transfer of the brachioradialis to improve wrist extension in high spinal cord injury. *J. Bone Joint Surg. Am.*
49:648–652.

Freehafer, A.A., et al. 1974. Tendon transfers to improve grasp after injuries to the cervical spinal cord. *J. Bone Joint Surg. Am.* 56:951–959.

Freehafer, A.A., et al. 1984. Tendon transfer for the restoration of upper limb function after a cervical spinal cord injury. *J. Hand Surg.* 9:887–893.

Hentz, V.R., et al. 1983. Upper limb reconstruction in quadriplegia: Functional assessment and proposed treatment modifications. *J. Hand Surg.* 8:119–130.

House, J.H., and M.A. Shannon. 1985. Restoration of strong grasp and lateral pinch in tetraplegia—A comparison of two methods of thumb control in each patient. *J. Hand Surg.* 10:21–29.

House, J.H., et al. 1976. Restoration of strong grasp and lateral pinch in tetraplegia due to cervical spinal cord injury. *J. Hand Surg.* 1:152–159.

Johnstone, B.R., et al. 1988. A review of surgical rehabilitation of the upper limb in quadriplegia. *Paraplegia* 26:317–339.

Lamb, D.W. 1963. "The management of upper limbs in cervical cord injuries." In *Proceedings of Symposium, Royal College of Surgeons of Edinburgh,* ed. Morrison and Gibb, Edinburgh, Scotland.

Lamb, D.W. 1987. "The upper limb and hand in traumatic tetraplegia." In *The paralyzed hand,* ed. D.W. Lamb, 136–152. New York, N.Y.: Churchill Livingstone.

Lamb, D.W., and K.M. Chan. 1983. Surgical reconstruction of the upper limb in traumatic tetraplegia. A review of 41 patients. *J. Bone Joint Surg. Br.* 65:291–298.

Lamb, D.W., and R. Landry. 1971. The hand in quadriplegia. *Hand* 3:31–37.

Lamb, D.W., and R.M. Landry. 1972. The hand in quadriplegia. *Paraplegia* 9:204–212.

Lipscomb, P.R., et al. 1958. Tendon transfers to restore function of hands in tetraplegia, especially after fracture dislocation of sixth cervical vertebra on the seventh. *J. Bone Joint Surg. Am.* 40:1071–1080.

McDowell, C.L., et al. 1979. International Conference on Surgical Rehabilitation of the Upper Limb in Tetraplegia. *J. Hand Surg.* 4:387–390.

McDowell, C.L., et al. 1986. The second International Conference on Surgical Rehabilitation of the Upper Limb in Tetraplegia (Quadriplegia). *J. Hand Surg.* 11:604–608.

Moberg, E. 1975. Surgical treatment for absent single hand grip and elbow extension in quadriplegia. *J. Bone Joint Surg. Am.* 57:196–206.

Moberg, E. 1987. The present state of surgical rehabilitation of the upper limb in tetraplegia. *Paraplegia* 25:351–356.

Waters, R.L., et al. 1985. Brachioradialis to flexor pollicis longus tendon transfer for active lateral pinch in tetraplegia. *J. Hand Surg.* 10:385–391.

Zancolli, E. 1975. Surgery for the quadriplegic hand with active strong wrist extension preserved—A study of 97 cases. *Clin. Orthop.* 112:101–113.

Zancolli, E. 1979. *Structural and dynamic basis of hand surgery.* 2d ed. Philadelphia, Pa.: Lippincott, 229–262.

Chapter 15

Pain in Spinal Cord Injury

Elliot J. Roth

"Phantom body pain in paraplegic patients is the most mysterious of all pain phenomena."

Melzack & Loeser 1978, p. 195

THE PROBLEM OF PAIN IN PATIENTS WITH SPINAL CORD INJURY

It is an unfortunate irony that many patients with spinal cord injury (SCI) experience pain because SCI is most often associated with sensory loss rather than an increase in sensory phenomena. Spontaneous or elicited painful sensations in individuals with SCI are frequent and enigmatic problems for patients, clinicians, and scientists.

Although precise figures of the prevalence of pain in these patients are difficult to specify, it is estimated that between at least 33% and as much as 95% of patients with SCI experience pain as a complicating feature of their injury. Fortunately, only a minority of patients experience severe, disabling, and persistent pain, but for that subgroup the pain may be as disabling as the direct physical consequences of the SCI or even more so. In addition, the pain syndrome may be refractory to medical management; it may cause considerable discomfort in the patients who are affected and require considerable effort by professionals who are involved in their care. The complexity of the problem is exacerbated by several other factors, including the subjective nature of the pain experience, the multiplicity of pain types that exist in these patients, and the paucity of controlled clinical trials to test the efficacy of various treatment methods. As a consequence, diagnostic assessment may be difficult, and management is empirically based.

A number of excellent reviews exist on the subject of pain in patients with SCI (Bedbrook 1985; Burke & Woodward 1976; Donovan et al. 1982; Pagni 1987; Tunks 1986). The present chapter synthesizes the current and evolving understanding of the prevalence, clinical features, mechanisms, and management approaches of the various types of pain syndromes in these patients.

SCOPE OF THE PROBLEM

Prevalence

Reported prevalence rates of pain vary widely, with published pain frequencies ranging between 3% (Bedbrook 1985; Burke & Woodward 1976; Kuhn 1947; Schwartz, H.G. et al. 1965) and 94% (Botterell et al. 1953) of all patients with SCI. It has been described as both one of the major complications (Richardson et al. 1980a) and not a prominent feature (Munro 1950) of SCI. A number of factors, all of which are widely disparate in studies of SCI pain, affect the specific reported prevalence rates: differences in pain definitions, pain type studied, pain severity, study sample inclusion criteria, specific reporting center studied, and others. The average range of pain reported in the literature and the average estimated prevalence based on extensive clinical experience probably fall between one third and one half of all patients with SCI.

Pain was reported in many of the early published reports of care experiences of patients with SCI. These early reports are important insofar as they rely on simple empirical observations and provide a background perspective on the natural history of the clinical problem. In one of the first reports of the results of a systematic experience with management of a large series of patients with SCI, Davis and Martin (1947) reported that 82% of their 471 patients had spontaneous complaints of pain; in two other classic reports, however, Munro (1948, 1950) found pain in only 34% of 99 patients and in 31% of 224 patients at discharge from the hospital. Most of those patients had pain of nerve root type.

Specific definitions and criteria for identifying pain are important for determining the exact prevalence in these studies. The inconsistency of definitions among these reports contributes to the variation in reported pain frequency. This is especially important in view of the highly subjective and variable nature of the pain experience. A particularly important aspect of the pain definition problem is distinguishing true pain from unpleasant sensory disturbances and from nonpainful sensory abnormalities.

In a landmark study, Bors (1951) found that all 50 patients with SCI whom he studied had a variety of abnormal body and limb phantom sensations (but not necessarily pain) in their legs, penis, and other structures. Weinstein (1962) also reported abnormal sensations below the level of injury in all of his patients with SCI. Both these investigators emphasized that these sensations were more often described as a discomfort than as pain but that sometimes they were painful. Evans (1962) carefully recorded the body image disturbances described by 7 patients with complete paraplegia who reported pain, heat, and pressure but without distress. In an excellent and thorough review, Burke and Woodward (1976) noted the distinction between phantom sensations and phantom pain and stated that it was their impression that nearly all patients experienced these sensations at some point after injury.

Botterell et al. (1953) documented that 94% of 125 patients with traumatic SCI had pain. This is the greatest prevalence rate reported in any of the literature. Nepomuceno et al. (1979) reported findings based on results of questionnaires mailed to patients with SCI. They found that 80% experienced abnormal sensations and that 48% described the sensation as painful.

Probably the most useful prevalence figure was noted by Kennedy (1946), who observed that between one third and one half of patients with SCI will have some form of unpleasant sensory disturbances that are more or less persistent. Other studies include those by Kaplan et al. (1962), who found that pain was present on admission in 43% of patients with SCI, and by Zankel et al. (1954), who reported an incidence of 42%.

Even with consistency of observers, different centers have reported disparate results. Burke (1973) reported on the differences in his observations of pain in patients with SCI among SCI centers in Australia and the United States. Significant pain occurred in 14% of the Heidelberg, Australia, patients with SCI and in 45% of the Los Angeles patients with SCI. The investigator ascribed the wide variation in reported frequency to differences in spinal stabilization techniques, but

cultural, age, gender, and geographical differences and etiological factors may have played a substantial role in the findings. Likewise, a single report enumerated pain frequencies among patients with SCI in four Veterans Administration hospitals as 12%, 15%, 17%, and 50% (Veterans Administration 1948). Variations among centers (even within the same system), cultural aspects, etiologies, and possibly management aspects of the injuries may have accounted for these differences. In addition, it is possible that methodological factors used to study the problem may have varied among centers. Obviously this is an important factor because many of the results are dependent on the way in which investigators define, elicit, and report pain.

Severity

Two key methodological issues contributing to the diversity of incidence rates for this syndrome are the use of different definitions of pain and inconsistent inclusion criteria. These research issues are related closely to the important clinical consideration of determining which patients have pain serious enough to treat. The resolution of this question depends on the criteria for severity.

Probably only a minority of patients with SCI have pain that is considered severe or excruciating (Tunks 1986). For example, Kennedy (1946) stated that less than 10% have pain persistent or severe enough to require surgical intervention, and Munro (1950) reported that only 6% of patients had disabling pain on discharge from the hospital. A series of 637 patients (Porter et al. 1966) with cauda equina injury included 6% who required surgical treatment for pain. Kaplan et al. (1962) observed that 5% of patients with SCI have pain interfering with function. On the other hand, in the Davis and Martin series (1947) 27% complained of pain severe enough to impair function and requiring consideration of steps to be taken for relief. Botterell et al. (1953) described 30% of their sample to have severe disabling pain; 9 of the 38 persons with severe pain required surgery.

One of the best measures or indicators of pain severity was used by Nepomuceno et al. (1979). In their study, 25% of patients described the pain as severe to extreme, and 44% stated that pain interfered with functional activities. Some of the most revealing findings in that study were that 37% of the patients with thoracolumbar injuries and 23% of the patients with cervical or high thoracic injuries would trade the possibility of neurologic recovery, gait, hand use, and sexual, bladder, or bowel function to obtain pain relief.

Overall Prevalence and Severity Findings

The ranges provided by early investigators of the frequency and intensity of pain in patients with SCI are broad, reflecting a number of factors. This wide variety of proportions cited by these observers fails to provide a meaningful perspective for clinicians on the exact extent to which this problem affects the day-to-day functioning of the patient with SCI. A more specific range of numbers, however, can be elicited from both clinical experience and a distillation of the literature. In general, it is reasonable to estimate that between one third and one half of all patients with SCI have pain and that about 10% to 20% of all patients have severe, disabling pain. Only about 5% of the patients or less undergo surgery for pain, and most of those were reported in the early literature.

CLASSIFICATION SYSTEMS

Probably the single most important reason for the profound diversity in figures estimating the prevalence of pain in patients with SCI is the disparity among studies in the systems utilized to classify pain in this group. These classification methods are important because they help investigators and clinicians organize their thinking about the pain phenomena, to specify and communicate more clearly with others the pain types being evaluated, and to more directly focus treatment efforts. Little organization exists among the organizational formats, and Bedbrook (1985) noted that the classifications are confusing. Pain may be described according to its regional distribution (Botterell et al. 1953; Davis, L. 1954; Maury 1977; Michaelis 1970), its underlying neurophysiological mechanism (Bedbrook 1985; Donovan et al. 1982; Freeman & Heimburger 1947; Kaplan et al. 1962; Munro 1950), its clinical presentation (Burke & Woodward 1976), its temporal course (Bedbrook 1985; Botterell et al. 1953; Melzack & Loeser 1978), or its pathological concomitants (Bedbrook 1985). The first three of these are discussed below.

Classification by Location

One of the most useful classification systems is also the simplest method and the one based on common sense. Some observers organize thinking about pain in patients with SCI based on location of the pain; the three categories of pain are above the level of the neurological lesion, at the lesion level, and below the lesion. Prototype clinical syndromes of each type include musculotendinous shoulder or neck pain above the lesion, hyperalgesic bandlike sensations at the lesion level, and diffuse burning or tingling discomfort below the injury level. Michaelis (1970) formally reported on the applicability of this system.

Maury (1977) also used this simple scheme, expanding it to provide more information and therefore making it more useful. Supralesional pains include acute shoulder pain referred from abdominal viscera, painful stiffness of the shoulder, and the headache of autonomic dysreflexia. Lesional pains can be divided into hyperesthesia at the border zone, radicular pain, and cauda equina injury pain. Sublesional pains are noted to be the most numerous and consist of three types: pain by over-stretching of the vascular envelopes (related to posture), visceral pain, and pain from spasticity.

Two early reports (Davis & Martin 1947; Pollock et al. 1951) differentiated three types of pain: pain referred to the lesion segments (typical root pain), visceral or visceral-referred pain (cramping, diffuse, and vague), and pain that occurs distal to the lesion (diffuse, poorly localized, burning, tingling, or stinging sensation). In later publications, Burke (1973), Guttmann (1973), and Burke and Woodward (1976) concurred and used this system. Burke and Woodward (1976) noted that the diffuse burning pain below the level of the lesion was the commonest pain syndrome, an observation frequently made by others (Botterell et al. 1953; Davis & Martin 1947; Pollock et al. 1951).

Guttmann's (1973) review of disturbances of sensibility in patients with SCI included disturbances below the transverse lesion, those above the lesion due to tendinous or articular contractures in the upper extremity, those at or above the injury level due to root or segmental irritation (which include the nociceptive border zone reactions and the paresthesias of cauda equina injury), phantom sensations, and pain arising from visceral hyperactivity.

Similarly, R. Davis (1975) described pain arising from three sites, separately or in combination: pain at the site of trauma (from tissue injury to the vertebral column, ligaments, muscles, and tendons), pain referred from damaged roots (described as sharp, shooting, aching, and burning), and pain experienced below the level of injury (spinal cord dysesthesias with numbness, burning, tingling, and aching).

Classification by Clinical Syndrome

In his comprehensive review of pain in patients with SCI, Tunks (1986) divided pain syndromes in SCI into pain located at or above the lesion level (the pain of the spinal fracture, myofascial pain syndrome, and the mechanical strain from repeated limb overuse), nerve root pain, hyperalgesic border zone reactions, and central pain syndromes. The central pain syndromes can be further divided into burning diffuse pains, phantom limb discomforts, and viscerallike pains.

One recent report (Frisbie & Aguilera 1990) identified three types of pain: central, musculoskeletal, and syringomyelic. Melzack and Loeser (1978) also had identified three pain types, as suggested in Guttmann's (1973) schema; these were root pain (or girdle pain), visceral pain, and phantom body pain.

Waisbrod et al. (1984) grouped pain into three categories: lesional area pain (occurs late and has a mechanical character), projected pain (occurs early, is in distal body parts, and is unrelated to position) and triggered pain (provoked by trigger zone stimuli).

Long (1982) identified only two forms of pain in patients with paraplegia: pain of mechanical origin (including pain arising from facet strain or localized nerve root compression) and diffuse dysesthetic pain below the level of injury corresponding to the area of sensory loss (spontaneously evoked or exacerbated by movement or light touch).

Bedbrook (1985) noted the practical utility of classifying pain according to its time of onset: early (less than 3 weeks), intermediate (between 3 and 6 weeks), and later (after 6 weeks). He also identified three areas of pathology as a means of specifying types of pain: musculoskeletal, neural, and complications. He attempted to relate each of the specific pathological pain substrates to a certain time course; thus musculoskeletal pain was considered the major cause of early pain. It is related to bony, joint, and muscle strain or injury, usually in the shoulder and hand but also in the vertebral facets and intervertebral disks. Neural pains include the phantom sensations associated with deafferentation. Complication-induced pains include those caused or exacerbated by contracture, spasm, pressure sores, urinary infection, or psychosocial problems.

In contrast to these systems, Kaplan et al. (1962) identified six types of pain: musculoskeletal (of a dull and aching character in the abdomen and lower back, including vertebral and sacroiliac syndrome), visceral (vague, deep, dull aching sensation of abdominal fullness), root (girdlelike radiating pain of a sharp and burning or dull and aching character), sympathetic (burning), psychic, and phantom.

A Clinical-Neurophysiological Classification System

Finally, an organization system that is both highly practical and intellectually satisfying was developed by Donovan et al. (1982). In this schema, five distinct categories of pain are enumerated:

1. peripheral segmental nerve (including cauda equina) pain: onset of days to weeks; burning, stabbing quality; duration of seconds; worsens with rest; improves with activity

2. central spinal cord pain: onset of weeks to months, tingling and numbness quality, timing is constant, worsens with activity, improves with rest

3. visceral pain: onset of weeks to months, burning quality, timing is constant

4. muscle tension or mechanical pain: onset of weeks to months, dull and aching quality, duration is variable, worsens with activity, improves with rest

5. psychogenic pain: onset, quality, duration, and precipitating and relieving factors are variable

This system is important because it matches clinical experience and is easy to apply in the clinical setting. Moreover, each category within this system has a neurophysiological basis, as discussed in the original report. This system is used in this chapter with one modification: The similarity in quality, character, presentation, and treatment strategies between central and segmental pain makes it easy to combine those two pain types into one category called the dysesthetic pain syndrome (Davidoff et al. 1987a). A fair amount of recent attention has been directed toward the description and treatment of this syndrome (Beric et al. 1988; Davidoff et al. 1987a, 1987b).

DYSESTHETIC PAIN SYNDROME

Of all pain types, dysesthetic pain is probably the most persistent and resistant to treatment. It also is arguably the most common (Botterell et al. 1953; Burke & Woodward 1976; Davis & Martin 1947; Pollock et al. 1951). Typical characteristics of dysesthetic pain syndrome are summarized in Exhibit 15–1.

Quality

The most distinguishing feature of the dysesthetic pain syndrome is its quality. For this reason, the best way to learn about and understand this pain is to listen to patients' verbal reports of the pain experience. Naturally, the descriptions of the sensations, and therefore our understanding of the clinical syndrome, are shaped by the words selected by patients to communicate their experience. It is typically burning, tingling, shooting, and stinging in nature. Other commonly used terms are stabbing, piercing, crushing, aching, cutting, dragging, and drilling (Davis & Martin 1947; Davis, R. 1975; Krueger 1960). It is usually continuous (Davis & Martin 1947).

Waisbrod et al. (1984) provided a simple listing of descriptive words identified by SCI patients with pain. In descending order, these descriptors are dragging, burning, cutting, tingling, drilling, tearing, pressing, and pounding.

Riddoch (1917 and 1918, 1938, 1941) probably was the first formally to report observations of pain in patients with SCI; he observed the occurrence of what were called phantom sensations. Another early and eloquent account of this type of pain in patients with SCI, which is frequently associated with hyperalgesia, was provided by Holmes (1919):

> Those pains are usually more or less constant; but they may be excited, and are increased by all peripheral stimuli. Even the light contact of a finger or the touch of a wisp of cotton-wool evokes or aggravates them, but it is movement of the affected parts which is particularly dreaded by the patients; his arms . . .

Exhibit 15–1 Typical Characteristics of SCI Dysesthetic Pain Syndrome

1. **Quality**
   - Burning, Tingling, Shooting, Stinging, Stabbing, Piercing, Crushing, Cutting, Dragging

2. **Onset**
   - Two Thirds Occur within One Year of Injury

3. **Timing**
   - Tends to Decrease over Time

4. **Location**
   - Diffuse, Poorly Localizing, Asymmetric, Patchy Legs, Perineum, Back, Abdomen, Arms in Quadriplegics, Hands and Feet
   - Hyperalgesic Border Zone Reactions

5. **Predisposing Factors**
   - Any SCI Level
   - More Common in:
     Cauda Equina Injuries
     Central Cord Syndrome
     Incomplete Injuries
     Gunshot Wounds
     Increasing Age
     Increasing Intelligence
     Increasing Anxiety
     Adverse Psychosocial Situation

6. **Exacerbating Factors**
   - Any Noxious Stimuli:
     Smoking
     Bladder or Bowel Complications
     Pressure Sore
     Spasticity
     Prolonged Sitting/Inactivity
     Fatigue
     Cold, Damp Weather
     Changes in Weather

lie motionless, and any change in their position produces such agony that he fears to bring them into a more comfortable posture. Even a slight jar to the bed may bring on a bout of intense pain. . . . I have not, I think seen . . . any condition associated with such intense suffering. (p. 235)

Several reports quote metaphors provided by patients to describe their pain. Many patients describe the sensation as pins and needles, viselike, streams of fire, knife-twisting, shooting like electricity, or tingling after frostbite (Davis & Martin 1947). Other vivid descriptions reported by Heyl (1956) were of naked legs hanging out of window on a freezing cold day and snakes squirming in the buttocks. A report by Krueger (1960) noted the pain similar to that felt in frostbite or pain like the pressure of a knife buried in the tissues. Another set of descriptions comes from Guttmann (1973), whose patients noted feeling as if their legs were blown off or swollen to twice their size. More recently, Tunks (1986) noted that the sensation could feel like a knife stabbing, twisting, and withdrawing all at the same time.

Onset

Onset of pain usually is early, generally occurring within the first year after injury in the majority of patients; late onset is possible, however. For example, Nepomuceno et al. (1979) found that two thirds of the patients who report pain have onset within the first 6 months after injury and 90% within 4 years. Similarly, Burke (1973) stated that 60% of patients have pain onset within 6 months. Most other authors (Davis & Martin 1947; Guttmann 1973; Holmes 1919) agree that the pain generally is an immediate or early phenomenon. These findings closely match clinical experience in which most, but not all, patients who ever develop pain do so in the first year after injury. In their classic study, however, Botterell et al. (1953) said that pain onset may be either immediate or late.

Late onset may suggest occurrence of a significant organic cause, and a search for spinal, visceral, or other pathology may be initiated. Furthermore, syringomyelia should be considered a potential cause of late-onset pain. It should be noted, however, that for the majority of SCI patients with dysesthesias of late onset, no organic cause is ever identified despite a thorough search. In that setting, late onset of the SCI dysesthetic pain syndrome is the likely origin of the symptoms, and treatment should be instituted accordingly.

Timing

In general, there is over time a decrease both in the frequency and intensity of pain complaints and in the number of patients who report pain (Botterell et al. 1953; Davis & Martin 1947; Davis, L. 1954; Davis, R. 1975), probably for a number of reasons.

L. Davis (1954) and Davis and Martin (1947) observed that pain diminished as time passed from an 82% prevalence in the hospital to an 18% prevalence at follow-up. They hypothesized that the diminution in pain perception over time resulted from either an increase in pain threshold or, more likely, a receding from consciousness of the pain sensation by the patients. Lamid et al. (1985) found a 60% incidence of pain among inpatients and a 17% incidence among outpatients. R. Davis (1975) stated that the intensity of the burning and tingling sensations gradually recede in time, which he associated with increasing level of activity. Botterell et al. (1953) stated that the pain does not remit spontaneously; rather, the patients learn to live with the pain.

Whether the pain tends to decrease over time because of neurophysiological or psychological reasons (or both) remains a controversial subject. There is no question that preoccupation with other activities and distractions may be extremely effective in reducing pain complaints. Patients often report that the pain sensation still exists but that they do not fixate on it as much as they had previously. In addition, many patients learn to avoid potential precipitating factors such as medical complications that may give rise to the pain problem. Furthermore, many achieve pain relief with medications or other modalities that help them control the pain. In some, the pain sensations may fade away by some neurological cause that allows the pain to subside. On the other hand, in their questionnaire study Nepomuceno et al. (1979) found that 41% of patients with SCI reported that pain increased over time. Kaplan et al. (1962) had similar findings; although pain was present in 43% at admission and 37% at discharge, it was noted in 56% at the 1-year follow-up.

In a few instances, the late onset of pain or the worsening of the pain syndrome over time may reflect organic pathology for which physiological causes should be sought. Examples include intraabdominal visceral disease, osteomyelitis or other infection, ectopic ossification, osteoarthritis, contracture, spasticity, or others. A particularly important potential cause of late onset of pain is syringomyelia, which may cause functional motor or sensory losses in addition to the pain syndrome. It is important to recognize, however, that in most situations in which late pain develops a clear pathological cause cannot be found, and the diagnosis is SCI dysesthetic pain syndrome.

Tunks (1986) provided the best overall summary of the changes in pain frequency and severity over time; he stated that some improve and most persist, but only a minority of patients will have intolerable suffering resulting from the pain.

Location

The pain is usually described as diffuse, poorly localized, asymmetrical, and patchy (Davis & Martin 1947), often in the soles, legs, abdominal wall, and perineum (Davis & Martin 1947; Kaplan et al. 1962; Michaelis 1970; Nashold & Bullitt 1981; Nepomuceno et al. 1979; Pollock et al. 1951). There are rarely any clearly demarcated boundaries (Tunks 1986).

In a study of paraplegic patients, Waisbrod et al. (1984) found that the most commonly identified areas of pain included the legs (seen in almost all the patients with high-level paraplegia and in nearly half those with low-level paraplegia), back, feet, thighs, and toes. Also noted to be involved were the buttocks, hips, upper back, fingers, abdomen, and neck.

Likewise, in the questionnaire study of Nepomuceno et al. (1979) the legs were the most common site of pain in patients with paraplegia, and the arms were the most common site in those with quadriplegia. The neck, trunk, and buttocks were involved less often in both groups, and about 10% of patients experienced pain in the viscera.

Several interesting specific pain distribution patterns have emerged in these patients. Occasionally seen is involvement of only the feet or of the hands and feet together in a stocking-and-glove distribution. Often patients will identify the burning sensation only in the back, with or without radiation to the buttocks and legs, which may prompt a search for a spinal or myofascial type of pain. Another unique and interesting variant is the specific complaint of many patients with central cord syndrome who experience tingling or coldness in only the hands.

Patients with complete thoracic SCI are at risk for the hyperpathologic border zone reactions, bandlike sensations of burning and tingling immediately at the level of injury. In a few patients with quadriplegia who experience the same syndrome, that bandlike sensation may occur across an upper extremity dermatome, often involving the neck, shoulder, or even the forearm. This distribution allows this pain sensation to be mistaken for an above the lesion mechanical or musculoskeletal pain sensation.

Predisposing Factors

Most investigators agree that, although the dysesthetic pain of SCI can occur at any level of injury (Botterell et al. 1953; Davis & Martin 1947; Kuhn 1947; Munro 1950), this syndrome is seen most commonly in patients with cauda equina lesions (Botterell et al. 1953; Burke 1973; Davis & Martin 1947; Guttmann 1973; Munro 1950; Nepomuceno et al. 1979). It may be somewhat more common in patients with incomplete SCI (Cohen et al. 1988; Davidoff et al. 1987a; Donovan et al. 1982; Richardson et al. 1980a; Tunks 1986). The early report by Holmes (1919) indicated that the pain sensation was more common in patients with cervical SCI, but this observation has not been fully corroborated since then; it is seen with considerable frequency in the central cervical cord syndrome, however (Bosch et al. 1971; Donovan et al. 1982; Hopkins & Rudge 1973; Roth et al. 1990). Holmes (1919) also pointed out that the pain appeared to be more common in patients whose injuries were caused by gunshot wounds, a finding that has been replicated in research (Davidoff et al. 1987a) and in clinical experience.

Certain other characteristics besides injury variables may be important predisposing features of the pain syndrome. Richards et al. (1980) systematically studied the relationship between persistent pain in patients with SCI and demographic, medical, and psychosocial factors. Higher levels of subjective pain were found to be associated with greater age, higher verbal IQ, higher anxiety levels, and more adverse psychosocial situations. Interference with daily activities by the pain tended to occur in patients who were older, of higher intelligence, more depressed, experiencing greater levels of distress, and involved with more negative psychosocial environments. One early study (Mueller 1962) used psychological test measures to predict success of surgical measures in relieving intractable pain in patients with SCI.

A more recent report of the psychological correlates of pain in patients with SCI was published by Cohen et al. (1988). In that investigation, the quality and intensity of pain in 49 SCI patients with pain and 95 able-bodied patients with chronic pain in a pain clinic were studied using the McGill Pain Questionnaire (MPQ; Melzack 1975; Melzack & Loeser 1978) and the Minnesota Multiphasic Personality Inventory (MMPI; McCreary et al. 1979; Naliboff et al. 1982). When compared with patients from a traditional chronic pain treatment program, SCI patients with pain scored differently than general pain patients. MPQ results indicated that patients with incomplete SCI had intensity and impact of pain similar to those patients with complete SCI, but that the latter patients reported less severe pain. On the other hand, the patients with incomplete SCI had a less disturbed MMPI profile than those with incomplete SCI or the general pain patients. The data suggested that, although the pain may have been severe or disturbing to them, the patients with complete SCI did not make it their major or central area of focus; this was probably because the functional disability caused by the injury itself rather than the pain limited these patients the most. Patients with incomplete SCI, on the other hand, were less limited by physical losses. This meant that the pain syndrome, although not as severe in these patients, had more of an impact as a disabling factor.

Exacerbating Factors

Some of the most interesting clinical observations reported in the literature about SCI dysesthesias are the descriptions of which internal or external factors or events may precipitate or exacerbate the problem. In addition to important preventive and therapeutic implications, an understanding of these helps one evaluate the etiology and mechanism of the pain.

Any noxious stimulus may induce the pain or heighten its intensity. These stimuli may be either internal or external, and many of them are preventable or at least amenable to reduction. One frequently cited exacerbating factor is smoking (Botterell et al. 1953; Burke 1973; Burke & Woodward 1976; Davis & Martin 1947; Krueger 1960; Melzack & Loeser 1978; Rossier 1964). Poole (1945) reported on two patients who developed their burning sensations only when they smoked. Krueger (1960) described a patient with complete paraplegia who had no sensation below his lesion level until he smoked, at which time he felt a "waking up" feeling in his legs and toes.

Other noxious stimuli are important contributing factors as well. Among the most common are those that are direct consequences of the physiological alterations induced by the SCI.

These include bladder and/or bowel distension, infections, urinary tract calculi, pressure sores, heterotopic ossification, thrombophlebitis, and extremity fractures (Botterell et al. 1953; Burke 1973; Melzack & Loeser 1978; Rossier 1964; Tunks 1986). These same factors may make spasticity more pronounced.

The interaction of spasticity and pain is interesting. Spasticity may exacerbate pain, and pain may exacerbate spasticity (Botterell et al. 1953; Burke 1973; Rossier 1964; Tunks 1986). Many patients note that it is the spasticity itself that is painful and that reduction of spasticity (by physical or pharmacologic means) results in relief of the dysesthesias.

Although it is most common for patients to report that prolonged sitting, positioning in the same situation, or inactivity may worsen pain, some patients state that body movement, activity, or overexertion makes the pain worse (Nepomuceno et al. 1979). Abnormal posture may also play a role; scoliosis or leaning while sitting may make pain worse.

Fatigue is a frequently reported exacerbating factor (Botterell et al. 1953; Burke 1973; Davis & Martin 1947; Krueger 1960; Rossier 1964), as are anxiety, hostility, and psychological stresses (Burke 1973; Burke & Woodward 1976; Davis & Martin 1947; Krueger 1960; Rossier 1964). Several investigators have reported that both depression and excitement may worsen the sensations (Botterell et al. 1953; Davis & Martin 1947; Rossier 1964). Cold, humid, or damp weather (Botterell et al. 1953; Burke 1973; Davis & Martin 1947; Krueger 1960; Melzack & Loeser 1978; Rossier 1964) or changes in weather (Botterell et al. 1953; Burke 1973; Burke & Woodward 1976; Davis & Martin 1947; Davis, R. 1975; Nepomuceno et al. 1979; Rossier 1964) may make the pain worse. Patients with this syndrome are particularly sensitive to sensory stimuli, so that any skin contact, even light touch or a jarring of the bed, may induce or exacerbate the pain (Davis & Martin 1947; Krueger 1960).

Recognition of these factors is critical in pain management because so many of them are preventable or remediable. Early identification of these exacerbating stimuli, together with avoidance of them and prompt institution of treatment, may prevent or minimize the pain.

Recent Reports

In a carefully designed study conducted at the Midwest Regional Spinal Cord Injury Care System at the Rehabilitation Institute of Chicago (Davidoff et al. 1987b), 19 SCI patients with function-limiting dysesthetic pain syndrome were studied. Patients were included only if they had a history of burning, stinging, and radiating pain below the level of injury of at least a 4-week duration with initial presentation within 1 year after injury. All patients had failed conventional treatment for the pain, including therapeutic exercise, physical modalities, over-the-counter analgesic medications, nonsteroidal anti-inflammatory agents, and narcotics. All patients also experienced functional impairment as a result of the pain. This impairment was defined as the presence of disturbance in the sleep–wake cycle because of pain, inability to complete activities of daily living because of pain, or inability to comply with a therapeutic exercise program because of pain. Compared with the general cohort of patients with SCI, those with pain were significantly more likely to have incomplete sensory injuries (74%), paraplegia (84%), gunshot wound etiology (53%), and nonsurgical spinal stabilization (34%).

Previous diagnostic procedures that the subjects had undergone included electromyography (42%), radiography (42%), myelography (21%), computed tomography of the spine (21%), diagnostic peripheral nerve block (21%), contrast gastrointestinal radiographic series (16%), and radionuclide bone scanning (11%). None of these showed abnormalities other than those attributable to sequelae of the SCI. Previously attempted therapeutic interventions for this group included transcutaneous electrical nerve stimulation (42%), epidural stimulator placement (11%), biofeedback training (11%), acupuncture treatment (6%), and therapeutic peripheral nerve block (6%). Previously used pharmacologic agents included narcotics (74%), tricyclic antidepressants (53%), anticonvulsants (47%), aspirin (47%), nonsteroidal antiinflammatory agents (16%), and neuroleptic medications (16%).

All patients in the study underwent a battery of pain assessment scales, which consisted of the MPQ (Melzack 1975), the Sternbach Pain Intensity Rating (Sternbach et al. 1974), and the Zung Pain and Distress Index (Zung 1983). The most frequently chosen MPQ terms to describe the pain were cutting (64%), burning (58%), piercing (47%), radiating (47%), tight (37%), cruel (37%), and nagging (37%). The most common locations were lower extremities (84%), posterior trunk (63%), anterior trunk (42%), and upper extremities (16%). The pain was internal in 84% and mixed internal and external in 16%.

Mean pain ratings were as follows: Rating Index (MPQ-PRI)–Total, 32.9; MPQ-PRI–Sensory, 23.7; MPQ-PRI–Affective, 7.1, MPQ-PRI–Evaluative, 2.6; MPQ–Present Pain Intensity, 2.1; MPQ–Number of Words Chosen, 13.4; Sternbach Pain Intensity on the examination day, 60.4; Sternbach Pain Intensity for the past week, 70.5; and Zung Pain and Distress Index, 59.6. The relevant and significant aspect of these results is that all values equaled or exceeded scores reported for other pain syndromes, including toothache pain (Grushka & Sessle 1984), labor pain (Melzack et al. 1981), cancer pain (Graham et al. 1980), and other pain syndromes (Melzack 1975). These findings underscore the potential intensity and impact of this dysesthetic pain syndrome.

Another report focused additional attention on spinal cord dysesthesias. Beric et al. (1988) performed quantitative sensory and neurophysiological testing in 13 patients who complained of diffuse, ongoing dysesthesias with a burning quality below the level of SCI. This group represented 13% of the 102 SCI patients with chronic pain and 5% of all 243 consecutive patients with SCI. Nine stated that their dysesthesias were present from the level of the lesion continuously downward, and the other 4 had a free zone immediately caudal to the lesion level with dysesthesias from the waist downward. Nine patients indicated that the pain interfered with functional activities.

Perhaps the most striking result of this study was the relative consistency of findings on neurologic sensory and electrophysiologic examination. In the majority of patients, there was relative preservation of proprioception, vibratory sense, and deep touch sensation with an absence of pain and temperature sensation. The investigators speculated that it was the imbalance between spinothalamic and dorsal column system function that may have been an underlying mechanism producing CNS misinterpretation of residual peripheral input. Interestingly, the results of this investigation are virtually identical to those of earlier studies, which noted that section of the spinothalamic tract alone caused sensory disturbances of central dysesthesias (Nathan & Smith 1979; Pagni & Maspes 1972a, 1972b; White 1963) and that posterior column lesions were not associated with persistent central pain (Cassinari & Pagni 1969; Riddoch 1938).

Pathogenesis

The pathogenesis of central pain has not been elucidated fully to date, although there have been numerous theories proposed. A major area of controversy is the precise location of the origin of the pain signals: the periphery within the spinal cord or higher centers.

Much of the data to support a central mechanism of the pain come from reports that burning sensations persist even after amputation (Catchlove 1983; Pollock et al. 1951), local anesthesia (Mihic & Pinkert 1981; Pollock et al. 1951), cordotomy, or known complete spinal cord transection (Melzack & Loeser 1978).

Bedbrook (1985) listed the pathologic findings that he considered significant in the determination of the etiology of central pain; proximal changes occurring in the posterior horn cells, neuronal regeneration, scarring and gliosis, canal stenosis, and cavitation are present, any or all of which may predispose to or directly cause pain. In attempting to elucidate a mechanism for pain, Bedbrook (1985) observed that section of nerves distal to the lesion does not reduce pain; that sources of pain may be proximal to the lesion, as occurs with neuronal regeneration; and that loss of sensory input may, in fact, cause pain.

In his thorough review, Pagni (1987) listed nine proposed mechanisms of central pain:

1. irritation of sensory pathways
2. irritation of the sympathetic system
3. hypothalamic origin
4. summation and wrong integration of nociceptive impulses on a few nociceptive neuromas spared by the lesion
5. loss of an inhibitory mechanism damping nociceptive afferents
6. activation of alternative secondary pathways
7. activation of the nonspecific polysynaptic pathways pertaining to the paleospinothalamic system
8. abnormal firing pattern of deafferented central sensory nuclei
9. hyperactivity of deafferented nonspecific reticulothalamic pathways

The author noted that there probably was not a unique pathophysiological mechanism but rather that many mechanisms probably combined to work simultaneously to generate the central pain phenomenon.

Of all these proposed mechanisms, several have received considerable early and recent attention and are of particular note. Krueger (1960) listed several possible origins for the burning pain sensations: from within the intraspinal contents, from either intact or partially injured nerve roots, or from neuroma formation in severed nerve roots or at the proximal stump immediately above the level of injury in the spinal cord. Nine years earlier, Pollock et al. (1951) had hypothesized that the site of origin of the burning pain was the distal end of the segment proximal to the level of the lesion, which they based on the observation that application of anesthetic immediately proximal to the cord lesion caused the painful phantom sensation to disappear. Many other investigators have proposed that irritation at the injured segment of the cord or a painful neuroma at the distal end of the segment of the spinal cord immediately proximal to the lesion level may have been the source of pain (Botterell et al. 1953; Pollock et al. 1951). Mathews and Osterholm (1972) observed small neuromas in some nerves after SCI.

Many investigators (Davis & Martin 1947; Freeman & Heimburger 1947; Gross 1974; Lawrence 1980; Pollock et al. 1951; Procacci & Zoppi 1983) have implicated central sympathetic fibers as the anatomic substrates for the pain mechanism. Proponents of this concept assert that the afferent signals arising below the level of the spinal cord lesion ascend the nervous system through the sympathetic nervous system along the vascular tree, thereby bypassing the central spinal cord lesion. These pain impulses then enter the CNS at levels above the lesion. This theory would explain the vague, poorly localized, burning nature of the pain sensation because that is the way that the sympathetic sensory system operates. Persistence of pain after sympathectomy, however, argues against this proposed mechanism (Melzack & Loeser 1978).

Other proposed theories have included neuronal sprouting at the lesion level as a cause of pain, utilization of surviving subclinical pain pathways across the lesion level, and sensation resulting from abnormal transmission patterns through nerves that cross the lesion at the level of injury.

The model for central pain that appears most consistent with observed clinical phenomena and that is currently enjoying the greatest amount of scientific support was first put forth by Melzack & Loeser (1978). They proposed that pools or nuclei of pain-generating neurons known as central pattern generating mechanisms normally exist at multiple levels within the spinal cord, brain stem, and brain. These centers are tonically active and normally send pain signals rostrally to the thalamus and cortex; under normal circumstances, however, the signals generated by these centers are modulated (enhanced, decreased, or completely turned off) by multiple inputs.

The stimuli to the pattern generating mechanisms come from a variety of sources, such as descending tonic influences originating in the brain (cultural, personality, memory, or experiential factors), phasic influences from the brain (anxiety, expectation, and other emotional, attentional, or visual factors), visceral inputs, autonomic stimuli, tonic somatosensory inputs (trigger points or scar tissue), phasic somatosensory inputs (injury or noxious stimuli), descending brain stem–derived central inhibition or stimulation, segmentally derived inhibitory or excitatory influences, and others. The loss of some or all of these central or peripheral influences, as occurs during the deafferentation of SCI, may result in an increase in the spontaneous abnormal neuronal activity of the central pattern generating mechanisms, giving rise to the perception of the pain experience. The loss of the descending supraspinally mediated inhibition of the pattern generating mechanisms, for instance, might make it easier for otherwise nonnoxious stimuli (such as light touch) to trigger and send abnormal pain impulse-bursting patterns (Melzack 1975; Melzack & Loeser 1978).

This theory appeared to contradict a prevailing notion that peripheral mechanisms are important in the generation of pain. The concept that deafferentation may provide the necessary conditions to allow abnormal bursting patterns that evoke pain, however, is consistent with a number of clinical observations and basic findings. Important observations explained by this theory include the persistence of pain despite amputation (Catchlove 1983; Pollock et al. 1951) or peripheral anesthesia (Mihic & Pinkert 1981; Pollock et al. 1951), the fact that lesions at any level of the nervous system may be associated with these pains (Cassinari & Pagni 1969; Melzack & Loeser 1978; Tunks 1986), the relatively consistent failure of pain relief (and even some pain exacerbation) after neurosurgical ablative procedures (Leriche 1938; Livingston 1943; Melzack & Loeser 1978; White & Sweet 1955), and some exciting central electrophysiological data produced by Levitt (1983) and Levitt and Levitt (1981).

Levitt (1983) and Levitt and Levitt (1981) studied macaque monkeys with bilaterally symmetrical deafferentation syndrome after spinal lesions. They were able to demonstrate foci of abnormal neural activity communicated to the brain from deafferented sensory neurons at segmented levels in the spinal cord of those animals. In a more recent study of the human pain syndrome, Lenz et al. (1987) recorded single unit activity in the somatosensory nuclei of the thalamus of a quadriplegic patient with central pain. Those investigators suggested that thalamic regions that lose their normal somatosensory input through the deafferentation of SCI contain groups of neurons that exhibit abnormal spontaneous and evoked activity. Similar work was conducted by Loeser et al. (1968).

Although the central pain generating mechanism is the most attractive of the purported theories of central dysesthesias, it is important to recognize that a number of other explanations exist as well. It is most likely that there are many origins or mechanisms and that the clinical central pain syndrome is the common end product of a variety of diverse pathophysiologic events (Pagni 1987).

SYRINGOMYELIA

The subject of posttraumatic syringomyelia is handled in more detail in Chapter 11 and is discussed here only in the context of its potential relationship to dysesthetic pain sensations.

Syringomyelia, or cystic cavitation of the spinal cord, may be a complicating feature of SCI in about 5% of patients (Alcazaren 1984; Barnett & Jousse 1973b; Barnett et al. 1966; Dworkin & Staas 1985; Eismont et al. 1984; Griffiths & McCormick 1981; Jensen & Reske-Nelsen 1977; Rossier et al. 1981, 1985; Shannon et al. 1981; Vernon et al. 1982; Watson 1981; Williams et al. 1981). The typical presentation consists of a picture of progressive loss of motor and/or sensory function in an ascending pattern together with increasing spasticity and hyperhydrosis.

In addition to the motor and sensory changes, spontaneous pain, often of a burning and tingling quality, or other sensory changes may occur (Alcazaren 1984; Barnett & Jousse 1973a, 1973b; Barnett et al. 1966; Rossier et al. 1985). Indeed, pain occurring spontaneously or with coughing is the most common symptom (Alcazaren 1984). At times, these sensory alterations and pain precede the other signs of the disease by many years (Pagni 1987; Riddoch 1938). Initially, the dysesthesias are intermittent and scattered, but later they may become continuous, persistent, and diffuse. Clinical features of syringomyelia are summarized in Exhibit 15–2.

Electrophysiologic abnormalities can be detected (DiBenedetto & Rossier 1977; Dyro & Rossier 1985; Fincham & Cape, 1968; Glatzel & Grunes 1976; Schwartz, M.S. et al. 1980; Veilleux & Stevens 1987), but definitive diagnosis is made by magnetic resonance imaging of the spinal cord (Grant et al. 1987a, 1987b) or myelography. Treatment of posttraumatic syringomyelia is controversial (Barbaro et al. 1984; Logue & Edwards 1981; Rossier et al. 1985; Schlesinger et al. 1981). Surgical treatment with syringoperitoneal or syringosubarachnoid shunts may be effective in some patients (Edgar 1976; Vernon et al. 1983), although conservative management may be more appropriate in some situations (Watson 1981). One report suggested that surgical management improved pain most consistently, motor power less, and sensation least (Anton & Schwegel 1986).

MUSCULOSKELETAL AND OTHER CAUSES OF EXTREMITY PAIN

Musculoskeletal complications are major contributing factors to the problem of pain in patients with SCI (Exhibit 15–3). Musculoskeletal pain, also known as muscle tension or mechanical pain, is of a dull, aching character. It is generally aggravated by activity and relieved by rest (Donovan et al. 1982; Tunks 1986).

Exhibit 15–2 Clinical Features of Syringomyelia

- Progressive Functional Motor Loss
- Progressive Sensory Loss
- Increasing Spasticity
- Hyperhydrosis
- Bowel and Bladder Function Changes
- Burning, Tingling Pain

Exhibit 15–3 Causes of Musculoskeletal and Soft Tissue Pain in SCI

- Long bone fractures
- Myofascial pain syndrome
- Ectopic ossification
- Compressive mononeuropathy (e.g., carpal tunnel syndrome)
- Reflex sympathetic dystrophy syndrome
- Degenerative bony changes (e.g., bone cysts, osteophytes)
- Shoulder dysfunction (e.g., inflammation, degenerative changes, overuse, impingement syndromes)

Any pain-causing clinical entity that occurs in noninjured patients may occur in patients with SCI as well. Examples include long bone fractures, myofascial pain syndrome, and others (Tunks 1986). In addition, there are certain clinical problems that are seen with increased frequency in patients with SCI. Examples include shoulder complications, sacroiliac and hip joint dysfunction, heterotopic ossification, and hand pain from a variety of causes, including compressive mononeuropathy and reflex sympathetic dystrophy syndrome. Only some of these painful syndromes are reviewed here. An excellent review of the musculoskeletal and rheumatologic manifestations of SCI was published by Rush (1989), and the reader is referred to this report for additional details concerning syndromes not discussed in the present chapter.

Early Shoulder Dysfunction

The clinical features of the shoulder pain experienced by patients with acute SCI can be distinguished from the shoulder problems in patients with long-term SCI. In individuals who have had a recent SCI, soft tissue and periarticular pain may occur around the shoulder joint (Nichols et al. 1979; Ohry et al. 1978; Scott & Donovan 1981). Subluxation, bursitis, tendinitis, and adhesive capsulitis are possible. Radiographs are usually normal in these patients, reflecting the soft tissue origin of the pain. This pain may occur in both spastic and flaccid lesions.

Some investigators attribute the pain to improper transferring, positioning, or patient handling techniques (Bedbrook 1985), although there is no evidence to support this assertion. Furthermore, other investigators suggest that immobility, lack of exercise, and onset of contracture cause the shoulder dysfunction (Scott & Donovan 1981; Tunks 1986). The precise pathogenesis of the pain is unknown, but shoulder problems probably result from a combination of factors. These might include preexisting degenerative abnormalities (as in the rotator cuff), local inflammation, repeated local trauma, excessive traction with movement, vigorous stretching, muscle imbalance, soft tissue compression, and contracture arising from paralysis, spasticity, flaccidity, disuse, and misuse (Ohry et al. 1978).

The pain can be severe and disabling. The shoulder discomfort can interfere with performance of a therapeutic exercise program with optimal positioning or, more commonly, with sleep; unlike many of the other pain syndromes in these patients, however, the shoulder problems in most patients with acute SCI are amenable to treatment. In particular, shoulder pain usually responds favorably to proper positioning and upper body handling, sling use, range of motion exercises, and especially therapeutic ultrasound and nonsteroidal antiinflammatory agents. Often a combination of approaches is most successful in relieving the discomfort. Scott and Donovan (1981) advocate the use of positioning the shoulder in abduction, external rotation, and extension to prevent pain and contracture.

Late Shoulder Dysfunction

A considerable amount of interest has been directed toward the musculoskeletal problems of patients with long-term SCI (Bayley et al. 1987; Gellman et al. 1988c; Nichols et al. 1979; Wing & Tredwell 1983; Wylie & Chakera 1988) in the context of studying the changes of these patients as they age. These chronic-stage shoulder problems may be significant because of the altered mechanical stresses placed on the body of the patient with SCI. These stresses are especially prominent in the upper limb, which carries out extensive and strenuous activities as a weight-bearing structure in the patient with SCI. These are activities that the upper limb is not well suited to perform. The design and form of the joints of the upper extremity are not optimal for the types of activities for which most patients with SCI use their arms and hands. Commonly performed activities include transfers, wheelchair propulsion, and push-up pressure reliefs, all of which cause repeated trauma to the articular surfaces of the shoulder joint, the elbow, the wrist, and the hand.

Increasing recognition of the frequency with which these problems have complicated the lives of patients with SCI has resulted in a number of studies on the subject and the identification of the clinical syndrome known as weight-bearing shoulder (Nichols et al. 1979) or wheelchair-user's shoulder (Bayley et al. 1987; Wing & Tredwell 1983).

Nichols and associates (1979) were the first to apply the term *wheelchair-user's shoulder*. That group found shoulder pain in 51% of patients with long-term SCI who responded to a mailed questionnaire. They stated that the pain occurred secondary to overuse, wheelchair use, transfers, other muscular strains, and myofascial pain. Some patients demonstrated classic myofascial pain syndrome with trigger points around the shoulder girdle and neck. The investigators noted that the pain tended to increase with increasing time after injury.

In a well-designed and comprehensive investigation of the weight-bearing shoulder, Bayley et al. (1987) found that 31% of patients with SCI had chronic shoulder problems. That group identified most of the problems as rotator cuff tears and found that 45% of the patients had abnormal shoulder arthrograms. The most striking finding in that study was the measurement of intraarticular shoulder pressure during transfers. Using manometers in the shoulder joint during the activity, it was found that transfers elevated the intraarticular pressures to 250 mm Hg, which is much greater than the normal intraarticular pressure. The investigators recommended conservative management.

Similarly, Gellman et al. (1988b) reported a 68% incidence of upper extremity pain in 84 patients with paraplegia and a 30% incidence of shoulder pain during transfer activities. That group also found that pain tended to increase with time after injury, from 52% in the first 5 years to 62% at 10 years, 72% at 15 years, and 100% at 20 years. The most common cause of shoulder pain was found to be bicipital tendinitis.

Likewise, Wylie and Chakera (1988) studied only paraplegic patients with disability of 20 years or more and found that 32% had shoulder pain. This group differed significantly from others, however, in that they attributed the pain problem to inactivity rather than overuse.

Despite these differences, a few common features of the long-term SCI mechanical shoulder pain problem can be listed. The pain is more common in patients with paraplegia than quadriplegia, and it increases in frequency with increased time after injury. It usually has a soft tissue or periarticular site of origin. There may be bursitis, tendinitis, or a rotator cuff tear associated with the pain. Impingement syndromes are also possible. Radiographs may or may not be normal. Rest tends to help somewhat but is extremely impractical to employ as treatment in these patients, who are dependent on their arms to carry out most of their physical activities.

Compressive Mononeuropathy

Carpal tunnel syndrome has been detected at an alarmingly high rate in individuals with SCI. This is not completely surprising in view of the fact that carpal tunnel syndrome symptoms are produced or aggravated by both a sudden increase in manual activity and persistent or recurrent hyperextension of the wrist (Tanzer 1959). Pressures within the carpal tunnel have been measured during hand and wrist activities and have been found to be elevated (Brain et al. 1947; Gelberman et al. 1981; Tanzer 1959). Most functional activities performed by patients with SCI are done with the carpal tunnel in a position of maximum stress, and the problem is compounded by the recurrent trauma to the area by the patient carrying out those activities.

Aljure et al. (1985) reported a 40% incidence of carpal tunnel syndrome based on clinical findings and a 63% incidence of carpal tunnel syndrome based on electrophysiological evidence. It should also be noted that this study reported a 40% incidence of concurrent ulnar neuropathy at the elbow. Notably, that study also reported that the incidence of pain was related directly to the duration of the paraplegia; the incidence rates were 0% at 1 year after injury, 30% at 1 to 10 years, 54% at 11 to 30 years, and 90% at 31 or more years.

Gellman et al. (1988a) also conducted a detailed investigation of carpal tunnel syndrome in patients with paraplegia. In that study, 49% of the patients were found to have signs and symptoms of carpal tunnel syndrome, and that prevalence was found to increase with increasing length of time after injury. Manometric studies indicated that pressures within the carpal tunnel during wrist extension of paraplegic patients with or without the syndrome were significantly higher than those of patients without SCI. These investigators agreed that repeated trauma to the palmar surface of the hand and wrist from the activities of wheelchair propulsion, transfers, and pressure reliefs, superimposed on the recurrent need to place the wrist in the maximum stress position of extension, probably contributed to the high tunnel pressures and the high prevalence rate of the syndrome. Another, more recent study of compressive mononeuropathies in the upper extremities of patients with paraplegia was conducted by Davidoff et al. (1991).

Symptoms of the syndrome in these patients are typical of carpal tunnel syndrome and include burning and tingling sensations in the hand, which are usually worse at night. The sensation often follows a median nerve distribution but may be felt throughout the hand. Often there will be an association with activity or wrist position. Diagnosis is based on a combined clinical and eletrophysiological approach. It is necessary to individualize treatment carefully because of the heavy emphasis that patients with paraplegia place on their hands for functional activities. Any treatment method used must be instituted with a sensitivity to the patient's need to carry out mobility and personal care activities. Management modalities include immobilization, resting hand splint use, power wheelchair use, steroid injections, and surgical carpal tunnel release.

Degenerative Bony Changes

Abnormalities in the upper limbs of 50 patients who used either wheelchairs or crutches for mobility were evaluated by Blankenstein et al. (1985). The sample included 24 with hand pain, 16 with elbow pain, and 19 with shoulder pain. On X-ray examination, these investigators found bony cysts in 19, joint space narrowing in 14, bony irregularity in 6, osteophytes in 6, joint destruction in 5, and bony sclerosis in 3. It was asserted that the repetitive impulse loading induced by the physical functional activities caused these destructive changes. In the study by Bayley et al. (1987), 5 patients in the sample of 31 paraplegic patients with shoulder pain were found to have aseptic necrosis of the humeral head on X-ray examination.

Although few other formally reported studies exist on degenerative upper extremity changes, these problems are much more common than previously believed and are likely to prove to be major disabling factors for individuals with SCI.

Reflex Sympathetic Dystrophy Syndrome

Several scattered case reports exist on the occurrence of reflex sympathetic dystrophy syndrome in patients with SCI (Andrews & Armitage 1971; Cremer et al. 1989; Ohry et al. 1978; Wainapel 1984; Wainapel & Freed 1984). Although not a common problem, it can be quite troubling and disabling. Wainapel (1984) reported on two patients with incomplete cervical lesions who demonstrated reflex sympathetic dystrophy syndrome as a cause of previously unexplained upper extremity pain. Cremer et al. (1989) studied five additional patients with SCI who met clinical and scintigraphic criteria for the syndrome. Gellman et al. (1988c) reported the incidence of reflex sympathetic dystrophy syndrome in patients with SCI to be 10%.

The pain of this syndrome may present with a burning and tingling quality. It is associated with swelling and loss of range of motion in the hand and shoulder. A major clinical problem is delay in diagnosis because of failure to recognize reflex sympathetic dystrophy syndrome as a potential problem in these patients. Prompt treatment often results in gratifying relief and resumption of active rehabilitation and exercise.

Lower Extremity Degenerative Changes

The lower extremities of patients with SCI undergo numerous degenerative changes. In some patients, this problem can be a source of pain in the low back, pelvis, and buttocks. In other patients, these problems are nothing more than radiographic findings without clinical symptoms. Studies of the problem are lacking, but some information does exist.

Sacroiliac joint changes were first noted in patients with SCI in 1949 (Abramson et al. 1949) and have been reported extensively since that time (Abel 1950; Bhate et al. 1979; Hunter et al. 1979; Khan et al. 1979; Liberson & Mihaldzic 1966; Lodge 1956; Pool 1974; Wright et al. 1965). The prevalence of sacroiliac joint abnormality ranges between 3% and 85% with an average reported frequency of about 50% (Rush 1989). The frequency and severity of sacroiliac joint abnormalities have been thought to be related to three potential factors: the level of spinal injury (Khan et al. 1979), urinary tract infection frequency (Khan et al. 1979), and reduced patient mobility (Pool 1974). On the other hand, Wylie and Chakera (1988) report that only 13% of patients who were disabled by SCI for 20 years or more demonstrated abnormal sacroiliac joints on X-ray examination and that there was no relationship between these changes and spinal injury level, urinary tract infection, or activity level.

Likewise, hip joint changes have been reported in a few studies of patients with SCI (Baird et al. 1986; Wylie & Chakera 1988). In the study by Wylie and Chakera (1988), 70% of patients with quadriplegia and 37% of those with paraplegia developed degenerative hip changes. Inactivity, but not age or urinary tract infection, was related to the onset of these changes.

It is likely that most of these abnormalities are not detected because of sensory changes resulting from the SCI and because of the difficulty in imaging these joints satisfactorily. For these reasons, the reported incidence rates probably are underestimates of the true disease frequency.

VISCERAL PAIN

Contrary to a common belief among many patients with SCI and professionals, individuals with SCI can in fact experience pain of visceral origin. Unfortunately, this often is felt much later in the course of the precipitating event and in a much more vague and diffuse fashion than might otherwise be appreciated, but the sensation usually does get transmitted. The late and altered nature of the presentation probably contributes to the finding in older literature that acute abdominal catastrophes were responsible for up to 10% of the deaths in patients with SCI (Breithaupt et al. 1961; Dietrick & Russi 1958). Visceral causes of pain in patients with SCI have been appreciated for many years and reported by many investigators (Berlly & Wilmot 1984; Charney et al. 1975; Davis & Martin 1947; Donovan et al. 1982; Kaplan et al. 1962; Michaelis 1970; Miller et al. 1975; Pollock et al. 1951).

Mechanism and Clinical Features of Visceral Pain

Understanding the mechanism by which intraabdominal pain is normally detected helps clarify the physiologic effects of SCI on visceral sensation. Visceral pain arises from distension, spasm, ischemia, perforation, or inflammation of internal organs or from traction on the intraabdominal supporting structures (Charney et al. 1975; Miller et al. 1975; Procacci & Zoppi 1983; Tunks 1986). Small-diameter autonomic visceral sensory nerve fibers, which receive stimuli from large, overlapping sensory fields, send the pain signals through a diffuse, multisynaptic pathway into the sympathetic chain and then into the spinothalamic tract of the spinal cord. Peritoneal sensation, on the other hand, is more specific and segmental in its spinal cord input. In SCI, many of the more specific segmental connections are lost, but the diffuse and overlapping structure of the visceral afferent nerves might allow some pain impulses to be detected (Charney et al. 1975; Miller et al. 1975; Procacci & Zoppi 1983; Tunks 1986).

Clinically, the diffuse and overlapping organization of these signals results in vague and dull periumbilical or diffuse sensations of pain, discomfort referable to the abdomen, a bloating sensation, or referred pain detected elsewhere, such as in the shoulder. Frequently in SCI it is the association with other symptoms that suggests the nature and origin of the pain; associated reactions include increased spasticity, malaise, anorexia, nausea, fever, abdominal distension, changes in bowel function, and others. Severe rebound tenderness may be elicited, as may abdominal muscle spasm and hyperpathia of the abdominal wall (Charney et al. 1975; Miller et al. 1975; Tunks 1986). Normally, the sensations of various types and sources of pain may be distinguished from each other; thus the deep epigastric pain of gastritis may be distinguished from the burning sensation of cystitis (Tunks 1986).

The ability to make the distinction between pain types and origins usually is altered after SCI. The loss of sensation in these patients frequently renders historical features of intraabdominal disease unreliable, and the motor changes make findings on physical examination suspect. These physiologic changes necessitate the use of specialized testing to elucidate the cause of the pain. These tests might include fluoroscopic contrast gastrointestinal series, endoscopic evaluation, ultrasonography, and computed tomography of the abdomen.

Visceral Causes of Abdominal Pain

Gastrointestinal complications of SCI are discussed in more detail in Chapter 4. They should be seriously considered as potential causes of abdominal pain syndromes in patients with SCI.

A study by Gore et al. (1981) of gastrointestinal complications in 567 consecutive patients with SCI found 87 episodes of gastrointestinal disease in 63 patients. Slightly more than half of these complications occurred after the first month following injury. Specific gastrointestinal complications included ileus, peptic ulcer disease, gastric dilatation, pancreatitis, fecal impaction, and others. Another study (Berlly & Wilmot 1984) of major abdominal disease identified intra-abdominal pathology in 5% of patients with SCI during the first 4 weeks after injury. These problems included upper gastrointestinal hemorrhage, perforated peptic ulcers, and pancreatitis. Peptic ulcer disease (El Masri et al. 1982; Epstein et al. 1981; Gore et al. 1981; Kewalramani 1979; Leramo et al. 1982) and pancreatitis (Carey et al. 1977; Charney et al. 1975; Gore et al. 1981; Young et al. 1982) have received considerable attention in the literature in recent years.

Still other studies (Charney et al. 1975; Hoen & Cooper 1948; Ingberg & Prust 1968; Tanaka et al. 1979; Tibbs et al. 1979) have reported a number of other potential abdominal problems in these patients: abdominal abscesses, appendicitis (with or without perforation), gastrointestinal obstruction, diverticulitis, bowel infarction, and others. It should also be recognized that urinary tract problems such as calculi, cystitis, epididymitis, pyelonephritis, and urinary tract fistulae are possible.

In addition, it has been observed that cholecystitis and cholelithiasis occur more commonly among patients with SCI than in noninjured individuals (Apstein & Dalecki-Chipperfield 1987). Furthermore, gallbladder problems occur frequently in patients with SCI who would otherwise be considered at low risk for gallbladder disease had they not been injured. In particular, men and younger patients with SCI may have cholecystitis and cholelithiasis. This is important to consider as a cause of visceral pain in SCI.

A recent publication by Roth et al. (1991) reported on the association of superior mesenteric artery (SMA) syndrome with SCI, adding three patients to the five patients with SCI already reported to have SMA syndrome (Gore et al. 1981; Ramos 1975; Raptou et al. 1964). Patients with SCI are somewhat more likely to have SMA syndrome (an otherwise rare condition) than noninjured persons because of the presence of common risk factors, including prolonged supine positioning, rapid weight loss, and use of a spinal orthosis. This syndrome may be a frequently unrecognized cause of persistent abdominal discomfort, vague postprandial pain, and a recurrent sensation of abdominal fullness.

Most important in the consideration of the causes of abdominal pain is the observation that constipation and fecal impaction are probably the most common problems associated with abdominal pain in patients with SCI. It can be felt as a vague or dull ache throughout the abdomen, or it may be periumbilical. At times the pain may be of a crampy or colicky nature. It is often felt as a sensation of fullness or bloating. Physical examination is often unreliable in detecting this problem, and radiographic examination may be necessary. Bowel evacuation and institution of a regimen to help bowel regulation can alleviate and prevent recurrence of the pain and discomfort.

Nonvisceral Causes of Abdominal Pain

Musculoskeletal problems resulting in abdominal pain may often be mistaken for visceral problems because of the similarity in pain location. One report focused attention on the myofascial pain syndrome as an etiology of abdominal pain in a patient with quadriplegia (Schwartz, R.G. et al. 1984).

In addition, abdominal wall spasticity can be excruciatingly painful and often mistaken for internal organ pathology. The chest and abdominal wall muscles are skeletal muscles and, as such, may have as great a likelihood of demonstrating spasticity as the muscles of the extremities. Frequently movement or sensory stimulation will trigger a sudden phasic spasm of the abdominal wall musculature. This can feel like a squeezing or sensation of tightness and often is mistaken for a sign of visceral disease. Of course, in the diagnostic approach abdominal wall spasticity should be a diagnosis of exclusion.

The problem of differential diagnosis is compounded by the fact that reflex abdominal wall spasm may, in fact, be a sign of intraabdominal disease (Miller et al. 1975; Tunks 1986). Naturally, the prudent clinical approach is first to rule out intraabdominal pathology as the cause with physical examination and advanced testing as appropriate. A relatively benign nature, together with findings of a spastic abdominal wall on examination and a successful trial of management with physical methods or pharmacologic agents used to treat spasticity, suggest that abdominal wall hypertonia is the cause of pain.

Another syndrome that may cause abdominal wall pain consists of spinal cord dysesthesias, as described earlier in this chapter. For patients with midthoracic injuries, the hyperpathic border reactions may be felt as a burning, pricking, or squeezing band around the abdomen and back. The diffuse pain of the dysesthetic pain syndrome in patients with SCI at any level may be particularly pronounced in the abdominal region in some patients. These sensations can be confused with intraabdominal sources of pain.

Diagnostic Approach

The differential diagnostic strategy for abdominal pain in these patients should include first an approach to determine whether there is, in fact, intraabdominal visceral disease and, if so, to determine next the site of origin of the discomfort. To do so requires a high clinical index of suspicion, careful and meticulous evaluation, and, as noted above, reliance on specialized imaging procedures.

DIAGNOSTIC CONSIDERATIONS

In general, most SCI pain syndromes are diagnosed on a clinical basis. Many of the syndromes are classified by characteristics reported by history, including quality, location, onset, timing, relieving and exacerbating factors, and associated symptoms. One report, for example, described an expedient approach to classifying SCI pain using only pain quality and location as criteria (Frisbie & Aguilera 1990). Pagni (1987) provided a detailed list of methods to assist in localization of the lesion based on the pain distribution alone. On the other hand, the altered recognition of sensory phenomena in these patients makes the historical features and physical examination findings unreliable and suspect, necessitating the use of specialized testing in certain situations.

History should focus extensively on a description of the quality of the sensation. If necessary, some suggested descriptor terms should be provided. As noted earlier, location, intensity, duration, onset, changes over time, precipitating factors, and prior treatment attempts should be recorded. Physical examination should focus not only on a careful neurologic evaluation but also on potential internal causes or contributing factors for the pain. These might include acute or subacute intraabdominal processes, infections, mechanical factors, and others.

Specialized testing used in selected patients based on clinical judgment includes electrodiagnostic studies, radiographs, gastrointestinal series, scintigraphic scans, myelography, computed tomographic scanning of the spine or abdomen, magnetic resonance imaging of the spine (especially to evaluate for the presence of syringomyelia), diagnostic peripheral nerve blocks, and others as appropriate.

There are two critical components of the clinical approach to the diagnosis of the pain syndrome, both of which are often overlooked by clinicians. The first is the heavy reliance on the patient's description of the pain. Management of the pain has to be done as a partnership between the physician or health care professional and the patient. This means that active listening, taking patient complaints seriously, and enlisting the cooperation and collaboration of the patient are keys to successful diagnosis and management. The second important element of the clinical approach to pain in patients with SCI is the need to exclude serious complications as a cause of or a contributing factor in the presentation of the pain. Evaluation of the pain in the overall context of the patient and his or her presentation, together with the use of some of the specialized diagnostic or imaging procedures listed here, may help clarify the etiology of the pain syndrome.

REFERENCES

Abel, M.S. 1950. Sacroiliac joint changes in traumatic paraplegics. *Radiology* 53:235–239.

Abramson, D.J., et al. 1949. Spondylitis: Pathological ossification and calcification associated with spinal cord injury. *J. Bone Joint Surg. Am.* 31:275–283.

Alcazaren, E.G. 1984. Post-traumatic cystic myelopathy: A late neurological complication of spinal cord injury. *Curr. Concepts Phys. Med. Rehabil.* 1:15–24.

Aljure, J., et al. 1985. Carpal tunnel syndrome in paraplegic patients. *Paraplegia* 23:182–186.

Andrews, L.G., and K.J. Armitage. 1971. Sudeck's atrophy in traumatic quadriplegia. *Paraplegia* 9:159–165.

Anton, H.A., and J.F. Schwegel. 1986. Post-traumatic syringomyelia: The British Columbia experience. *Spine* 11:865–868.

Apstein, M.D., and K. Dalecki-Chipperfield. 1987. Spinal cord injury is a risk factor for gallstone disease. *Gastroenterology* 92:966–968.

Baird, R.A., et al. 1986. Non-septic hip instability in the chronic spinal cord injury patient. *Paraplegia* 24:293–300.

Barbaro, N.M., et al. 1984. Surgical treatment of syringomyelia; favourable results with syringoperitoneal shunting. *J. Neurosurg.* 61:531–538.

Barnett, H.J.M., and A.T. Jousse. 1973a. "Nature, prognosis and management of post-traumatic syringomyelia." In *Syringomyelia*, ed. H.J.M. Barnett et al., 154–164. Philadelphia, Pa.: Saunders.

Barnett, H.J.M., and A.T. Jousse. 1973b. "Syringomyelia as late sequel to traumatic paraplegia and quadriplegia—Clinical features." In *Syringomyelia*, ed. H.J.M. Barnett et al., 129–152. Philadelphia, Pa.: Saunders.

Barnett, H.J.M., et al. 1966. Progressive myelopathy as sequel to traumatic paraplegia. *Brain* 89:159–174.

Bayley, J.C., et al. 1987. The weight-bearing shoulder. *J. Bone Joint Surg. Am.* 59:676–769.

Bedbrook, G.M. 1985. "Pain in paraplegia and tetraplegia." In *Lifetime care of the paraplegic patient*, ed. J.M. Bedbrook, 245–256. Edinburgh, Scotland: Churchill-Livingstone.

Beric, A.L., et al. 1988. Central dysesthesia syndrome in spinal cord injury patients. *Pain* 34:109–116.

Berly, M.H., and C.B. Wilmot. 1984. Acute abdominal emergencies during the first four weeks after spinal cord injury. *Arch. Phys. Med. Rehabil.* 65:687–690.

Bhate, D.V., et al. 1979. Axial skeletal changes in paraplegics. *Radiology* 133:55–58.

Blankenstein, A., et al. 1985. Hand problems due to prolonged use of crutches and wheelchairs. *Orthop. Rev.* 12:29–34.

Bors, E. 1951. Phantom limbs of patients with spinal cord injury. *Arch. Neurol. Psychiatry* 66:610–631.

Bosch, A., et al. 1971. Incomplete traumatic quadriplegia, a 10-year review. *J.A.M.A.* 216:473–478.

Botterell, E.H., et al. 1953. Pain in paraplegia: Clinical management and surgical treatment. *Proc. R. Soc. Med.* 47:281–288.

Brain, W.R., et al. 1947. Spontaneous compression of both median nerves in the carpal tunnel: Six cases treated surgically. *Lancet* 1:277–282.

Breithaupt, D.J., et al. 1961. Late causes of death and life expectancy in paraplegia. *Can. Med. Assoc. J.* 85:73–77.

Burke, D.C. 1973. Pain in paraplegia. *Paraplegia* 10:297–313.

Burke, D.C., and J.M. Woodward. 1976. "Pain and phantom sensation in spinal paralysis." In *Handbook of clinical neurology*, ed. P.J. Vinken & G.W. Bruyn, 489–499. Vol. 26. New York, N.Y.: Elsevier.

Carey, M.E., et al. 1977. Pancreatitis following spinal cord injury. *J. Neurosurg.* 47:917–922.

Cassinari, V., and C.A. Pagni. 1969. *Central pain: A neurological survey.* Cambridge, Mass.: Harvard University Press.

Catchlove, R.F.H. 1983. Phantom pain following limb amputation in a paraplegic: A case report. *Psychother. Psychosom.* 39:89–93.

Charney, K.J., et al. 1975. General surgery problems in patients with spinal cord injuries. *Arch. Surg.* 110:1083–1088.

Cohen, M.J., et al. 1988. Comparing chronic pain from spinal cord injury to chronic pain of other origins. *Pain* 35:57–63.

Cremer, S.A., et al. 1989. The reflex sympathetic dystrophy syndrome associated with traumatic myelopathy: Report of five cases. *Pain* 37:187–192.

Davidoff, G., et al. 1987a. Function-limiting dysesthetic pain syndrome among traumatic spinal cord injury patients: A cross-sectional study. *Pain* 29:39–48.

Davidoff, G., et al. 1987b. Trazodone hydrochloride in the treatment of dysesthetic pain in traumatic myelopathy: A randomized, double-blind, placebo-controlled study. *Pain* 29:151–161.

Davidoff, G., et al. 1991. Compressive mononeuropathies of the upper extremities in chronic paraplegia. *Paraplegia* 29:17–24.

Davis, L. 1954. Treatment of spinal cord injury. *Arch. Surg.* 69:488–495.

Davis, L., and J. Martin. 1947. Studies upon spinal cord injuries. II. The nature and treatment of pain. *J. Neurosurg.* 4:483–491.

Davis, R. 1975. Pain and suffering following spinal cord injury. *Clin. Orthop. Relat. Res.* 112:76–80.

DiBenedetto, M., and A.B. Rossier. 1977. Electrodiagnosis in posttraumatic syringomyelia. *Paraplegia* 14:286–295.

Dietrick, R.B., and S. Russi. 1958. Tabulation and review of autopsy findings in 55 paraplegics. *J.A.M.A.* 166:41–44.

Donovan, W.H., et al. 1982. Neurophysiological approaches to chronic pain following spinal cord injury. *Paraplegia* 20:135–146.

Dworkin, G.E., and W.E. Staas. 1985. Post-traumatic syringomyelia. *Arch. Phys. Med. Rehabil.* 66:329–331.

Dyro, F.M., and A.B. Rossier. 1985. Electrodiagnosis abnormalities in 15 patients with post-traumatic syringomyelia: Pre- and postoperative studies. *Paraplegia* 23:233–245.

Edgar, R.E. 1976. Surgical management of spinal cord cysts. *Paraplegia* 14:21–27.

Eismont, F.J., et al. 1984. Post-traumatic spinal-cord cyst: A case report. *J. Bone Joint Surg. Am.* 66:614-618.

El Masri, W., et al. 1982. Gastrointestinal bleeding in patients with acute spinal cord injuries. *Injury* 14:162–167.

Epstein, N., et al. 1981. Gastrointestinal bleeding in patients with spinal cord trauma: Effects of steroids, cimetidine and mini-dose heparin. *J. Neurosurg.* 54:16–20.

Evans, J.H. 1962. On disturbance of the body image in paraplegia. *Brain* 85:687–700.

Fincham, R.W., and C.A. Cape. 1968. Sensory nerve conduction in syringomyelia. *Neurology* 18:200–201.

Freeman, L.W., and R.F. Heimburger. 1947. Surgical relief of pain in paraplegic patients. *Arch. Surg.* 55:433–440.

Frisbie, J.H., and E.J. Aguilera. 1990. Chronic pain after spinal cord injury: An expedient diagnostic approach. *Paraplegia* 28:460–465.

Gelberman, R.H., et al. 1981. The carpal tunnel syndrome: A study of carpal canal pressures. *J. Bone Joint Surg. Am.* 63:380–383.

Gellman, H., et al. 1988a. Carpal tunnel syndrome in paraplegic patients. *J. Bone Joint Surg.* 70-8:517–519.

Gellman, H., et al. 1988b. Late complications of the weight-bearing upper extremity in the paraplegic patient. *Clin. Orthop. Relat. Res.* 233:132–135.

Gellman, H., et al. 1988c. Reflex sympathetic dystrophy in cervical spinal cord injury patients. *Clin. Orthop. Relat. Res.* 233:126–131.

Glatzel, W., and J.V. Grunes. 1976. Results of electromyographical and electroneurographical investigations concerning syringomyelia. *Eur. Neurol.* 14:60–67.

Gore, R.M., et al. 1981. Gastrointestinal complications of spinal cord injury. *Spine* 6:538–544.

Graham, C., et al. 1980. Use of the McGill Pain Questionnaire in the assessment of cancer pain: Replicability and consistency. *Pain* 8:377–387.

Grant, R., et al. 1987a. MRI measurement of syrinx size before and after operation. *J. Neurol. Neurosurg. Psychiatry* 50:1685–1687.

Grant, R., et al. 1987b. Syringomyelia: Cyst measurement by magnetic resonance imaging and comparison with symptoms, signs and disability. *J. Neurol. Neurosurg. Psychiatry* 50:1008–1014.

Griffiths, E.R., and C.C. McCormick. 1981. Post-traumatic syringomyelia. *Paraplegia* 19:81–88.

Gross, D. 1974. "Pain and autonomic nervous system." In *Advances in neurology*, ed. J.J. Bonica, 93–103. Vol. 4. New York, N.Y.: Raven.

Grushka, M., and B.J. Sessle. 1984. Applicability of the McGill Plain Questionnaire to the differentiation of "toothache" pain. *Pain* 19:49–57.

Guttmann, L. 1973. "Disturbances of sensibility." In *Spinal cord injuries: Comprehensive management and research*, 2d ed., ed. L. Guttmann, 280–292. Oxford, England: Blackwell Scientific.

Heyl, H.L. 1956. Some practical aspects in the rehabilitation of paraplegics. *J. Neurosurg.* 13:184–189.

Hoen, T.I., and I.S. Cooper. 1948. Acute abdominal emergencies in paraplegia. *Am. J. Surg.* 75:19–24.

Holmes, G., ed. 1919. "Pain of central origin." In *Contributions to medical and biological research*, 235–246. New York, N.Y.: Hoeber.

Hopkins, A., and P. Rudge. 1973. Hyperpathia in the central cervical cord syndrome. *J. Neurol. Neurosurg. Psychiatry* 36:637–642.

Hunter, T., et al. 1979. Histocompatibility antigens in paraplegic and quadriplegic patients with sacroiliac joint changes. *J. Rheum.* 6:92–95.

Ingberg, H.O., and F.W. Prust. 1968. The diagnosis of abdominal emergencies in patients with spinal cord lesions. *Arch. Phys. Med. Rehabil.* 49:343–348.

Jensen, F., and E. Reske-Nelsen. 1977. Post-traumatic syringomyelia—Review of the literature and two new autopsy cases. *Scand. J. Rehabil. Med.* 9:35–43.

Kaplan, L.I., et al. 1962. Pain and spasticity in patients with spinal cord dysfunction: Result of a follow-up study. *J.A.M.A.* 182:918–925.

Kennedy, R.H. 1946. The new viewpoint toward spinal cord injuries. *Ann. Surg.* 124:1057–1065.

Kewalramani, L.S. 1979. Neurogenic gastroduodenal ulceration and bleeding associated with spinal cord injuries. *J. Trauma* 19:259–265.

Khan, M.A., et al. 1979. Sacroiliac joint abnormalities in paraplegics. *Ann. Rheum. Dis.* 38:317–319.

Krueger, E.G. 1960. Management of painful states in injuries of the spinal cord and cauda equina. *Am. J. Phys. Med.* 39:103–110.

Kuhn, W.G. 1947. The care and rehabilitation of patients with injuries of the spinal cord and cauda equina: Preliminary report on 113 cases. *J. Neurosurg.* 4:40–68.

Lamid, S., et al. 1985. Chronic pain in spinal cord injury: Comparison between inpatients and outpatients. *Arch. Phys. Med. Rehabil.* 66:777–778.

Lawrence, R.M. 1980. Phantom pain: A new hypothesis. *Med. Hypotheses* 6:245–248.

Lenz, F.A., et al. 1987. Abnormal single-unit activity recorded in the somatosensory thalamus of a quadriplegic patient with central pain. *Pain* 31:225–236.

Leramo, O.B., et al. 1982. Massive gastroduodenal hemorrhage and perforation in acute spinal cord injury. *Surg. Neurol.* 17:187–190.

Leriche, R. 1938. *The surgery of pain.* Baltimore, Md.: Williams & Wilkins.

Levitt, M. 1983. The bilaterally symmetrical deafferentation syndrome in macaques after bilateral spinal lesions: Evidence for dysesthesias resulting from brain foci and considerations of spinal pain pathways. *Pain* 16:167–184.

Levitt, M., and J.H. Levitt. 1981. The deafferentation syndrome in monkeys: Dysesthesias of spinal origin. *Pain* 10:129–147.

Liberson, M., and N. Mihaldzic. 1966. Sacro-iliac changes and urinary infection in patients with spinal cord injuries. *Br. J. Venereal Dis.* 42:96–99.

Livingston, W.K. 1943. *Pain mechanisms.* New York, N.Y.: Macmillan.

Lodge, T. 1956. Bone, joint and soft tissue changes following paraplegia. *Acta Radiol.* 46:435–445.

Loeser, J.D., et al. 1968. Chronic deafferentation of human spinal cord neuron. *J. Neurosurg.* 29:48–50.

Logue, V., and M.R. Edwards. 1981. Syringomyelia and its surgical treatment: An analysis of 75 patients. *J. Neurol. Neurosurg. Psychiatry* 44:273–284.

Long, D.M. 1982. "Pain of spinal origin." In *Neurological surgery,* 2d ed., ed. J.R. Youmans, 3613–3626. Philadelphia, Pa.: Saunders.

Mathews, G.J., and J.L. Osterholm. 1972. Painful traumatic neuromas. *Surg. Clin. North Am.* 51:1313–1324.

Maury, M. 1977. About pain and its treatment in paraplegics. *Paraplegia* 15:349–352.

McCreary, C., et al. 1979. The MMPI as a predictor of response to conservative treatment for low back pain. *J. Clin. Psychol.* 35:278–284.

Melzack, R. 1975. The McGill Pain Questionnaire: Major properties and scoring methods. *Pain* 1:277–299.

Melzack, R., and J.D. Loeser. 1978. Phantom body pain in paraplegics: Evidence for a central pattern generating mechanism for pain. *Pain* 4:195–210.

Melzack, R., et al. 1981. Labour is still painful after prepared childbirth training. *Can. Med. Assoc. J.* 125:357–363.

Michaelis, L.S. 1970. The problem of pain in paraplegia and tetraplegia. *Bull. N.Y. Acad. Med.* 46:88–96.

Mihic, D.N., and E. Pinkert. 1981. Phantom limb pain during peridural anesthesia. *Pain* 11:269–272.

Miller, L.S., et al. 1975. Abdominal problems in patients with spinal cord lesions. *Arch Phys. Med. Rehabil.* 56:405–408.

Mueller, A.D. 1962. Pain study of paraplegic patients. *Arch. Neurol.* 7:117–120.

Munro, D. 1948. Rehabilitation of veterans paralyzed as the result of injury to the spinal cord and cauda equina. *Am. J. Surg.* 75:3–17.

Munro, D. 1950. Two-year end-results in the total rehabilitation of veterans with spinal-cord and cauda-equina injuries. *N. Engl. J. Med.* 242:1–10.

Naliboff, B.D., et al. 1982. Does the MMPI differentiate chronic illness from chronic pain? *Pain* 13:333–341.

Nashold, B.S., and E. Bullitt. 1981. Dorsal root entry zone lesions to control central pain in paraplegics. *J. Neurosurg.* 55:414–419.

Nathan, P.W., and M.C. Smith. 1979. "Clinico-anatomical correlation in anterolateral cordotomy." In *Advances in pain research and therapy,* ed. J.J. Bonica et al., 921–926, Vol. 3. New York, N.Y.: Raven.

Nepomuceno, C., et al. 1979. Pain in patients with spinal cord injury. *Arch. Phys. Med. Rehabil.* 60:605–609.

Nichols, P.J.R., et al. 1979. Wheelchair user's shoulder? Shoulder pain in patients with spinal cord lesions. *Scand. J. Rehabil. Med.* 11:29–32.

Ohry, A., et al. 1978. Shoulder complications as a cause of delay in rehabilitation of spinal cord injured patients. *Paraplegia* 16:310–316.

Pagni, C.A. 1987. "Central pain due to spinal cord and brainstem damage." In *Textbook of pain,* 2d ed., ed. P.D. Wall and R. Melzack, 634–655. Edinburgh, Scotland: Churchill-Livingstone.

Pagni, C.A., and P.E. Maspes. 1972a. "A new approach to the surgical treatment of phantom limb pain." In *Pain: Basic principles—Pharmacology—Therapy,* ed. R. Janzen et al., 215–217. Stuttgart, Germany: Thieme.

Pagni, C.A., and Maspes, P.E. 1972b. "The relief of intractable pain in malignant diseases of the head and neck by stereotactic thalamotomy or sensory root section." In *Pain: Basic principles—Pharmacology—Therapy,* ed. R. Janzen et al., 204–207. Stuttgart, Germany: Thieme.

Pollock, L.J., et al. 1951. Pain below the level of injury of the spinal cord. *Arch. Neurol. Psychiatry* 65:319–322.

Pool, W.H. 1974. Cartilage atrophy. *Radiology* 112:47–50.

Poole, J.L. 1945. "Spinal cord injuries." *Conference on Spinal Cord Injuries.* J.L. Poole, ed. Atlantic City, N.J.: Army Service Forces, Second Service Command, Thomas M. England General Hospital, 149.

Porter, R.W., et al. 1966. Cordotomy for pain following cauda equina injury. *Arch. Surg.* 92:765–770.

Procacci, P., and M. Zoppi. 1983. "Pathophysiology and clinical aspects of visceral and referred pain." In *Advances in pain research and therapy,* ed. J.J. Bonica et al., 643–658. Vol. 5. New York, N.Y.: Raven..

Ramos, M. 1975. Recurrent superior mesenteric artery syndrome in a quadriplegic patient. *Arch. Phys. Med. Rehabil.* 56:86–88.

Raptou, A.D., et al. 1964. Intermittent arteriomesenteric occlusion of the duodenum in a quadriplegic patient. *Arch. Phys. Med. Rehabil.* 45:418–423.

Richards, J.S., et al. 1980. Psychosocial aspects of chronic pain in spinal cord injury. *Pain* 8:355–366.

Richardson, R.R., et al. 1980a. Neurostimulation in the modulation of the intractable paraplegic and traumatic neuroma pains. *Pain* 8:75–84.

Richardson, R.R., et al. 1980b. Transcutaneous electrical neurostimulation in musculoskeletal pain of acute spinal cord injuries. *Spine* 5:42–45.

Riddoch, G. 1917 and 1918. The reflex functions of the completely divided spinal cord in man compared with those associated with less severe lesions. *Brain* 40:617 and 41:264–402.

Riddoch, G. 1938. The clinical features of central pain. *Lancet* 234:1093–1098, 1150–1156, 1205–1209.

Riddoch, G. 1941. Phantom limbs and body shape. *Brain* 64:197–222.

Rossier, A.B. 1964. Rehabilitation of the spinal cord injury patient. *Doc. Geigy Acta Clin. North Am. Ser.* 3:80–82.

Rossier, A.B., et al. 1981. Progressive late post-traumatic syringomyelia. *Paraplegia* 19:96–97.

Rossier, A.B., et al. 1985. Post-traumatic cervical syringomyelia: Incidence, clinical presentation, electrophysiological studies, syrinx protein and results of conservative and operative treatment. *Brain* 108:439–461.

Roth, E.J., et al. 1990. Traumatic central cord syndrome: Clinical features and functional outcomes. *Arch. Phys. Med. Rehabil.* 71:18–23.

Roth, E.J., et al. 1991. Superior mesenteric artery syndrome in acute traumatic quadriplegia: Case reports and literature review. *Arch. Phys. Med. Rehabil.* 72:417–420.

Rush, P.J. 1989. The rheumatic manifestations of traumatic spinal cord injury. *Semin. Arthritis Rheumatol.* 19:77–89.

Schlesinger, E.B., et al. 1981. Hydromyelia: Clinical presentation and comparison of modalities of treatment. *Neurosurgery* 9:356–365.

Schwartz, H.G., et al. 1965. "Definitive treatment." In *Neurological surgery of trauma*, ed. I.N. Coates and A.L. Marowsky, 123–144. Washington, D.C.: Department of the Army.

Schwartz, M.S., et al. 1980. Pattern of segmental motor involvement in syringomyelia: A single fibre EMG study. *J. Neurol. Neurosurg. Psychiatry* 43:150–155.

Schwartz, R.G., et al. 1984. Abdominal pain in quadriparesis: Myofascial syndrome as unsuspected cause. *Arch. Phys. Med. Rehabil.* 65:44–46.

Scott, J.A., and W.H. Donovan. 1981. The prevention of shoulder pain and contracture in the acute tetraplegia patient. *Paraplegia* 19:313–319.

Shannon, N., et al. 1981. Clinical features, investigation, and treatment of post-traumatic syringomyelia. *J. Neurol. Neurosurg. Psychiatry* 44:35–42.

Sternbach, R.A., et al. 1974. "Measuring the severity of clinical pain." In *Advances in neurology*, ed. J.J. Bonica, 281–288. Vol. 4. New York, N.Y.: Raven.

Tanaka, M., et al. 1979. Gastroduodenal disease in chronic spinal cord injury. *Arch. Surg.* 114:185–187.

Tanzer, R.C. 1959. The carpal tunnel syndrome: A clinical and anatomical study. *J. Bone Joint Surg. Am.* 41:626–634.

Tibbs, P.A., et al. 1979. Problem of acute abdominal disease during spinal shock. *Am. Surg.* 45:366–368.

Tunks, E. 1986. "Pain in spinal cord injured patients." In *Management of spinal cord injuries*, eds. R.F. Bloch and M. Basbaum, 180–211. Baltimore, Md.: Williams & Wilkins.

Veilleux, M., and J.C. Stevens. 1987. Syringomyelia: Electrophysiologic aspects. *Muscle Nerve* 10:449–458.

Vernon, J.D., et al. 1982. Post-traumatic syringomyelia. *Paraplegia* 20:339–364.

Vernon, J.D., et al. 1983. Post-traumatic syringomyelia: Results of surgery. *Paraplegia* 21:37–46.

Veterans Administration. 1948. *Veterans Administration technical bulletin TB10-503: Spinal cord injuries.* Washington, D.C.: Veterans Administration.

Wainapel, S.F. 1984. Reflex sympathetic dystrophy following traumatic myelopathy. *Pain* 18:345–349.

Wainapel, S.F., and M.M. Freed. 1984. Reflex sympathetic dystrophy in quadriplegia: Case report. *Arch. Phys. Med. Rehabil.* 65:35–36.

Waisbrod, H., et al. 1984. Chronic pain in paraplegics. *Neurosurgery* 15:933–934.

Watson, N. 1981. Ascending cystic degeneration of cord after spinal cord injury. *Paraplegia* 19:89-95.

Weinstein, S. 1962. Proceedings of the 11th Annual Spinal Cord Injury Conference. *Veterans Admin.* 11:138.

White, J.C. 1963. Anterolateral chordotomy—Its effectiveness in relieving pain of non-malignant disease. *Neurochirurgia* 6:83–102.

White, J.C., and W.H. Sweet. 1955. *Pain—Its mechanisms and neurosurgical control.* Springfield, Ill.: Thomas.

Williams, B., et al. 1981. Syringomyelia as a sequel to traumatic paraplegia. *Paraplegia* 19:67–80.

Wing, P.C., and S.J. Tredwell. 1983. The weightbearing shoulder. *Paraplegia* 21:107–113.

Wright, V., et al. 1965. Bone and joint changes in paraplegic men. *Ann. Rheum. Dis.* 24:419–430.

Wylie, E.J., and T.M.H. Chakera. 1988. Degenerative joint abnormalities in patients with paraplegia of duration greater than 20 years. *Paraplegia* 26:101–106.

Young, J.S., et al. 1982. *Spinal cord injury statistics: Experience of the Regional Spinal Cord Injury Systems.* Phoenix, Ariz.: Good Samaritan Medical Center.

Zankel, H.T., et al. 1954. A paraplegic program under physical medicine and rehabilitation: One year's experience. *Arch. Phys. Med. Rehabil.* 35:296–302.

Zung, W.M. 1983. A self-rating pain and distress scale. *Psychosomatics* 24:887–894.

Chapter 16

Practical Pain Management Strategies

Elliot J. Roth

Pain syndromes commonly experienced by patients with spinal cord injury (SCI) are discussed in Chapter 15. Management of pain syndromes is a challenging clinical undertaking. The pain often is persistent and refractory to most commonly used treatment modalities. Consequently, both the patient and professional must exercise sensitivity, perseverance, open-mindedness, and goal directedness; a true desire to find effective treatment, together with patience and the application of sound scientific principles, may result in gratifying relief. An important component of successful pain management is collaboration between the patient and the professional.

This pain can be persistent. A number of treatment modalities have been attempted in the past, with various results. Several problems exist in the clinical and scientific study of pain in patients with SCI. First, some of the difficulty in studying the efficacy of potential interventions for this clinical problem results from the subjective nature and the diversity of personal experiences that make up the outcome variable (pain) under investigation. This difficulty is seen in both clinical settings and research work. Furthermore, there is a major lack of consistency in both the definitions of pain employed and the specific types of pain syndromes being studied. This area is clouded even further by the paucity of controlled and carefully conducted studies of various treatment methodologies. For all these reasons, successful treatment of the SCI patient with pain relies heavily on the patience, cooperation, collaboration, and ingenuity of the patient and the professional alike. It takes a combination of a sincere desire to find the effective treat-ment and persistence in continuing the search for appropriate management. At times, the search may seem as if it relies on an empirical trial and error approach to treatment, but that, unfortunately, is the state of the art in SCI pain management, with some scientific principles being applied as well.

There are some excellent reviews of a number of different modalities used for these pain syndromes. Readers are referred to work by Krueger (1960), Burke and Woodward (1976), Donovan et al. (1982), Tunks (1986), and Pagni (1987). Briefly stated, potential methods of management of SCI pain can be divided into general nursing or therapeutic measures, psychological methods, physiatric modalities, pharmacologic agents, neurolytic injections, peripheral and central electrical stimulation, and neurosurgical procedures.

GENERAL MEASURES: DISEASE PREVENTION AND HEALTH PROMOTION

General measures refer to those commonsense techniques to prevent complications and maintain good general physical health. As noted in Chapter 15, pain may be triggered or exacerbated by infections, pressure sores, bladder and bowel distension, temperature extremes or changes, smoking, emotional distress, spasticity, and any other noxious stimulus to the system. Avoiding these problems in the first place and treating them promptly, appropriately, and aggressively when they do occur are the mainstays of good, effective pain prevention and management. Other general measures include maintenance of good nutrition and hydration, appropriate spine fracture and alignment management, passive range of motion exercises to prevent contracture, proper positioning, and avoidance of the complications of prolonged immobilization and deconditioning. Use of proper splints and positions can be extremely helpful in preventing pain.

Prevention also is considered the best management technique for the problems of adhesive capsulitis and periarthritis of the shoulders. Early and properly performed mobilization and rehabilitation constitute the major preventive techniques used. Scott and Donovan (1981) advocated a specific position of the upper extremities as a means of preventing pain and contracture in the shoulders when patients are lying supine. It calls for the shoulders to be abducted to 90° and slightly extended with both arms supported on pillows on specially made boards that slip under the mattress. Cautious body handling during turns and transfers also is beneficial.

PSYCHOLOGIC MEASURES

Also beneficial in pain prevention and treatment are reassurance, psychological support, training in relaxation techniques, hypnosis, biofeedback, and other psychological measures. In many ways, the psychological support and assistance to the patient toward achieving optimal psychosocial adaptation are integral components of the rehabilitation program. Pain complaints often are associated with certain psychosocial variables and attributes (Botterell et al. 1953; Richards et al. 1980), as noted earlier in Chapter 15.

One report formally investigated (but only in four patients) the use of relaxation techniques in SCI patients with chronic pain and found them efficacious (Grzesiak 1977). The study used the method of selective inattention. This method usually emphasizes muscular relaxation, becoming more sensitive to one's inner feelings, breathing training, and imagery using pleasant thoughts. Another recent presentation (Alden 1990) advocated hypnosis as a routine treatment modality to be used on an SCI unit for patients with pain. Hypnosis generally is considered effective in pain relief in about 10% of patients (Tunks 1986). These methods may be especially useful as adjunctive measures, to be used in combination with other modalities.

Tunks (1986) stated,

> . . . the patient may be encouraged to know that with increased activity as rehabilitation progresses, the usual pattern is for pain to decrease or become more tolerable and manageable . . . the degree of pain depends in part on the success of rehabilitation, the level of physical activity, and the morale and other psychosocial factors. (p. 205)

Pagni (1987) and others (Albe-Fessard 1972) point out that the cerebral cortex exerts a powerful inhibitory influence on the activity of the spinal cord brain pathways. These findings help account for the strong effect that psychological factors play in the genesis and treatment of pain.

Clinically, emotional well-being appears to exert a great positive effect on pain relief. In addition, psychological stress, hostility, anxiety, or depression may precipitate or exacerbate pain. Emphasizing positive or favorable attributes and focusing on abilities rather than limitations, together with the specific functional training program that is the hallmark of the rehabilitation program, may be effective in pain control. Engaging patients in outside activities such as work, school, recreation, and others allows their attention to be focused toward an external function and away from dwelling on the inner pain. This can be a most useful tool in treatment.

PHYSICAL MODALITIES

Physical modalities have been advocated and described by only a few published studies, but many clinicians use them in practice. Naturally, functional training, mobilization, and therapeutic exercise provided in the form of physical therapy and occupational therapy may help improve range of motion, tone, strength, and movement patterns. Some early investigators advocated the use of massage, Hubbard tank, ultrasound, short-wave diathermy, acupuncture, and biofeedback (Kaplan et al. 1962; Zankel et al. 1954). Many patients find great benefit in using many of these modalities. In particular, various methods of hydrotherapy have proved beneficial in a variety of circumstances.

MEDICATIONS

Although analgesic medication use is common in patients with SCI, the efficacy of these agents may vary, and scientific support for their use is lacking. Medication use is limited by the adverse effects of the drugs. For this reason, medications are prescribed only if the expected effectiveness is thought to outweigh the potential side effects. Even so, medications represent a mainstay of the interventions for pain in patients with SCI. In particular, medications should be used only if the pain is disabling. Pain that interferes with the sleep–wake cycle, prohibits participation in a therapeutic exercise program, and limits functional capabilities represents the major indication for pharmacologic intervention.

It is important to avoid the tendency to overlook the use of simple, common analgesic agents such as acetaminophen and aspirin. Often, these drugs alone result in adequate relief with a minimum of side effects. Nonsteroidal antiinflammatory agents such as ibuprofen, naproxen sodium, sulindac, tolmetin sodium, diflunisal, and others have been tried, but with mixed success. There are no controlled studies of their efficacy. These medications generally are well tolerated but have the potential to cause fluid retention or gastrointestinal disturbances such as peptic ulcer disease or gastritis.

Many patients take narcotic analgesic agents if the pain is extreme and function limiting. These agents are limited by their adverse effects, however, including clouded thinking, overdose and abuse potential, constipation, and multiple drug interactions. For this reason, these medications, which include codeine, oxycodone, propoxyphene, Dilaudid, and others, are reserved for those patients and situations that are extreme and unusual and, ideally, only for the short term.

A number of psychotropic drugs have been used successfully to treat neuropathic pains. The major class of medications associated with central or peripheral dysesthetic pain consists of the tricyclic antidepressant drugs. There is a plethora of open and closed trials investigating and reporting on the efficacy of these agents for a variety of pain syndromes (Clarke 1981; Cough & Hassanein 1979; Davis, J.L. et al. 1977; Diamond & Baites 1971; Gomersall & Stuart 1973; Hameroff et al. 1982; Johansson & Knorring 1979; Kvinesdal et al. 1984; Lance & Curran 1964; Merskey & Hester 1972; Pilowsky et al. 1982; Taub 1973; Ward et al. 1979; Watson et al. 1973).

In SCI pain, the literature on tricyclic antidepressant drugs is considerably more limited. Although these medications, which include amitriptyline, desipramine, imipramine, trazodone, doxepin, and fluoxetine, have been put to fairly extensive clinical use recently, there are few clinical trials testing their efficacy and usefulness. There are two early reports of open studies of psychotropic medications for the pain of SCI.

Heilporn (1977) studied 11 SCI patients with the central dysesthetic pain syndrome to whom low doses of tricyclic antidepressant medications were given. The patients received a combination of melitracin (50 mg) and flupenthixol (3 mg) daily. Three patients reported long-lasting relief, but the investigator did not use any formal pain measurement scales to determine outcome or efficacy. Maury (1977) recommended use of tricyclic antidepressant agents for the treatment of radicular and dysesthetic pain after SCI but presented no data to support his recommendations. There is only one randomized, double-blind, placebo-controlled study testing the efficacy of a tricyclic antidepressant agent for this difficult to treat pain syndrome. Davidoff et al. (1987b) at the Rehabilitation Institute of Chicago investigated the use of trazodone for the treatment of the dysesthetic pain syndrome in 18 patients with SCI. Subjects were given either trazodone or placebo and were studied at 2-week intervals for a total of 8 weeks using the McGill Pain Questionnaire, the Sternbach Pain Intensity Index, and the Zung Pain and Distress Index. The study revealed no significant changes in any of the reported pain measures between patients allocated to the active drug group and those given the placebos or between week 1 and week 8 on the randomized drug. There were significantly more patients who were randomized to trazodone, however, who complained of side effects and prematurely terminated their participation.

The rationale for this study was based on the finding that serotonin and other catecholamine neurotransmitters mediate the endogenous descending analgesia pathways. Selective inhibition of the presynaptic reuptake of serotonin from the synaptic cleft, as occurs with trazodone and other tricyclic antidepressant medications, might be expected to enhance the activity of the descending pain control structures and to reduce central pain (Akil & Mayer 1972; Riblet & Taylor 1981). Failure of trazodone to provide adequate pain relief in the SCI patients with central dysesthetic pain syndrome probably was related to a number of factors. It is possible that more recently introduced agents such as fluoxetine or other serotonin-specific presynaptic reuptake blockers at different dosages might be effective for this difficult to treat syndrome.

Despite the fact that carefully controlled clinical trials of these medications are lacking, there is still a sufficient theoretical rationale and enough empirical clinical evidence to use these agents with caution. These medications generally are well tolerated at the low doses at which they are prescribed for pain. Potential side effects that may limit their use include drowsiness, clouded sensorium, dry mouth, urinary retention, bowel program alteration, and other anticholinergic effects. Other psychotropic medications, including major tranquilizers such as phenothiazines, may be used. Anticonvulsant medications such as carbamazepine and phenytoin have been advocated for central pain (Davis, R. 1975). Gibson and White (1971) noted the best results while treating the pain of paraplegia with carbamazepine. The rationale for the use of anticonvulsant medications rests on their neuronal membrane stabilizing properties. Results are mixed, however. Often a combination of two or more of these medications, such as amitriptyline and carbamazepine, may be effective when one or the other agent alone is not. Only clinical empiricism and cautious testing of different regimens will optimize the pharmacologic management of these patients.

The common theme discussed with each of these pharmacologic approaches is that outcomes of their use are variable. Nepomuceno et al. (1979) reported that 38% of the patients in their series used medications for pain but that only 22% obtained consistent relief from their use. Pagni (1987) stated that pharmacological treatment is generally ineffective. From a practical clinical perspective, medications offer some pain relief in some patients, but usually only after a considerable effort is made and time is allowed to optimize the pharmacologic regimen.

NEUROLYTIC INJECTIONS

The pain associated with SCI is most commonly considered central in origin, rendering neurolytic injections unlikely to afford significant pain relief. Some peripheral nerve injections have been attempted with variable results, however, and other injection types may be used. At times, temporary relief may be secured.

Peripheral nerve blocks may be useful in the pain of cauda equina injury. Cain (1965) reported on and advocated the use of injections of phenol solutions into the subarachnoid space for relief of pain and spasticity of SCI, describing them as an extremely valuable therapeutic approach to the problem but noting the potential complications of increased muscle weakness, sensory loss, and genitourinary dysfunction. R. Davis (1975) recommended the use of steroid injections into painful apophyseal facet joints to treat localized pain at the site of trauma.

A particularly exciting new method was reported recently by Glynn et al. (1986) in 15 patients with deafferentation pain from SCI. Epidural injections of 150 µg of clonidine were found to be more effective in treating this pain than epidural morphine or buprenorphine. These results may have significant scientific implications in that they may indicate a role of the spinal noradrenergic system in the transmission of pain in patients with SCI. More important, however, these findings suggest a new, previously unrecognized, and potentially useful treatment modality.

ELECTROSTIMULATION

Electrical stimulation of nerves in a variety of locations within the nervous system has been attempted in a number of painful states, with good effectiveness in many. In the specific problem of pain in SCI, the reports are more limited and the results mixed.

Since its introduction by Wall and Sweet (1967), transcutaneous electrical nerve stimulation (TENS) has been used for a variety of acute and chronic pain states, including postoperative pain, neurogenic pain, and musculoskeletal pain (Andersson 1979; Augustinsson et al. 1977; Hymes et al. 1974; Loeser et al. 1975; Picazza et al. 1975; Shealy 1974a, 1974b; Sweet & Wepsic 1974; Taub 1974). This technique temporarily abolishes chronic pain by electrically stimulating peripheral nerves using skin surface electrodes. Its attractiveness is partly a result of its noninvasive nature. It has been attempted in SCI patients with pain from a variety of sources with mixed success. Significantly more clinicians have used it than have published results of their trials.

Davis and Lentini (1975) used TENS to treat chronic pain complaints in 31 patients with SCI. They found a difference in the type of response based on the type of pain experienced. Seven of 11 patients with musculoskeletal or lesional pain responded well to TENS, but only 2 of 11 patients with root pain or central dysesthesias had any lasting relief. Richardson et al. (1980b) successfully applied TENS specifically for musculoskeletal and soft tissue pain complaints in patients with acute SCI. They reported significant pain relief in 75% of pa-

tients. Hachen (1977) reported on the use of prolonged sessions of TENS in 7 quadriplegic and 32 paraplegic patients with pain. After 1 week of use, 49% had complete or almost complete relief, and 41% had slight to moderate relief. At the 3-month follow-up, 28% had complete or nearly complete relief, and 4% had partial relief. Other anecdotal reports of personal experiences with superficial stimulation (Banerjee 1974; Stonnington et al. 1976) also have confirmed the mixed results obtainable with TENS for SCI pain.

Despite these practical successes in certain pain states and under certain circumstances, it is important to understand that a subgroup of patients may experience an exacerbation of their pain from the stimulation. This is especially true of patients with central pain. In addition, Florante et al. (1979) observed that the use of TENS by patients with quadriplegia was associated with detrusor-sphincter dyssynergy and bladder dysfunction. These findings suggest a relative contraindication for the use of TENS in patients with quadriplegia who are on intermittent catheterization programs, and they highlight the need for careful supervision and follow-up of such patients using these techniques.

Epidural dorsal column electrical stimulation is a much more invasive procedure. Implanted stimulators have been used for chronic pain and spasticity since their introduction by Shealy et al. (1970). Like the peripheral stimulators, however, these epidural stimulators have had mixed successes in relieving pain in patients with SCI. Early enthusiasm for these procedures gave way to a realization of their potential complications and to an understanding of the importance of careful and proper patient selection for the procedure. A few transient and long-term successes have resulted, but the general effects of dorsal column stimulation have been disappointing (Nashold & Friedman 1972; Sweet & Wepsic 1969; Urban & Nashold 1978).

Long and Erickson (1975) followed patients who received dorsal column stimulator implants for a variety of painful neurologic conditions, including SCI. Only 19% of the patients had any pain relief after 1 year of implantation. Richardson et al. (1980a) studied the efficacy of an implantable epidural neurostimulator for the treatment of intractable pain in 10 patients with paraplegia and compared these results with those of 9 patients with intractable postamputation or posttraumatic neuroma pain. Of the 10 patients with SCI, only 5 underwent a permanent stimulator implantation, with only 1 patient still reporting significant pain relief at 1 year after implantation. In contrast, 6 of the 9 patients with neuroma or amputation pain reported continued pain relief 1 year after implantation of the stimulator. Today these stimulators are used only rarely in patients with SCI.

Deep brain electrical stimulation for pain relief has received some recent neurosurgical attention (Levy et al. 1987); patients with SCI often have poor results from this procedure, however. In one report, none of 11 patients with paraplegic pain obtained pain relief with deep brain stimulation (Levy et al. 1987).

NEUROSURGICAL PROCEDURES

Invasive neurosurgical procedures have been used to treat severe intractable pain in patients with SCI for many decades. Much of the early enthusiasm for these procedures has given way to recent disappointment, however. Currently, ablative or destructive procedures are seldom used, partly because of lack of efficacy at intermediate or long-term follow-up and partly because of the desire by many patients and professionals to avoid permanent destruction of existing anatomical structures. Older literature contains numerous reports of the indications, usefulness, technique, and outcome of a number of procedures. Davis and Martin (1947) reported relatively disappointing results and several complications of cordotomies in SCI patients with pain, but Munro (1950) noted that more than half the patients in his series who underwent surgical procedures to ameliorate pain had either complete or adequate relief of pain. These procedures included exploratory laminectomy with cauda equina neurolysis, lumbar sympathectomy, and cordotomy. Porter et al. (1966) and Freeman and Heimburger (1947) were major advocates of cordotomy. The latter investigators noted that the procedure was the best answer to the problem of pain. Other proponents included Druckman and Lende (1965), DeSaussure (1950), and Krueger (1960).

Other early investigators suggested that anterolateral cordotomy (which involves removal of the lateral spinothalamic tract) provides some benefit of pain relief (Bors 1951; Botterell et al. 1953; Davis, L. 1954; Davis & Martin 1947; DeSaussure 1950; Freeman & Heimburger 1947; Kahn & Peet 1948; Krueger 1960; Porter et al. 1966). On the other hand, Melzack and Loeser (1978) stated that the failure of these procedures and the later exacerbation of the pain were predictable. White and Kjellberg (1973) found that only half their 62 subjects (SCI and non-SCI) followed for 10 to 20 years obtained permanent relief with cordotomy but that 65% of the patients who underwent selective posterior rhizotomy had long-term success.

Percutaneous radiofrequency cordotomy resulted in a pain-free state in 40% of patients with a variety of chronic, intractable pain syndromes, according to Rosomoff (1974). Some good results have been obtained from facet rhizotomy in patients with damaged, arthritic, or chronically unstable facet joints (Davis, R. 1975; Long 1982).

The procedure that has received the most extensive recent interest is the dorsal root entry zone (DREZ) lesion. DREZ ablation has also been advocated by several groups for the treatment of SCI pain (Friedman & Nashold 1986; Richter & Seitz 1984). In the largest reported treatment experience with DREZ lesions (Friedman & Nashold 1986), 56 SCI patients with intractable pain were studied. Overall, 50% of the pa-

tients reported good relief for 6 months to 6 years after the DREZ ablation procedure, but results varied according to pain type. Patients with diffuse distal pain had the poorest success rate (20% reported good outcome), and patients with significant burning pain had slightly better results (38% reported good outcome). Complications included cerebrospinal fluid leak, increased motor weakness, and new sensory loss. Similar findings have been noted by Richter and Seitz (1984).

In another report on the use of DREZ lesion in central pain, Nashold and Bullitt (1981) described their experience while following 13 patients with intractable chronic pain of paraplegia for 5 to 38 months after the procedure. Their findings were more favorable than those in the previous reports. Many other reports exist on the applicability, surgical technique, and outcomes of these procedures (Friedman & Nashold 1986).

PAIN MANAGEMENT IN PERSPECTIVE

The problem of pain in patients with SCI is complicated by a wide variety of factors, and a systematic approach to its management is necessary to achieve a successful outcome. It is important first and above all else to identify and carefully characterize the specific type of pain that a patient is experiencing and then to direct its management appropriately. On initial inspection, this may appear to be an obvious treatment principle, but it is often overlooked in clinical practice. It is critical to determine clearly the type and characteristics of pain under study.

Donovan et al. (1982) advocated specific management directed toward amelioration of the specific pain categories outlined in their report. Thus peripheral segmental nerve pain (including pain associated with cauda equina injury) is best treated with peripheral nerve blocks, oral carbamazepine use, or, rarely, TENS or epidural stimulation. Results may be variable, however. Regarding central spinal cord pain, this group noted that treatment of this condition remains difficult. Pharmacotherapy is thought to be ineffective, although some improvement may occur with tricyclic antidepressant medications for the central form of pain. Naturally, visceral pain is best treated by alleviating the pathological problem, muscle tension or mechanical pain is treated by addressing the mechanical factors, and psychogenic pain is managed with psychological methods of treatment.

It is also important to recognize that abnormal sensations, even pain, may be an extremely common (if not universal) finding in patients with SCI. Not all these patients require medical intervention, however, and in view of the potential for adverse effects of some of these modalities treatment should be entered into with care and caution. The general guideline is that only pain that interferes with function (however defined) necessitates treatment.

The refractory nature of the pain experience means that patience, perseverance, and ingenuity are key ingredients of the

Exhibit 16–1 Practical Management Strategies for SCI Pain

1. **Prevention and Treatment of Complications**

   - Pressure Sores
   - Bowel and Bladder Dysfunction
   - Infection
   - Temperature Extremes
   - Spasticity
   - Emotional Distress
   - Prolonged Immobilization/Deconditioning
   - Contractures

2. **Health Promotion**

   - Smoking Cessation
   - Maintain Nutrition and Hydration
   - Spine Fracture Management
   - Passive Range of Motion Exercises
   - Proper Positioning
   - Activity and Exercise

3. **Psychological Interventions**

   - Reassurance, Psychologic Support
   - Relaxation Training; Hypnosis
   - Biofeedback

4. **Physical Modalities**

   - Exercise
   - Massage
   - Hydrotherapy
   - Ultrasound, Short Wave Diathermy
   - Acupuncture
   - Biofeedback

5. **Medications**

   - Mild Analgesics
   - Nonsteroidal Antiinflammatory Agents
   - Narcotics
   - Tricyclic and Other Antidepressants
   - Anticonvulsants
   - Phenothiazines
   - Clonidine, Mexiletine, Other Newer Drugs

6. **Neurolytic Injections**

7. **Electrical Stimulation**

   - Transcutaneous Electrical Nerve Stimulation
   - Epidural Dorsal Column Stimulation
   - Deep Brain Electrical Stimulation

8. **Neurosurgical Procedures**

   - Laminectomy
   - Sympathectomy
   - Cordotomy
   - Myelotomy
   - Selective Posterior Rhizotomy
   - Dorsal Root Entry Zone Lesion

treatment regimen. The patient and SCI professional should consider the treatment program a partnership.

It is important to treat the pain within the context of the total patient and not in isolation. The individual's life style, coping style, past experiences, locus of control, and life outlook play a role in determining results from pain management, as they do in determining outcome after SCI rehabilitation.

The multitude of treatment methods is summarized in Exhibit 16–1. The treatment strategy of choice is the adoption of a multidisciplinary approach utilizing a combination of the methods outlined in this chapter (health promotion, psychological methods, pharmacologic agents, electrotherapy, neurolytic injection, and surgical procedures). Only a conglomeration of diverse management techniques can be expected to address adequately the multifactorial nature of the pain problem. In this light, it is the interdisciplinary team of experienced rehabilitation professionals practicing the rehabilitation model that is in the optimal position to manage effectively the SCI patient with pain. The rehabilitation program provides a coordinated team effort designed to maximize the acquisition of new knowledge and skills; to facilitate psychological adaptation; to encourage the resumption of previous family, work, and community life roles; to promote community reintegration; and to enhance the likelihood of achieving maximum functional and social outcomes. To this end, the rehabilitation program allows the opportunity to enlist the patient as partner in overcoming multiple obstacles, one of which might be pain. In this way, the rehabilitation team and program provide the ideal context to optimize the management of the SCI patient with pain.

REFERENCES

Akil, H., and D.J. Mayer. 1972. Antagonism of stimulation-produced analgesia by p-CPA, a serotonin synthesis inhibitor. *Brain Res.* 44:692–697.

Albe-Fessard, D.G. 1972. "Central pain pathways for noxious stimuli." In *Cervical pain,* ed. C. Hirsch and Y. Zotterman, 179–193. Oxford, England: Pergamon.

Alden, P. 1990. The use of hypnosis in the management of pain in spinal cord injured patients. *Proc. Int. Med. Soc. Paraplegia* 29:6.

Andersson, S.A. 1979. "Pain control by sensory stimulation." In *Advances in pain research and therapy,* ed. J.J. Bonica et al., 569–585. Vol. 3. New York, N.Y.: Raven.

Augustinsson, L.R., et al. 1977. Pain relief during delivery by TENS. *Pain* 4:59–66.

Banerjee, T. 1974. Transcutaneous nerve stimulation for pain after spinal injury. *N. Engl. J. Med.* 291:796 (letter).

Bors, E. 1951. Phantom limbs of patients with spinal cord injury. *Arch. Neurol. Psychiatry* 66:610–631.

Botterell, E.H., et al. 1953. Pain in paraplegia: Clinical management and surgical treatment. *Proc. R. Soc. Med.* 47:281–288.

Burke, D.C., and J.M. Woodward. 1976. "Pain and phantom sensation in spinal paralysis." In *Handbook of clinical neurology*, ed. P.J. Vinken and G.W. Bruyn, 489–499. Vol. 26. New York, N.Y.: Elsevier.

Cain, H.D. 1965. Subarachnoid phenol block in the treatment of pain and spasticity. *Paraplegia* 3:152–160.

Clarke, I.A.M. 1981. Amitriptyline and perphenazine (triptaphen DA) in chronic pain. *Anesthesia* 36:210–212.

Cough, J.R., and R.S. Hassanein. 1979. Amitriptyline in migraine prophylaxis. *Arch. Neurol.* 36:695–699.

Davidoff, G., et al. 1987a. Function-limiting dysesthetic pain syndrome among traumatic spinal cord injury patients: A cross-sectional study. *Pain* 29:39–48.

Davidoff, G., et al. 1987b. Trazodone hydrochloride in the treatment of dysesthetic pain in traumatic myelopathy: A randomized, double-blind, placebo-controlled study. *Pain* 29:151–161.

Davis, J.L., et al. 1977. Peripheral diabetic neuropathy treated with amitriptyline and fluphenazine. *J.A.M.A.* 238:2291–2292.

Davis, L. 1954. Treatment of spinal cord injury. *Arch. Surg.* 69:488–495.

Davis, L., and J. Martin. 1947. Studies upon spinal cord injuries. II. The nature and treatment of pain. *J. Neurosurg.* 4:483–491.

Davis, R. 1975. Pain and suffering following spinal cord injury. *Clin. Orthop. Relat. Res.* 112:76–80.

Davis, R., and R. Lentini. 1975. Transcutaneous nerve stimulation for treatment of pain in patients with spinal cord injury. *Surg. Neurol.* 4:100–101.

DeSaussure, R.L. 1950. Lateral spinothalamic tractotomy for relief of pain in cauda equina injury. *Arch. Neurol. Psychiatry* 64:708–714.

Diamond, S., and B.J. Baites. 1971. Chronic tension headache, treated with amitriptyline: A double-blind study. *Headache* 6:110–116.

Donovan, W.H., et al. 1982. Neurophysiological approaches to chronic pain following spinal cord injury. *Paraplegia* 20:135–146.

Druckman, R., and R. Lende. 1965. Central pain of spinal cord origin: Pathogenesis and surgical relief in one patient. *Neurology* 15:518–522.

Florante, J., et al. 1979. Effects of transcutaneous nerve stimulation on the vesicourethral function in spinal cord injury patients. *J. Urol.* 121:635–639.

Freeman, L.W., and R.F. Heimburger. 1947. Surgical relief of pain in paraplegic patients. *Arch. Surg.* 55:433–440.

Friedman, A., and B.S. Nashold. 1986. Dorsal root entry zone lesions for relief of pain related to spinal cord injury. *J. Neurosurg.* 65:465–469.

Gibson, J.C., and L.E. White. 1971. Denervation hyperpathia: A convulsive syndrome of the spinal cord responsive to carbamazepine therapy. *J. Neurosurg.* 35:287–290.

Glynn, C.J., et al. 1986. Role of spinal noradrenergic system in transmission of pain in patients with spinal cord injury. *Lancet* 2:1249–1250.

Gomersall, J.D., and A. Stuart. 1973. Amitriptyline in migraine prophylaxis; changes in pattern of attacks during a controlled clinical trial. *J. Neurol. Neurosurg. Psychiatry* 36:684–690.

Grzesiak, R.C. 1977. Relaxation techniques in treatment of chronic pain. *Arch. Phys. Med. Rehabil.* 58:270–272.

Hachen, H.J. 1977. Psychological, neurophysiological and therapeutic aspects of chronic pain: Preliminary results with transcutaneous electrical stimulation. *Paraplegia* 15:353–367.

Hameroff, S.R., et al. 1982. Doxepin effects on chronic pain, depression and plasma opioids. *J. Clin. Psychiatry* 43:22–26.

Heilporn, A. 1977. Two therapeutic experiments on stubborn pain in spinal cord lesions: Coupling melitracen-flupenthixen and the transcutaneous nerve stimulation. *Paraplegia* 15:368–372.

Hymes, A.C., et al. 1974. Acute pain control by electrostimulation: A preliminary report. *Adv. Neurol.* 4:761–767.

Johansson, F., and L.V. Knorring. 1979. A double-blind controlled study of a serotonin reuptake inhibitor (zimelidine) versus placebo in chronic pain patients. *Pain* 7:69–78.

Kahn, E.A., and M.M. Peet. 1948. The technique of anterolateral cordotomy. *J. Neurosurg.* 5:276–283.

Kaplan, L.I., et al. 1962. Pain and spasticity in patients with spinal cord dysfunction: Result of a follow-up study. *J.A.M.A.* 182:918–925.

Krueger, E.G. 1960. Management of painful states in injuries of the spinal cord and cauda equina. *Am. J. Phys. Med.* 39:103–110.

Kvinesdal, B., et al. 1984. Imipramine treatment of painful diabetic neuropathy. *J.A.M.A.* 251:1727–1730.

Lance, J.W., and D.A. Curran. 1964. Treatment of chronic tension headache. *Lancet* 1:1236–1239.

Levy, R.M., et al. 1987. Treatment of chronic pain by deep brain stimulation: Long-term follow-up and review of the literature. *Neurosurgery* 21:885–893.

Loeser, J.D., et al. 1975. Relief of pain by transcutaneous stimulation. *J. Neurosurg.* 42:308–314.

Long, D.M. 1982. "Pain of spinal origin." In *Neurological surgery*, 2d ed., ed. J.R. Youmans, 3613–3626. Philadelphia, Pa.: Saunders.

Long, D.M., and D.E. Erickson. 1975. Stimulation of the posterior columns of the spinal cord for relief of intractable pain. *Surg. Neurol.* 4:134–141.

Maury, M. 1977. About pain and its treatment in paraplegics. *Paraplegia* 15:349–352.

Melzack, R., and J.D. Loeser. 1978. Phantom body pain in paraplegics: Evidence for a central pattern generating mechanism for pain. *Pain* 4:195–210.

Merskey, H., and R.A. Hester. 1972. The treatment of chronic pain with psychotropic drugs. *Postgrad. Med. J.* 48:594–598.

Munro, D. 1950. Two-year end-results in the total rehabilitation of veterans with spinal-cord and cauda-equina injuries. *N. Engl. J. Med.* 242:1–10.

Nashold, B.S., and E. Bullitt. 1981. Dorsal root entry zone lesions to control central pain in paraplegics. *J. Neurosurg.* 55:414–419.

Nashold, B.S., and H. Friedman. 1972. Dorsal column stimulation for control of pain; preliminary report on 30 patients. *J. Neurosurg.* 36:590–597.

Nepomuceno, C., et al. 1979. Pain in patients with spinal cord injury. *Arch. Phys. Med. Rehabil.* 60:605–609.

Pagni, C.A. 1987. "Central pain due to spinal cord and brainstem damage." In *Textbook of pain*, 2d ed., ed. P.D. Wall and R. Melzack, 634–655. Edinburgh, Scotland: Churchill Livingstone.

Pagni, C.A., and P.E. Maspes. 1972a. "A new approach to the surgical treatment of phantom limb pain." In *Pain: Basic principles—Pharmacology—Therapy*, ed. R. Janzen et al., 215–217. Stuttgart, Germany: Thieme.

Pagni, C.A., and P.E. Maspes. 1972b. "The relief of intractable pain in malignant diseases of the head and neck by stereotactic thalamotomy or sensory root section." In *Pain: Basic principles—Pharmacology—Therapy*, ed. R. Janzen et al., 204–207. Stuttgart, Germany: Thieme.

Picazza, J.A., et al. 1975. Pain suppression by peripheral nerve stimulation: 1. Observations with transcutaneous stimuli. *Surg. Neurol.* 4:105–114.

Pilowsky, I., et al. 1982. A controlled study of amitriptyline in the treatment of chronic pain. *Pain* 14:169–179.

Porter, R.W., et al. 1966. Cordotomy for pain following cauda equina injury. *Arch. Surg.* 92:765–770.

Riblet, L.A., and D.P. Taylor. 1981. Pharmacology and neurochemistry of trazodone. *Clin. Pharmacol.* 1:175–225.

Richards, J.S., et al. 1980. Psycho-social aspects of chronic pain in spinal cord injury. *Pain* 8:355–366.

Richardson, R.R., et al. 1980a. Neurostimulation in the modulation of the intractable paraplegic and traumatic neuroma pains. *Pain* 8:75–84.

Richardson, R.R., et al. 1980b. Transcutaneous electrical neurostimulation in musculoskeletal pain of acute spinal cord injuries. *Spine* 5:42–45.

Richter, H.P., and K. Seitz. 1984. Dorsal root entry zone lesions for the control of deafferentation pain: Experience in 10 patients. *Neurosurgery* 15:956–959.

Rosomoff, H.L. 1974. "Percutaneous radiofrequency cervical cordotomy for intractable pain." In *International symposium on pain: Advances in neurology,* ed. J.J. Bonica, 603–688. Vol. 4. New York, N.Y.: Raven.

Scott, J.A., and W.H. Donovan. 1981. The prevention of shoulder pain and contracture in the acute tetraplegia patient. *Paraplegia* 19:313–319.

Shealy, C.N. 1974a. Electrical control of the nervous system. *Med. Prog. Technol.* 2:71–80.

Shealy, C.N. 1974b. Transcutaneous electrical stimulation for control of pain. *Clin. Neurosurg.* 21:269–277.

Shealy, C.N., et al. 1970. Dorsal column electroanalgesia. *J. Neurosurg.* 32:560–564.

Stonnington, H.H., et al. 1976. Transcutaneous electrical stimulation for chronic pain relief. *Minn. Med.* 59:681–683.

Sweet, W.H., and J.G. Wepsic. 1969. Treatment of pain by chronic electrical stimulation of large axons. *Excerpta Med. Int. Congr. Ser.* 193:81 (abstract).

Sweet, W.H., and J.G. Wepsic. 1974. Stimulation of pain suppressor mechanisms: A critique of some current methods. *Adv. Neurol.* 4:737–747.

Taub, A. 1973. Relief of post-herpetic neuralgia with psychotropic drugs. *J. Neurosurg.* 39:235–239.

Taub, A. 1974. Percutaneous local electrical analgesia, origin, mechanism and clinical potential. *Minn. Med.* 57:172–175.

Tunks, E. 1986. "Pain in spinal cord injured patients." In *Management of spinal cord injuries,* ed. R.F. Bloch and M. Bausbaum, 180–211. Baltimore, Md.: Williams & Wilkins.

Urban, B.J., and B.S. Nashold. 1978. Percutaneous epidural neurostimulation of the spinal cord for relief of pain: Long-term results. *J. Neurosurg.* 48:323–328.

Wall, P.D., and W.H. Sweet. 1967. Temporary abolition of pain in man. *Science* 155:108–109.

Ward, N.G., et al. 1979. The effectiveness of tricyclic antidepressants in the treatment of coexisting pain and depression. *Pain* 7:331–341.

Watson, C.P., et al. 1973. Amitriptyline versus placebo in post-herpetic neuralgia. *Neurology* 32:671–673.

White, J., and R. Kjellberg. 1973. Posterior spinal rhizotomy: A substitute for cordotomy in the relief of localized pain in patients with normal life-expectancy. *Neurochirurgia* 16:141–146.

Zankel, H.T., et al. 1954. A paraplegic program under physical medicine and rehabilitation: One year's experience. *Arch. Phys. Med. Rehabil.* 35:296–302.

Chapter 17

Wheelchairs

Linda Yasukawa, Sue Stevens, and Jennifer Ueberfluss

Wheelchairs are the primary means of mobility for most individuals with spinal cord injury (SCI). Their level of functional independence is related directly to their ability to complete a variety of wheelchair mobility skills either with or without the use of special options or adaptations. Each individual has specific needs that must be addressed when a wheelchair is chosen. The prescription for a wheelchair should be as precise as one for medication. The wheelchair must be of sufficient quality to withstand the activities of day-to-day living and mobility while at the same time offering the individual appropriate support and protection.

Ordering a wheelchair for your client is an important part of the client's reintegration into his or her previous home and life style. Because there are so many manufacturers and options available, your patient must be allowed a large part in the decision-making process.

The wheelchair seat depth is measured laterally along the femur from the most posterior aspect of the buttocks to the back of the knee. Two inches is subtracted to allow for clearance of the hamstring tendons. A seat depth too short or too long will result in improper leg positioning and possible deformities or pressure areas.

Measurements for footrest length are taken from the fibular head to the bottom of the shoe. Remember to add in the height of the cushion, or, for greater accuracy, measure the patient on the cushion. Improperly fitted footrests will increase the likelihood of pressure sores due to unevenly distributed seated pressures.

Back height is measured with the patient seated on the cushion. Measure from the bottom of the patient's cushion to the inferior angle of the scapula. A firm backrest is important for posturing, decreasing deformities, improving respiratory status, and providing stability during functional activities. Sling upholstery provides inadequate support, does not prevent deformities, and enhances a kyphotic posture. Table 17–1 lists other features of the backrest that are important to consider.

Armrest height should allow the shoulders to be relaxed with elbows flexed to 90°. Armrests that are too high will cause muscle tightness and decreased range of motion. Low armrests may lead to upper trapezius strain and shoulder subluxation. See Table 17–1 for other features of armrests.

Push handle height usually is related to backrest height. The push handles should be reached easily but should not interfere with functional activities, such as pushing and reaching.

When one is ordering a wheelchair, proper fit is the most important factor. The previously mentioned options should be decided upon primarily by the patient through an informed decision-making process.

The decision to get a power wheelchair for a person with SCI is based on diagnosis, functional ability, and life style. Generally, persons with SCI at C-6 or below do not need or want a power wheelchair. People with C-6 quadriplegia and below are most functional in a lightweight manual wheelchair unless they have other limiting factors, such as age, obesity, upper extremity contractures, asymmetrical upper extremity muscle function, arthritis, or pulmonary and cardiovascular diseases. This list is not all inclusive. If a patient has SCI and one or more of these limiting factors, he or she may need a power wheelchair to reach maximum level of function even though the injury is at C-6 or below. See Table 17–1 for important features of lightweight frames for manual wheelchairs.

Life style must also be considered when one is determining the need for a power wheelchair. For example, a patient with C-6 quadriplegia may be functional in a manual wheelchair until he or she has to push for long distances or if there are time constraints, such as on a college campus or job site. Other life-style questions that need answers are the following: Is the person's living environment accessible to a power chair? Are there resources to obtain ramps or lifts to get the wheelchair in and out of the home? Is there a reliable support system that can provide the care required to keep a power wheelchair functioning safely and appropriately?

Functional abilities must also be evaluated to determine whether a patient can propel a manual wheelchair both indoors and outdoors on various surfaces (e.g., grass, carpet, sidewalks, ramps, curbs, and cutouts). If a person cannot handle these surfaces safely or needs too much time to do so, a power wheelchair should be considered. The goal is for the person to be as independent as possible with the least amount of equipment.

If a power wheelchair is recommended based on the foregoing criteria, the next consideration would be whether a power recline system is needed. The deciding factor for a power recline system is whether the person can perform an adequate pressure relief while in the wheelchair. All persons with C-4 quadriplegia and above should have a power recliner. Some with C-5 and even C-6 quadriplegia may also benefit from a power recline system, especially if they have some of the limiting factors cited above and they cannot perform independent pressure reliefs.

Another consideration for persons with SCI is the need for a manual wheelchair even if they get power wheelchairs. A manual wheelchair is still needed for those times when the power wheelchair is not working or is unavailable during times of routine maintenance. Another reason why a manual wheelchair is needed is that it provides access to areas not accessible to a power wheelchair.

Table 17–1 lists other features that must be considered when one is ordering a wheelchair. Appendix 17–A provides a glossary of wheelchair accessories.

Table 17–1 Features To Be Considered When Ordering a Wheelchair

Type	Advantages	Disadvantages
Backrests		
Fixed	Strong, durable.	More difficult to transport.
Folding	Easier to transport.	May release accidentally.
Armrests		
Padded tubular	Easily moved/removed. Allows easier access to tables/desks. Lighter weight.	Minimal height adjustability. Does not protect clothing or skin or keep cushion in place. Comparatively not as stable. May not provide appropriate positioning for high tetraplegics.
Height adjustable		
Single post	Provides support and positioning options for upper extremities. Protects clothing and skin, and keeps cushion in place.	Less stable than a double post. Not durable. May be difficult for tetraplegics to manage.
Full length	Allows for support and positioning options. Helpful during sit-to-stand transfers.	Difficult to access work/table surfaces closely.
Desk length	Easier to access work surfaces.	May not provide enough support or positioning options.
Double post (height adjustable or standard model)	Greater stability. Some models help protect clothing and skin and keep cushion in place.	May be difficult to remove and insert.
Pivot arm	Easy to swing away. Stable.	Some styles are not height adjustable. May be difficult to manage with decreased hand function.
No armrest	Ease of transfers. Cosmesis.	No upper extremity support. Not recommended for higher-level injuries because of safety and posture concerns.
Lightweight Frames		
Rigid	Greater push efficiency. Greater strength and durability.	Overall folded size is bulkier.
Folding	Folded size is compact to increase ease of transport. Increased play in frame allows it to fit in tighter spaces.	Decreased durability. Less push efficiency.
Front Rigging		
Rigid	Strong, durable. Advantageous for wheelchair sports.	May interfere with transfers and ambulation. May limit access to tight spaces. May not provide adequate foot support.
Swing away	Can be moved out of the way for transfers and ambulation. Can be removed for easier access in tight spaces.	May add weight. Less durable than rigid type. Release mechanism may not be accessible to user.
Elevating	May decrease edema in elevated position. Minimizes orthostatic hypotension in elevated position.	Increases overall length of chair. Adds weight. Length of leg rest needs adjustment each time hanger angle is changed.
Fixed front rigging with flip-up foot plates	Strong, durable. Foot plates can be flipped up for transfers and ambulation.	May limit access to tight spaces.
Fixed hanger angles*		
Closer to 60°	Allows for more foot plate clearance.	Increases overall length of chair.
Closer to 90°	More anatomically correct sitting posture. Decreases overall length of chair.	May not allow adequate foot plate clearance. Need adequate knee range of motion.
Tapered	Cosmesis. Can get closer to furniture.	May touch the legs.

*Wheelchair manufacturers produce different hanger angles. Check with the manufacturers for the specific angles they provide.

continues

Table 17–1 continued

Type	Advantages	Disadvantages
Back Posts		
Angled	More comfortable.	—
Straight	—	Person may feel as if he or she is falling forward.
Brakes		
High mount	Easy to reach.	May interfere with pushing.
Low mount	Does not interfere with pushing.	Hard to reach. Need good hand function to use.
Front Casters (2 to 8 inches)**		
Small	Small turning radius.	Less stable. Less shock absorption.
Large	More stable. More shock absorption.	Less maneuverable.
Pneumatic	Good ride.	Gets flat tires. Needs maintenance.
Semipneumatic	No flat tires.	Better ride than poly, not as good as pneumatic.
Poly	No flat tires.	Less shock absorption.
Rear Wheels (24 inches)		
Spoke	Lighter.	Needs maintenance.
MAG	No maintenance.	A few ounces heavier than spokes.
Tires (Rear)		
Pneumatic	Good ride. Absorbs shocks.	Gets flat tires. Needs maintenance.
Pneumatic with solid inserts	No maintenance. Ride is better than with poly.	Ride is not as good as with pneumatic.
Poly	No flat tires.	Hard ride. Less shock absorption.

**Sizes available vary among manufacturers.

Anti-tippers

Also called wheelie bars. These devices prevent the wheelchair from tipping over backward. They usually are found on the back of the wheelchair near the floor. Most have tiny wheels on the ends.

Brake extension

An attachment to extend the brake applicator arm. Allows the patient to reach and apply brakes with increased ease. Available from approximately 6 to 9 inches; usually removable for transfers.

Camber

An angling of the wheel from top to bottom, usually done by inserting washers between the axle plate and the wheelchair frame. The angling increases the base of support (BOS) of the wheelchair and its stability and push efficiency; also increases the width of the wheelchair.

Caster pin lock

Located just over the caster housing, its purpose is to keep the caster in a forward position. It must be removed to turn a corner. This device is useful when propelling over a slanted surface.

Clothing guards

Guards sit on each side of the seat to protect the user from debris on the wheels. Guards can be made of any number of fabrics or plastic. Guards can be fixed (nonremovable) or removable.

Grade aid

Usually located near the brake, this device, when applied to the wheel, will allow the wheel to roll forward but not backward. It helps the individual on inclines. Also referred to as a hill holder.

Heel loop

Usually present as a cloth strap placed across the back of a single foot plate. It prevents the feet from sliding off the back of the foot plate.

Leg strap

Any type of strap used across the front rigging to prevent legs from getting caught underneath the wheelchair.

Push handles

Found on the back of the wheelchair, either attached to the back posts or mounted separately. They are used by a non–wheelchair user to push or manipulate the wheelchair. The push handles also are useful to hook with a user's arm as a point of stability while doing functional activities.

Rear wheel sizes

Sizes range from 20- to 26-inch diameters. The standard is 24 inches. Smaller sizes usually are used for hemiheight wheelchairs. With increased wheel diameter, the turning radius of the wheelchair is larger, so that the wheelchair may be harder to maneuver for some users.

Retractable armrests

Useful on wheelchairs that will recline because they recline with the backrest. This provides constant support for the user's upper extremities.

Seat belts

Depending upon the attachment (45° or 90°), seat belts can be for safety and/or positioning of the individual in the wheelchair. Clasp styles include wraparound, auto style, and airline style.

Spoke guard

This device rests over the spoked part of the wheel to prevent an individual's fingers from getting caught in the spokes.

Chapter 18

Functional Electrical Stimulation for Spinal Cord Injury

Alojz Kralj and Robert Jaeger

Practitioners have used electricity therapeutically for centuries (Liberson et al. 1961; McNeal 1977; Reswick 1979). A relatively new application of electricity in the medical field is using electrical currents to evoke functional movements in upper motor neuron lesion–paralyzed muscles. This process is called functional electrical stimulation (FES), functional neuromuscular stimulation, or neuromuscular stimulation. The goals of FES application for rehabilitation are to increase the patient's mobility, skills in activities of daily living (ADLs) at home and in the community, and independence.

THE HISTORY OF FES

The history of FES is interesting and extensive (Liberson et al. 1961; Reswick 1979). In 1956, Giamo proposed using a portable electrical stimulator for paralyzed leg muscles. In 1956, Browner proposed the first FES aid for ambulation. At the appropriate point of the gait cycle, the stimulator synchronously stimulated the muscles for ankle dorsiflexion. During subsequent years, similar and improved devices were proposed (Browner 1962; Keegan 1963; Liberson et al. 1961). All these FES orthotic devices used surface electrodes. In 1969, Wilemon (McNeal 1977; Wilemon et al. 1970) introduced the first FES system with implanted electrodes and radiofrequency transmission of stimulus. These initial systems were replicated and adapted by many other investigators, and many foot drop correction devices were designed.

During the early 1960s and 1970s, investigators applied FES as a rehabilitation technique to patients with different etiologies, such as stroke, head injury, cerebral palsy, and spinal cord injury (SCI). It is believed that during the years 1850 to 1870, Duchenne may have applied electrical stimulation to patients with SCI, but detailed citations have yet to be found.

The first short report concerning the use of FES with a paraplegic patient with a complete lesion at T-7 was published by Kantrowitz in 1963 (Vodovnik et al. 1981). No detailed description of the results and set-up are available, but it is known that the patient was able to stand for several minutes. Surface electrodes were used. Later, in 1968 and 1969, Wilemon and colleagues (1970) implanted bilateral electrodes for FES of the femoral and gluteal nerves in a patient with T-5 paraplegia. This enabled the patient to stand and walk with locked knees with crutches and ankle-foot orthoses.

In 1973, Kralj and Grobelnik reported data concerning 50 paraplegics with different etiologies and their responses to FES of various muscles. Their findings demonstrated that stimulated muscles behave dynamically in a manner similar to normal muscles. These investigators also found that daily FES exercising helped recondition the muscle with respect to force, endurance, bulk, and general condition. Rising from a sitting to a standing posture and quiet standing by means of FES also were described (Kralj & Grobelnik 1973).

Concurrently, Cooper et al. (1973) performed implants in two patients with lower thoracic paraplegia for bilateral FES of the femoral and sciatic nerves. Standing and crude locomotion using a roller seat were accomplished. In addition, histochemical and morphological studies revealed interesting changes in the muscles caused by prolonged electrical exercising (Cooper et al. 1973). Brindley et al. (1978) reported the results obtained in two patients with FES implants of the femoral and inferior and superior gluteal nerves. Both patients were able to perform a swing-to or swing-through gait using crutches and FES. Kralj et al. (1980) reported FES-induced bipedal reciprocal gait with the assistance of parallel bars. In 1981, roller walker–assisted FES-induced reciprocal gait was achieved, and in 1983 the biomechanical characteristics were documented. Bajd et al. (1983) reported crutch-assisted FES-enabled reciprocal gait in patients with paraplegia (Kralj & Bajd 1989). Thoma et al. (1983) described the implantation of a 16-channel FES system for gait assistance in patients with paraplegia. The implanted system provided bilateral FES for the inferior gluteal and femoral nerves. Standing and swing-to or swing-through crutch-assisted gait were achieved (Holle et al. 1984, Thoma et al. 1983). Marsolais and Kobetic (1983) reported FES-enabled reciprocal gait using percutaneous electrodes for nonambulating patients with stroke and head injury. In 1984, FES-induced stair walking was achieved in patients with paraplegia using percutaneous wire electrodes (Marsolais & Kobetic 1983; Marsolais et al. 1984). Petrofsky and Phillips (1983) also reported FES-induced reciprocal gait using surface electrodes and parallel bars for assistance. Petrofsky et al. (1984) utilized closed-loop control for improving walking. Interestingly, all these reports happened 20 years after Vodovnik's 1965 proposal (Vodovnik & McLeod 1985) for controlled electrical stimulation of extremities.

FES AND MUSCLE FATIGUE

Electrical stimulation reverses the natural recruitment order of muscle fibers. As a result, fatigue is accelerated and severe compared with that induced by voluntary muscle contraction. Therefore, research efforts have been directed to this problem (Fang & Mortimer 1987). In an attempt to simulate the natural activation at low stimulation frequencies (Peckham et al. 1976), low frequency FES is delivered via percutaneous helical coil electrodes placed in a muscle. Attempts to alleviate fatigue have also been made by sequentially stimulating the different heads of the quadriceps muscles (Brindley et al. 1978). Posture switching has been proposed to provide the required resting and recovery time for the muscles by cyclically activating different muscles (Kralj et al. 1986).

Fatiguing rate has been found to increase in proportion to the stimulation frequency, activation time, and peak force. Therefore, FES-initiated movement should minimize excessive muscular efforts and consequently reduce the associated fatiguing of the muscles. Investigators have therefore ex-

plored different FES control modes, of which there are two major types: closed-loop and open-loop. In the closed-loop mode, a sensor measures the performance while the control circuitry provides the feedback. This feedback is delivered in such a way that output deviates minimally from the input specified by the patient. Most of the attempts to use closed-loop controlled FES in patients with SCI for gait have not provided the expected improved results.

Currently, open-loop control is more frequently used in two modes. In the first mode, the patient provides the control and feedback, which in effect closes the loop (Kralj & Bajd 1989). The patient's brain and all preserved proprioception are thus used, providing good synchronization between voluntarily controlled upper body movements and the FES. This control is simple and does not put high demands on the external control circuitry. The second mode has the patient selecting the computer-stored sequences (called menus) and providing only the triggers. All the rest is done by the computer. This computer-controlled FES (Marsolais & Kobetic 1983; Petrofsky & Phillips 1983; Thoma et al. 1983) relies on prestored programs that the patient is unable to modify.

BALANCE

Attempts have been made to introduce closed-loop control for balance in patients with SCI, which would enable them to reduce or minimize dependence on hand-balancing aids. There is also research in progress for using the electromyographic signature discrimination of preserved voluntary trunk musculature (Graupe 1989). This control mode seems attractive because no learning is necessary, but it requires extremely complicated hardware. Also, no distinction has yet been made between regular trunk movement and movements that trigger stimulation.

FES-ASSISTED HAND MOVEMENT

Long and Masciarelli (1963) applied FES to patients with SCI for rehabilitation and restoration of hand function. Peckham et al. (1979) reported the use of multichannel FES for the hands of patients with quadriplegia. The use of closed-loop feedback for improving control of grasping and force exertion using FES in patients with quadriplegia has been proposed (Crago et al. 1980, 1986). Percutaneous wire electrodes are used in all these multichannel FES orthoses for hand function restoration. Additional corrective and restorative hand surgery is sometimes performed to augment the FES performance. Control of two degrees of freedom is provided via shoulder movements that are picked up by a joystick transducer. These FES systems for patients with quadriplegia are functional at present to the level of enabling patients to perform most of their simple ADLs. Rudel et al. (1982) proposed a surface electrode FES system for hand function restoration in patients with quadriplegia using a hand control. Similar work also has been performed in Japan (Handa & Hoshimiya 1987).

CURRENT CLINICAL USE OF FES OF LOCOMOTION REHABILITATION

For patients with incomplete SCI, the selection criteria and modalities of FES application concentrate on two issues: the augmented therapeutic effects of FES for muscle restrengthening during the recovery period, and FES-enabled locomotion patterning with the goal of converting wheelchair users into independent crutch walkers. For these patients, the rehabilitation goal is to obtain gait without reliance on the chronic use of FES. Therefore, the use of FES typically is limited to simple therapeutic gait training requiring one but not more than two channels of stimulation. This is dictated by practicality and the currently available hardware. In this respect, current research efforts for FES of patients with incomplete SCI are concentrated in the following areas: modes of FES-fitting procedures, tailoring and selecting the optimal number of channels, and determining implantation procedures for the system. For patients with complete SCI, the muscle restrengthening, standing, and gait phases are well defined from a rehabilitation point of view but still require modifications with regard to design and application of the FES systems.

Currently, FES is not widely applied in SCI rehabilitation on a routine clinical basis. Among the numerous hospitals and rehabilitation centers applying FES are Rancho Los Amigos Hospital and Rehabilitation Center, California (clinical use of FES), University Rehabilitation Center in Ljubljana, Slovenia (function restoration by use of FES), and Cleveland Metro General Hospital (application for hand function rehabilitation). Space limitations prevent us from presenting all the current work of many other research groups, such as the Cleveland Veterans Administration Hospital, the University of Vienna, and Wright State University.

In principle, all SCI patients with lesions between T-4 and T-12 with preserved lower motor neurons to the main extensor and flexor muscles are candidates. In practice, however, the suitable population of patients for FES is reduced dramatically because of additional complications caused by multiple trauma at the time of injury or secondary complications such as contractures or urinary tract infection. The major factors that exclude patients from FES are lower motor neuron lesions and joint contractures of the hip, knee, or ankle. Spasticity, sensory sparing that makes FES painful, and severe osteoporosis may prevent the use of FES. In addition, patients are excluded for psychological reasons (substance abuse or mental problems), inadequate cardiopulmonary function, inadequate hand function, obesity, age, autonomic dysreflexia, skin problems, and/or inadequate balance or trunk function.

The protocol for FES for locomotion may be divided into three phases:

1. FES-augmented restrengthening
2. FES-enabled standing
3. FES-assisted gait training

These phases differ with respect to patient selection, goals, application protocols, and expected outcome, according to the level of SCI and the completeness of the lesion.

FES-Augmented Restrengthening

Muscles are restrengthened by cyclical, isotonic FES activation. The goals for restrengthening are increasing force and endurance and retaining or increasing the range of motion. FES restrengthening may increase muscle force, bulk, and fatigue resistance. The possible side effects of restrengthening are modified or decreased spasticity and improved blood flow due to augmented venous pumping during muscle contraction. Owing to this, skin condition may also improve. The effects of progressive loading while restrengthening with FES are still under investigation. In patients with incomplete SCI, FES restrengthening may also increase sensory awareness and muscle facilitation for augmentation of voluntary control. Muscle tone and reflex organization may also be influenced.

FES restrengthening should be started as soon as possible after the SCI. Cyclical FES for restrengthening is performed over a limited time and is stopped after observable fatigue takes place. At the point of fatigue, the restrengthening session should be stopped because overexercising effects currently are not completely understood and may be contraindicated. For practical reasons, the total restrengthening time should not exceed more than several hours per day. Normally, two sessions are administered, one in the morning and one in the evening. To minimize the required doffing and donning, the sessions are carried out before rising or upon going to bed. Eight to 12 weeks of FES restrengthening will sufficiently restrengthen paralyzed muscles. This schedule has been determined by practical experience and is not yet fully supported by scientific data. The best tailored and optimal restrengthening modalities with respect to increased force, endurance, and duration have not yet been determined.

FES-Enabled Standing

After muscle restrengthening, FES-enabled standing is the second most practiced clinical use of FES in patients with SCI. Standing is a prerequisite for walking. Only patients mastering good and safe standing are able to continue to FES-initiated gait training.

FES-enabled standing is biomechanically similar to standing with knee-ankle-foot orthoses (KAFOs). FES is applied bilaterally to the quadriceps for knee joint locking. The hands are used for balancing the body across the ankle joint and assisting in maintaining a lordotic C posture. The patient must be introduced to limited standing time to avoid tiring the muscles. If the imposed gravitational torque overcomes the locking torque, jack-knifing may occur. Therefore, the patient's muscular endurance will determine standing time. Also, the patient is instructed to maintain standing for short periods on one leg because knee buckling frequently takes place first on the weaker side.

The incorporation of additional extensor muscles results in easier and better maintenance of posture, increased trunk stability, and prolonged standing time. Standing time for FES of the quadriceps alone should last for an average of 10 to 20 minutes. Some patients with good posture may stand for 40 minutes or more. Patients standing for 5 minutes or less are considered "bad standers." If posture switching is introduced, standing times may increase by a factor of 3 to 5.

Patients with safe and good standing can be trained to use FES standing to assist in various ADLs, such as transfers or grasping of high objects. For standing and hand support, different objects in the house can be used. Figure 18–1 shows a wheelchair-attached folding frame (produced and marketed by the University Rehabilitation Institute of Ljubljana, Slovenia). Such a folding frame allows a patient to stand via FES for short periods of time throughout the day. The frame may assist in performing tasks in, for instance, a library, kitchen, or shop or in transferring in narrow spaces such as toilets.

For patients with incomplete SCI requiring FES for standing assistance, standing training is similar to training for patients with complete SCI. For those with incomplete SCI who are able to stand on one sound leg, FES should be used only as a therapeutic modality when standing training is first taught. Later, one-leg standing using the sound leg is enforced.

In some patients with SCI, several muscles are lost because of lower motor neuron lesions. Such lesions will not respond

A

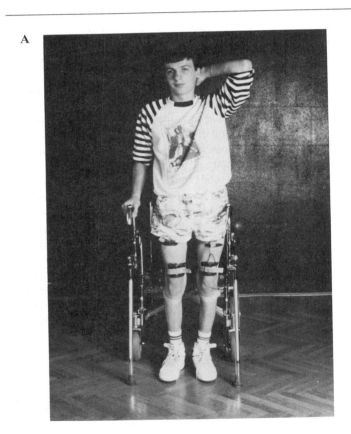

B

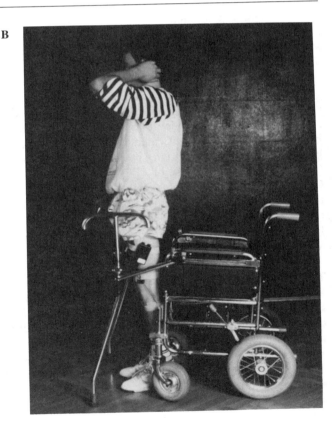

Figure 18–1 Frontal (**A**) and side (**B**) views of a paraplegic patient standing by bilateral electrical stimulation of quadriceps. A wheelchair-attached balance aid is used. When not in use, this balance aid is folded and moved to the side of the wheelchair. Pairs of large surface electrodes can be seen over the quadriceps. In the side view, the stimulator can be seen clipped to the strap of the upper electrode. The photo was taken at the Institut za Rehabilitacijo in Ljubljana, Slovenia.

to FES. The lost functions can be augmented by external classic orthotic bracing while the preserved upper motor neuron–paralyzed muscles are controlled by FES to provide the remaining functions. The combination of external bracing with FES creates the so-called hybrid system; recent versions have been described by Popovic et al. (1989) and Andrews et al. (1988).

FES-Assisted Gait

Four essential biomechanical elements make up FES-assisted gait: the FES-enabled single- and double-stance phase, the leg flexion phase for the swing, the balance provided by upper body movements (governed by the hands), and the propulsion provided by the hands and trunk adjustments. FES-generated gait can be made up of swing-to or swing-through gait, reciprocal bipedal gait, and possibly stair walking. In principle, any neural control preserved below the level of the lesion can be used along with FES to improve function and reduce hardware requirements and will result in more natural activation of muscles. Therefore, the swing phase can be synthesized either by efferent FES of the main leg flexors or by using the flexion reflex synergistic withdrawal movement. The flexion reflex can be triggered synchronously with the gait by sensory stimulation of the peroneal nerve in the region of the caput fibulae. This stimulation results in activation of hip and knee flexion along with ankle dorsiflexion and eversion. The synergistic flexion reflex movement provides better swing phase than direct motor stimulation of the main flexor muscles. It also results in reduced and simplified hardware.

Each of the possible gait synthesis modes has its advantages and disadvantages regarding the resulting flexion movement, repeatability, and hardware complexity. For balance and partial body support during weight transfer and generation of the propulsion forces, mechanical supportive devices such as parallel bars, walkers, or crutches are used. The majority of patients master roller walker–supported ambulation; only a few well-motivated patients with sufficient trunk balance master crutch-assisted walking, which is physically demanding. For stair ascending and descending, bimanual hand rails or single hand rails and a crutch can be used. In the latter case, the storing of the unused crutch represents a problem.

With respect to controlling the gait timing and events, two approaches are used: the menu approach and the autonomous on-line control. In the menu mode, the different gait modes are stored in the memory of the stimulator's on-board computer. The patient only triggers the events in the order in which they are stored. A characteristic of the on-line control approach is that the patient autonomously controls the timing and selects the order of events. For the menu principle, the FES sequences are firm, and the patient has no access to change them. The patient first selects the desired menu. Subsequent events are

ordered by a program and timed for segments between the triggers, such as an entire swing phase; the stored program determines the duration and amount of flexion in each joint.

Autonomous control requires the patient to compose and trigger the events. This mode provides complete freedom in movement selection and timing, but the patient must plan the events and master how to control the stimulation for a particular locomotion mode.

So far, the best results obtained in FES walking demonstrate that only rarely does a patient master community walking for 40 to 90 minutes but that many are able to use FES at home with a walker for 10 to 20 minutes daily. Also, the obtained speed of progression is low at present, being on the order of 0.1 to 0.4 m/sec. At this point we should remark that FES walking is still in its early development stage. In the near future, FES systems will be faster, more functional, and less tiring to the user. An FES system (Parastep® System, Sigmedics, Inc.) is now commercially available and is used by many patients with paraplegia for walking short distances. It is not yet able to replace the wheelchair for community activities.

THE STATUS OF FES AT THE REHABILITATION INSTITUTE OF CHICAGO AND THE PRITZKER INSTITUTE OF MEDICAL ENGINEERING, CHICAGO, ILLINOIS

The current research at the Rehabilitation Institute of Chicago and the Pritzker Institute has four goals. The first goal is to develop criteria to predict the outcome of electrically induced muscle restrengthening in individuals with paraplegia. The second is to implement limited periods of standing with FES in a laboratory setting. The third goal is to measure and evaluate the postural stability of a paraplegic individual's standing by both KAFOs and FES. Fourth, we wish to attain the widespread use of FES on a daily basis for mobility enhancement outside the laboratory.

To date, a total of 21 individuals with paraplegia have demonstrated standing by bilateral quadriceps stimulation using surface electrodes in our laboratory. Six of 14 have units for standing in their homes and use them outside of the laboratory. Also, 4 of these 14 have demonstrated crude bipedal gait within parallel bars.

The following is an outline of the protocol currently being used. The initial step in this study is a medical examination. Acceptable participants usually have thoracic lesions between T-3 and T-12. A lesion above T-3 results in considerable truncal instability and limits the ability to achieve a standing posture. Obviously, these criteria are not absolute. For example, a patient with a C-7 Brown-Séquard lesion was able to stand with FES in our laboratory, but his poor trunk control combined with diminished grasp made him quite unstable. Nonetheless, this patient was being fitted with long leg braces for standing at his rehabilitation hospital.

Some patients with lesions at or below T-12 may have lower motor neuron damage to the nerves of the lower extremities and, therefore, may not be suitable for FES. Thus excitability testing is an essential part of the screening program. Additional criteria of an otherwise unremarkable physical examination include absence of severe contractures and osteoporosis and psychological stability. Most of the patients participating in this study are at the end of their rehabilitation program.

Individuals are then prescribed stimulators and are instructed in their use for exercising atrophied muscles. The purpose of the stimulation is to increase muscle bulk and strength. Subjects are allowed to stimulate on the ward or at home without supervision after they are thoroughly instructed as to the proper restrengthening protocol to follow. At a minimum, this entails 1 hour spent with the investigator for teaching proper protocol and answering any questions. Follow-up visits are made to monitor patient compliance at least twice per month.

The stimulators used are designed locally and constructed for research purposes in our laboratory. Stimulation parameters are pulses of 0 to 120 V at 20-Hz frequency and 0.4-msec pulse width. The electrodes are carbon rubber. Thin, water-soaked sponges are used instead of electrode gel. Elastic straps are used to hold the electrodes in place. Stimulation begins with a 30-minute daily session that progresses to a 60-minute session.

Because the optimal procedure for muscle restrengthening is not yet known, we are using a 1:1 duty cycle of on/off stimulation. Our primary emphasis is the quadriceps because they are the most important muscle group for standing. During restrengthening, the subject either sits or lies recumbent with the knees elevated about 25 to 30 cm.

The main emphasis in the standing portion of this study is to gather data on the utility of and the problems associated with standing by FES. Although it might appear that this technique would be eagerly anticipated by individuals with paraplegia, this must be supported by data and experience. Concern with this issue is justified by the rejection rate of KAFOs. It is important that as many subjects as possible be evaluated in this regard. The basic difference between standing with FES and standing with KAFOs lies in timing and especially in the use of the arms. Standing by FES uses the leg muscles to achieve an upright posture. The patient therefore relies less on the upper extremities than when standing with KAFOs.

Standing by FES can be achieved with a minimum of two channels of stimulation. The knee joints are stabilized by bilateral quadriceps stimulation. A pair of surface electrodes is applied to each quadriceps femoris muscle and is held in place by straps. The electrodes are then connected to a single locking connector on the rear of the stimulator. In practice, we have found that essentially the same stimulus intensity for both the right and the left legs will produce acceptable standing; therefore, a single cable that does not differentiate right

and left legs is acceptable. The stimulator is then turned on by the off-on/amplitude knob on the front panel. The stimulation amplitude is adjusted by this front panel control and can be continuously varied from 0 to 120 V. This knob has two LEDs above it that indicate the presence of stimulation current through the electrodes. The stimulation frequency is kept constant at 20 Hz.

To effect standing, the postural change button on the right side of the panel is depressed. A 2-second delay occurs while the patient prepares for standing, an audible warning is sounded, and the stimulation begins. Pulse amplitude is increased linearly over the first 2 seconds to the level set by the amplitude control, and the pulse width is kept constant at 0.4 msec. This causes a smooth onset of quadriceps contraction and transition to a standing posture. Upon assuming upright posture, the hips are kept in hyperextension in a C-curve posture. The ankle joints are essentially unstable, necessitating reliance on external balance aids such as parallel bars or walkers. To sit, the postural change button again is depressed. After a 2-second delay, the warning is sounded, and the stimulation amplitude is decreased over the next 2 seconds to effect a smooth transition to a seated posture.

Once standing has been achieved, assuming the appropriate posture and using the balance aid must be practiced. When the patient has demonstrated expertise in standing in the physical therapy clinic, he or she may begin the transition to standing in the home. After an individual with paraplegia has experienced successful standing according to this protocol, evaluation for a permanent implantable stimulator may be considered, but this is still years from being clinically realized.

OTHER ISSUES PERTAINING TO FES RESEARCH

The psychological issues pertinent to conducting research with or introducing new devices to the individual with disability should not be overlooked. In particular, individuals who perceive FES as a cure or device that will allow them to regain use of much of their lower extremities may be at considerable psychological risk.

FES must be both effective and convenient to use if it is to be accepted. Therefore, an implantable system of electrodes and stimulator must be developed. The technology must be refined for safe, durable electrodes, and the necessary electronics must be miniaturized and encapsulated. Thus fabrication and clinical trials of implanted systems should be carried out in the future.

A number of fundamental questions concerning muscle physiology, safety, and sensory feedback must be solved before a truly effective FES system can be designed. Under normal conditions, the neuromuscular system is fatigue resistant because of the asynchronous activation of motor units. FES-induced muscle contraction reverses the natural order of muscle fiber recruitment. Also, all fibers are activated at once.

This leads to rapid fatigue and muscle ischemia. A number of strategies have been devised in an attempt to circumvent this problem, one being the principle of posture switching.

Safety is another consideration. The risks involved with using FES for standing and mobilization should not exceed the risk involved in using conventional KAFOs. Recently we measured the center of pressure and sway path in patients with paraplegia using both devices and found the results to be comparable.

Another important problem is that of sensory feedback or the provision of some appreciation of leg or arm position during FES without the need for constant visual attention. Patients with SCI who can walk have more difficulty doing so than patients with comparable motor deficits who have intact proprioception, as in those with poliomyelitis. In the paraplegic individual with a complete or nearly complete lesion, loss of proprioception is a major deficit. The penalties of loss of sensation are great even if traditional orthotic devices such as KAFOs are used. This is due to the general lack of sensory input from these devices unless they extend above the sensory deficit level. If FES is to succeed where traditional orthoses have failed, a strategy must be devised to interface remaining sensory systems in such a way as to provide sensory feedback from the lower extremities.

The use of FES to produce standing and rudimentary gait in patients with paraplegia has been demonstrated. Whether this use of FES can approach the success of a device such as the cardiac pacemaker remains to be determined. A system for standing and walking for patients with paraplegia is now available commercially in the United States. It uses technology similar to that developed by Kralj in Ljubljana. This system will be implemented and studied at the Rehabilitation Institute of Chicago for use by individuals with paraplegia for standing and walking.

REFERENCES

Andrews, B.J., et al. 1988. Hybrid FES orthosis incorporating closed-loop control and sensory feedback. *J. Biomed. Eng.* 10:189–195.

Bajd, T., et al. 1983. The use of a four-channel electrical stimulator as an ambulatory aid for paraplegic patients. *Phys. Ther.* 63:1116–1120.

Bajd, T., et al. 1986. FES rehabilitative approach in incomplete SCI patients. Paper presented at the RESNA 9th Annual Conference, Minneapolis, Minnesota.

Brindley, G.S., et al. 1978. Electrical splinting of the knee in paraplegia. *Paraplegia* 16:428–437.

Browner, W.J. 1962. Ambulatory electrical muscle stimulating device. U.S. Patent #3,025,858 (March 20, 1962).

Cooper, E.B., et al. 1973. Effects of chronic human neuromuscular stimulation. *Surg. Forum* 24:477–479.

Crago, P.E., et al. 1980. Closed-loop control of force during electrical stimulation of muscle. *Trans. Biomed. Eng.* 27:6:306–312.

Crago, P.E., et al. 1986. Open- and closed-loop control of FNS hand grasp. Paper presented at the I.E.E.E. Conference, Dallas/Fort Worth, Texas.

Fang, Z.P., and J.T. Mortimer. 1987. A method of activating natural recruitment order in artificially activated muscles. *Proc. 9th Ann. Conf. I.E.E.E. Eng. Med. Biol. Soc.*, New York, N.Y., 657–658.

Giamo, C.V. 1956. Electrical control of partially denervated muscles, U.S. Patent #2,737, 183 (March 6, 1956).

Graupe, D. 1989. EMG pattern analysis for patient-responsive control of FES in paraplegics for walker-supported walking. *I.E.E.E. Trans. Biomed. Eng.* 36:711–719.

Handa, Y., and N. Hoshimiya. 1987. Functional electrical stimulation for the control of the upper extremities. *Med. Prog. Technol.* 12:51–63.

Holle, J., et al. 1984. Functional electrostimulation of paraplegics: experimental investigations and first clinical experience with an implantable stimulation device. *Orthopedics* 7:1145–1155.

Keegan, J.R. 1963. Device for producing electrical muscle therapy. U.S. Patent #3,083, 712 (April 2, 1963).

Kralj, A., and S. Grobelnik. 1973. Functional electrical stimulation—A new hope for paraplegic patients? *Bull. Prosthet. Res.* 75:102.

Kralj, A., et al. 1980. Electrical stimulation providing functional use of paraplegic patients' muscles. *Med. Prog. Technol.* 7:3–9.

Kralj, A., et al. 1983. Gait restoration in paraplegic patients, a feasibility demonstration using multi-channel surface electrode FES. *J. Rehabil. Res. Dev.* 20:3–20.

Kralj, A., et al. 1986. Posture switching for prolonging functional electrical stimulation standing in paraplegic patients. *Paraplegia* 24:221–230.

Kralj, A.R., and T. Bajd. 1989. *Functional electrical stimulation: Standing and walking after spinal cord injury.* Boca Raton, Fla.: CRC.

Liberson, W.T., et al. 1961. Functional electrotherapy stimulation of the peroneal nerve synchronized with the swing phase of the gait of hemiplegic patients. *Arch. Phys. Med. Rehabil.* 42:101.

Long, C., and V.D. Masciarelli. 1963. An electrophysiologic splint for the hand. *Arch. Phys. Med. Rehabil.* 44:449.

Marsolais, E.B., and R. Kobetic. 1983. Functional walking in paralyzed patients by means of electrical stimulation. *Clin. Orthop.* 175:3036.

Marsolais, E.B., et al. 1984. "Improved synthetic walking in the paraplegic patient using implanted electrodes." In *Proceedings of the second International Conference on Rehabilitation Engineering,* Ottawa, Canada.

McNeal, D.R. 1977. "2000 years of electrical stimulation." In *Functional electrical stimulation,* ed. F.T. Hambrecht and J.B. Reswick. New York, N.Y.: Dekker.

Peckham, P.H., et al. 1976. Alteration in the force and fatiguability of skeletal muscle in quadriplegic humans following exercise induced by chronic electrical stimulation. *Clin. Orthop.* 114:326–334.

Petrofsky, J.S., and C.A. Phillips. 1983. Computer-controlled walking in the neurological-paralysed individual. *J. Neurol. Orthop. Surg.* 4:153.

Petrofksy, J.S., et al. 1984. Feedback control system for walking in man. *Comput. Biol. Med.* 14:135.

Popovic, D., et al. 1989. Hybrid assistive system—The motor neuroprosthesis. *I.E.E.E. Trans. Biomed. Eng.* 36:729–737.

Reswick, J.B. 1979. "A brief history of functional electrical stimulation." In *Neural organization and its relevance to prosthetics,* ed. W.S. Fields. Chicago, Ill.: Symposia Specialists.

Rudel, D., et al. 1982. Surface functional electrical stimulation of the hand in quadriplegics. Paper presented at the fifth Annual Conference on Rehabilitation Engineering, Houston, Texas.

Thoma, H., et al. 1983. First implantation of a 16-channel electric stimulation device in the human body. *ASAIO Trans.* 29:301–306.

Vodovnik, L., and W.D. McLeod. 1985. Electronic detours of broken nerve paths. *Electronics* 20:110–116.

Vodovnik, L., et al. 1981. Functional electrical stimulation for control of locomotor systems. *C.R.C. Crit. Rev. Bioeng.* 63:131.

Wilemon, W.K., et al. 1970. Surgically implanted peripheral neuroelectric stimulation (Internal report of Rancho Los Amigos Hospital, Los Angeles, Calif.).

Chapter 19

Home Modifications for People with Disabilities

Robert Harold Jackson

American society is shifting from an industrial labor–intensive existence to an informational and technological one. As U.S. businesses shift to accommodate these changes, many companies are paying closer attention to the disabled segment of the population because they have discovered an untapped resource of dedicated workers. In 1990 the Americans with Disabilities Act (ADA) was passed. The ADA is divided into five sections developed to eliminate discrimination against people with disabilities, to enable independent growth and development by individuals with disabilities, and to state a proper national goal for individuals with disabilities. Title I eliminates discrimination in employment, Title II concerns public services such as transportation, Title III addresses accommodations in public buildings and facilities and services operated by private entities, Title IV provides telecommunication services for individuals with hearing and speech impairment, and Title V establishes provisions for legal recourse and attorneys' fees and identifies other miscellaneous issues not covered under the body of the act. The ADA has had a major part in influencing thinking in American business; many corporations are tailoring their facilities, services, and products to address the needs of people inconvenienced through disability. These new employment opportunities have necessitated the need for home environments to be designed from the viewpoint of a disabled person competing in society.

As a result of this new trend of accommodating people with disabilities, architects and rehabilitation providers must alter their approach to planning. Modification of both home and work environments must be designed to reduce wasted time and motion while simultaneously addressing job-related issues such as stress. Making environmental changes is not always as complex as it appears. Simple selection of a product can solve an otherwise difficult or expensive problem. In many instances, simple devices such as a properly positioned grab bar, sound-activated switching devices, or household timers are all that are necessary. Larger problems can be resolved without making major structural changes while containing cost. For example, installing a mechanical wheelchair lift may eliminate the need for additional floor space for a ramp that might otherwise require structural modification, and a power door operator can eliminate the need for additional maneuvering space at entryways. The following is a basic operating guideline for considering modification of the home and work environments.

ENVIRONMENTAL PLANNING

Design Standards

Accessibility standards traditionally have focused on access to and around public facilities; therefore, they should be considered minimal guidelines to begin the planning process when one is modifying the home and work environment. These standards provide useful information about space dimensions and areas of concentration to be considered in home design. Existing standards tend to be more applicable to new construction or major alteration in public buildings to suit a broad range of disabilities and limitations in the general public. They do not always consider the functional abilities of the individual in the workplace, modification costs or design restrictions in the home environment that limit the person with a disability to compete equally for employment opportunities. It is highly recommended, however, that a copy of the standards be obtained when one is planning environmental modifications.

Four of the most widely used sources for standards are the following:

Illinois Accessibility Code
Capital Development Board
Third Floor, William G. Stratton Building
401 South Spring Street
Springfield, IL 62706
(217) 782-2864

Accessible and Usable Buildings and Facilities
(CABO/ANSI A 117.1-1992)
Sales Department
American National Standards Institute
1430 Broadway
New York, NY 10018
(212) 642-4900

Accessibility Guidelines for Buildings and Facilities and *Uniform Federal Accessibility Standards*
U.S. Architectural and Transportation Barriers Compliance Board
1331 F Street NW, Suite 1000
Washington, DC 20004-1111
(800) 872-2253

Planning

Whether a person's home is a house, apartment, condominium, or townhouse, it is seldom designed with reasonable space or facilities to accommodate a person with a disability, especially one in a wheelchair. In many cases, major modifications or new construction is required to accommodate the disabled individual and his or her family. Care should be taken to provide maximum utility and minimum inconvenience while maintaining family unity. All phases of evaluation and planning should be developed to stimulate motivation and personal achievement and to avoid psychological setbacks. Often the process of design, permit, and construction can exceed the total rehabilitation time. Early notification and action are imperative to begin the process. When delays are anticipated, short-range goals must be developed to allow transition from the rehabilitation unit to home with reasonable access and comfort. Long-range goals are then developed for permanent residency.

Photographs can be utilized to illustrate significant areas of concern that arise during the course of evaluation and will provide valuable input for architectural design. Often existing plans can be obtained from the owner, architect, or local building departments that will assist in the planning process and help minimize costs in design.

Evaluation

Because the home environment is the base of operations for daily living and vocational pursuits, it is one of the most important aspects to be considered in the course of rehabilitation. When one is evaluating daily functions, space requirements, and modification or design of the home, seven areas must be considered: general access, circulation, eating, sleeping, bathing, recreation, and transportation. Once the evaluation is completed and reviewed with the architect and/or contractor, recommendations can be made and design requirements established. Generally there are four possibilities available for consideration: modifying the existing home, providing independent access and a comfortable, usable environment in a reasonable time frame and a cost-efficient manner; expanding the existing home to achieve the desired results; relocating to an existing home that is easily modified; or designing and building a new home to suit the individual's needs. If relocation is indicated, temporary housing must be provided to allow time to complete the necessary planning and construction.

Design

After a comprehensive evaluation has been completed, conceptual sketches, drawings, and budgets can be developed. These are discussed and altered to suit the recommendations of the rehabilitation staff and are submitted to the owner for review of final design and cost. From these drawings and specifications, the working plans are completed and submitted for final changes and approval. Final adjustments are made, and the project is ready to be solicited for bid to contractors. The disabled individual and family should review all aspects of the project with the design architect and/or contractor before proceeding with construction.

Budget

Once a decision has been made about the type of home environment that will be developed, research should be conducted to determine costs of special appliances, fixtures, and equipment to ensure the most suitable manufacturer and to approximate the cost. A list of these products should be specified as part of the final plans that are submitted to contractors for bid. A detailed budget reflecting these special items and listing each trade should be developed. This budget is an important tool to be used for evaluating construction bids, maintaining consistency among the bidders, and monitoring the progress of construction.

Equipment

When one is evaluating a person's daily activities and future life style, it is important to develop an understanding of the adaptive equipment to be utilized. These devices provide ability where physical limitations exist. Careful consideration must be given to equipment recommendations to provide maximum independence. All too often, we tend not to realize that this equipment can make the difference between a person who becomes an active, participating member of society and an individual who becomes dependent on others for basic needs. Additionally, considerations must be made for equipment changes, replacement, and maintenance, with specifications being flexible to compensate for adjustments. Space to maneuver and to store these devices and supplies in the home environment will be required. Although standards have been developed for space utilized by equipment, modern day devices have a broad range of diversity in design and options. Therefore, the clear floor space required by a wheelchair, for example, may exceed the recommended standard (see Figure 19–1).

Medical equipment is divided into five principal categories: disposable products (urinary and medical supplies), daily living products (personal hygiene and self-help devices), prosthetics (prostheses and splints), durable medical products (wheelchairs, canes, crutches, cushions, and bathing devices), and accessibility products (lifts, showers, elevators, ramps, van lifts, and hand controls). Mechanical devices become a vital part of a person's life when he or she is inconvenienced by disability.

Rental Units

Through the process of hospitalization, rehabilitation, and transition to the home environment, the individual with a disability becomes expert in his or her needs. Whether the person

will live alone or with someone providing assistance, he or she usually chooses to live the most independent life style possible. The process of achieving independent living often begins by leasing the home environment. It is best to begin thinking of a rental unit from the perspective of life style and functions to be accomplished in daily living: eating, sleeping, bathing, socializing, general access, safety, and vocational pursuits. Developing a needs list of equipment and fixtures and researching sources and costs will assist the lessor and contractor in making modifications specified to individual needs. Often financial assistance can be obtained by contacting municipal, state, and federal agencies to determine available programs. A good place to begin is the department of human services or social services workers in the municipality.

By watching daily newspapers, an individual can become aware of preferential geographic areas, costs of rents in those areas, and projects being planned or in construction. Driving around different geographic locations will assist in evaluating the area for convenience, resources, and safety. Consideration should be given to leasing ground-floor units or units in elevator buildings. Contemporary designs are preferred because they provide open space with ample maneuvering room. Once a building has been identified, a personal visit is important to assess its compatibility with individual needs. Marketing brochures, floor plans, and sales personnel are helpful but do not provide specific information to address special needs of the individual.

The process of evaluation should begin outside the front door. A notebook and tape recorder are handy tools to list observations to be discussed before signing a lease. Note any curbs or obstructions in parking lots or approach walks. Evaluate the foyer and entry for ample maneuvering space and pressure of door closers. Once inside the unit, evaluate the bathroom for usability, efficiency, and maneuverability. Wall-hung plumbing fixtures instead of pedestal-mounted types can provide additional maneuvering space. Determine maneuverability in the kitchen. Floor plans that offer access and egress at opposite ends of the kitchen are preferable. When evaluating use of space, consider utilizing the living room for bedroom purposes if necessary because this room is usually larger. Wheel-in closets with doors removed can provide better flow with fewer obstructions. Using floor tile or carpeting breaks and furniture to define spaces will eliminate the need for walls that obstruct vision and maneuverability. Negotiate parking areas with lessor and fellow lessees for better usability and convenience to elevators or entryways. Insist on balconies in high-rise buildings to provide a safe area in case of emergency. Develop an emergency evacuation plan as soon as possible, and include notifying neighbors and local police and fire departments. An emergency alert system can be installed using regular telephone lines.

Whether an individual is modifying an apartment or a freestanding home, the guidelines provided in this chapter are

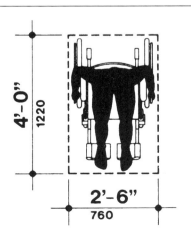

Figure 19–1 Wheelchair clear floor space.

similar. It is important to be creative and use common sense when addressing problems that are encountered in making the home environment usable for the disabled individual.

BATHROOMS

Bathroom Styles

There are two different styles of bathrooms for persons with disabilities. One is the modification of the existing bathroom with the adaptation of a shower chair, grab bars, shower wand, tub lift, or shower bench. Generally, these modifications are used for people who have the ability to transfer themselves in and out of the wheelchair (Figure 19–2). The other style of bathroom is a redesign in which a wheelchair shower is installed, allowing the person to wheel directly into the shower or, in some cases, an attendant to wheel him or her in. Space limitations should be considered when one is deciding to modify or redesign an existing bathroom (Exhibit 19–1).

When designing bathroom space for a person with a disability, we tend to design from the perspective of the able-bodied user, making the space simply usable. Bathroom space should be designed for the efficiency of the person so as to allow him or her to be competitive. Careful consideration should be given to safety and the amount of time spent in transferring and maneuvering. This time could be utilized more efficiently by the person with a disability, which is made possible with proper planning and design considering the entire family. Bathrooms generally are designed in minimal space and can be better utilized by having doors that swing out. Additionally, the doorway will not be blocked to outside assistance in case of accidental fall.

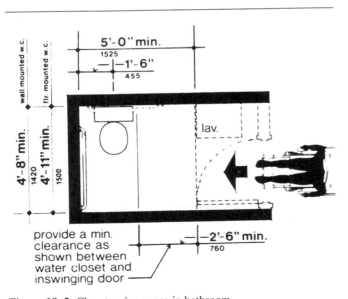

Figure 19–2 Clear turning space in bathroom.

Exhibit 19–1 Helpful Bathroom Checklist

Water Controls and Valves

Single-handle control
Lever or blade shape
Shut-off valve easy to use
Pressure balance and thermostatic control
Insulated pipes
105°F delivery temperature

Counters and Sinks

27 inches deep
Securely bracketed
Within reach of toilet
Knee space

Toilets

Raised toilet 20 inches
Raised toilet seat with cutout front and back
Ample space for transfer
Grab bars properly positioned
Water level and rim 7³/₄ inches
Easily used flushing device
Toilet paper and sink within reach

Grab Bars

Suitable height for individual ability
Positioned in bath tub and shower

Medicine Cabinets and Storage

Positioned for easy use
Bottom edge 36 inches high
Narrow shelves with single-row storage

Mirrors

Bottom edge 36 inches high
Full-length mirror

Bath Tubs

Grab bars positioned for individual use and ability
Bath seats or benches
Lifts and hoists
Bath mat or friction tape
Shower wand
Recessed shelf

Showers

Roll-in
Transfer with fixed bench
Roll-in with removable bench
Grab bars positioned for individual use and ability
Adequate space for transfer
Recessed shelf
Shower wand
Single-lever handle
Thermostatic control valve

Towel Racks and Soap Dishes

No more than 40 inches high
Withstanding 250 pounds of pressure

Water Controls and Valves

The use of single-handle control with a lever or blade shape that mixes the water to control temperature and adjusts the flow is recommended. A clear width is necessary between handles and the wall. When needed, remote control and electric valves can be used. Shut-off valves should be easy to use and accessible. Pressure balance and thermostatic control valves are used for safety and are best used at the point of supply instead of at individual fittings. A thermostatic valve should be used in the shower to allow for the variance of water temperatures when other sources of water are being used at the same time. Temperatures should be set between 110° and 120°F at the point of supply so that the delivery temperature will be approximately 105°F. All hot water feed and drainage pipes should be insulated to prevent scalding.

Counters and Sinks

The counter top for a sink should be 27 inches deep. Most standards call for wheelchairs to move under a securely bracketed sink. When there is knee space under the sink, drain pipes should be insulated (Figure 19–3). Quadriplegics with minimum hand function could use a counter to the left or right of the sink to move under, thus giving a work surface to manipulate self-help devices and personal hygiene products. If space will allow, consider a sink with storage underneath for easy access and convenience of position within reach of the toilet.

Toilets

Standards call for raised toilets 20 inches high for people in wheelchairs. In many cases, it is better to use a standard-height toilet and a raised toilet seat with a cutout front and back to allow an individual or attendant access for digital stimulation and hygiene purposes. The area around the toilet should be designed to provide ample space for wheelchair transfer. Grab bars should be placed at a height to maximize the person's ability. Specially designed seats with securely attached supporting arms may be useful for some people. The space between the water level and bowl rim should be 7¾ inches, the flushing device should be operated easily, and toilet paper and the sink should be within easy reach (Figure 19–4).

Grab Bars

Although standard height for grab bars or hand rails is 33 inches (Figures 19–5 and 19–6), many individuals may not have the ability to grasp a grab bar at that height for transferring into the wheelchair. Grab bars at wheelchair height of 24 inches may be more suitable for a person who has minimal ability in arm function and cannot push down from a higher bar. Grab bars in the shower may have to be positioned in various areas to assist in different functions such as transferring to and from wheelchair and shower seat and for stabilizing while in the shower.

Medicine Cabinets and Storage

These cabinets are used for medications and personal cosmetics. Cabinets should be positioned for easy access. In most cases, the bottom of the cabinet should be 36 inches from the floor. Narrow shelves with single-row storage are useful. Cabinets should be mounted close to the leading edge of the sink or vanity and recessed in the wall if possible.

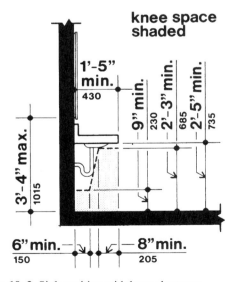

Figure 19–3 Sink position with knee clearance.

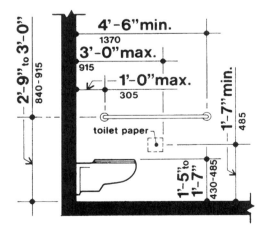

Figure 19–4 Toilet, grab bar, and paper dispenser mounting.

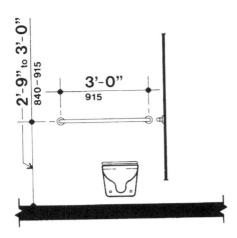

Figure 19–5 Rear wall grab bar mounting.

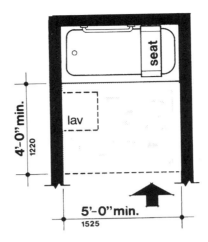

Figure 19–7 Floor space with in-tub seat, 90° turn.

Mirrors

Mirrors should be positioned so that the bottom edge is 36 inches from the floor and should extend high enough to be utilized by other family members. Full-length mirrors should be installed if possible.

Bath Tubs

To facilitate transfer to the bath tub, benches, bath tub seats, portable seats, built-in seats, and hydraulic seats can be used. Bath mats or friction strips should be used to provide a safe, nonslip surface, and grab bars should be used for transferring and stabilizing (Figures 19–7 through 19–9). A shower wand can be used and should be positioned for the convenience of the person. A recessed shelf can be used to hold soap, shampoo, and the like.

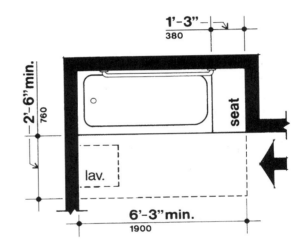

Figure 19–8 Floor space with tub ledge seat.

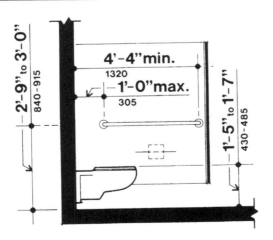

Figure 19–6 Side wall grab bar mounting.

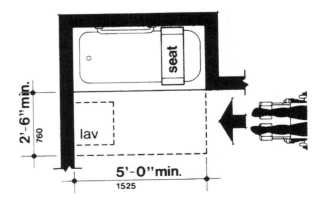

Figure 19–9 Floor space with in-tub seat, straight entry.

Showers

Basically there are three types of showers used by persons in wheelchairs: roll-in (Figures 19–10 and 19–11), transfer with fixed bench (Figures 19–12 and 19–13), and roll-in with removable bench. Preformed fiberglass shower units can be purchased and installed. Grab bars should be installed on three sides of the shower stall for convenience with regard to the individual's needs and abilities. Adequate space is necessary for transfer to the shower bench. A freestanding bench can be placed to suit individual needs and removed for a wheelchair shower. A recessed shelf for soap, shampoo, and so forth is useful. Shower wands should be positioned for the convenience of the person. A single-lever type handle should be used. A thermostatic shower valve is recommended even

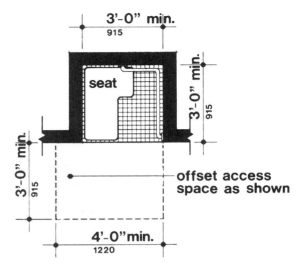

Figure 19–12 Transfer shower stall.

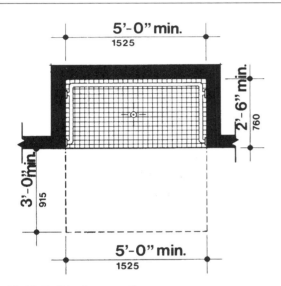

Figure 19–10 Roll-in shower stall.

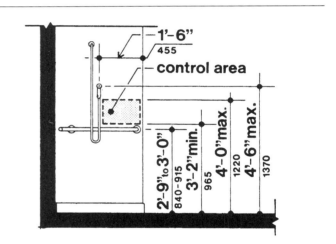

Figure 19–13 Transfer shower control wall.

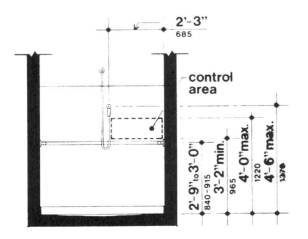

Figure 19–11 Roll-in shower control wall.

when hot water is controlled at the supply point to avoid overheated shower water due to varying requirements in the kitchen sink or laundry room.

Towel Racks and Soap Dishes

Towel racks, soap dishes, and shelves should be positioned no more than 40 inches from the floor. These items should be secured to the wall to withstand 250 pounds of pressure.

KITCHENS

Floor Space and Design

It is necessary that people in wheelchairs have unobstructed space in the kitchen around the refrigerator, stove, sink, and table (Exhibit 19–2). The floor should be of a smooth, nonskid surface. An L- or U-shaped design is the most efficient and requires the least amount of turning and moving (Figures 19–14 and 19–15).

Exhibit 19–2 Helpful Kitchen Checklist

Counters

  30- to 33-inch height
  Pullout work counter, 30-inch height

Sinks

  6 inches deep
  Rear drain
  Knee space under sink
  Spray attachment
  Insulated sink and pipes
  Temperature control hardware
  Mixing type faucet
  Shallow shelf over sink
  Garbage disposal

Refrigerators

  Side-by-side doors allow for most variation
  Standard one-door top freezer for ambulatory disabled
  Bottom freezer for person in wheelchair
  Self-defrosting

Ovens

  Side-hung or drop door
  Door strong enough to support food
  Cabinet space under oven
  Pullout board under oven
  Easily used, safe shelves

Cooktops

  No knee space under cooktop
  Burners in single row
  Burners flush to adjacent surface
  Range hood vent
  Controls in front
  Lip or drain along front edge

Cabinets and Shelves

  Easily used cabinet door pulls
  Cabinet space under counters and wall oven
  Full-height storage for variety of access
  High cabinet storage for those not in wheelchair
  High recessed base under cabinets to accommodate wheelchair
    footrests
  Narrow shelves for single-row storage

Miscellaneous

  Smooth, nonskid floor surface
  Open spaces for wheelchair passage
  Round table with pedestal base to allow for wheelchair
  Lighting under cabinets
  Bulb replacement within easy reach
  Strip plugs and accessible receptacles for small appliances
  Securely fixed drop ironing board with receptacle for iron
  Lap tray to help in carrying food and dishes
  Front-loading dishwasher, washing machine, and dryer

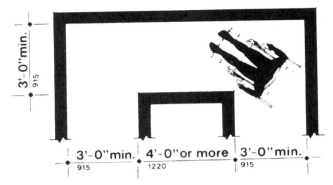

Figure 19–14 Cabinet turning clearance.

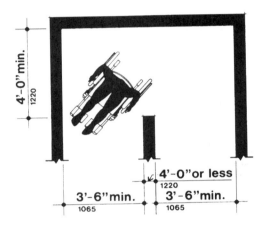

Figure 19–15 Cabinet turning clearance.

Counters

Counter height of 30 to 33 inches with undercounter clearance is preferred by most people in wheelchairs. A standard 36-inch counter height can be utilized for other people using the kitchen. To modify an existing 36-inch counter, a pullout shelf of 30 inches can be installed.

Sinks

Sinks should be no deeper than 6 inches, have drainage at the rear, and allow for knee space underneath. The underside and exposed pipes should be insulated. A reinforced cutting board can be utilized over the sink for convenient use of water for food preparation.

The kitchen sink should have an insulated swivel arm faucet, possibly capable of swinging over the adjacent counter top to have a convenient place for filling pots, kettles, and so forth. A spray attachment is a convenient means of cleaning the sink and can be used for filling pots with water. Instant hot water sink attachments are available. For persons with limited reach, levers can be placed below the counter rim to one side of the sink bowl. Adjustable-height sinks are available.

A sink garbage disposal is essential. It should be set back in one corner with the switch easily used and accessible. The unit and waste outlet must not obstruct knee approach. Trash compactors can be utilized for paper and can refuse. Although this process creates a bag that may be cumbersome to remove, it also is convenient in terms of minimizing the need for frequent removal of trash.

Refrigerators

A two-door, side-by-side refrigerator-freezer is best for both the person in a wheelchair and the ambulatory person with a disability because it allows for variation in areas of reach; if the standard one-door refrigerator is provided, however, the freezing compartment should be at the bottom for the wheelchair user or at the top for the ambulatory person with a disability. The self-defrosting models are the most convenient.

Ovens

A built-in oven with a side-hung door allows the person in a wheelchair good accessibility, especially when the door opens to 180°. The oven door should open away from the light source. A pullout board installed under the oven can be useful for transferring food to counters and for food preparation. When a drop door is used, care should be taken to minimize the risk of burns to hands, arms, and legs. If the drop door is strong enough, it can be used to transfer food from oven to counter, and it can also protect the legs from splatters and spills. Oven shelves should pull out easily and have nontip stops to ensure that they cannot be accidentally pulled out completely.

Cooktops

Burners should be arranged in a single row and can be designed at the back section of the cooktop so that the front section can be used for food preparation. Burners should be flush to adjacent surfaces to allow for easy sliding of pots and pans. Cooktop controls should be located at the front and easily used. No knee space should be allowed under the cooktop because of the danger of hot spills. A lip along the front edge or a slot with a drain pan below can reduce the danger from spilled hot liquid or food. A range hood vent above the cooktop can be operated by positioning the switch within easy reach.

Cabinets and Shelves

Cabinet door pulls, pullout boards, and drawers should be easy for the individual to use and have built-in stops. Narrow pullout shelves for single-row storage are useful and can be installed inside cabinet doors. A portable shelf unit on casters may be used to modify a kitchen when more accessible storage is needed. A high recessed base under the cabinets is necessary to accommodate wheelchair footrests.

GENERAL HOME CONSTRUCTION

Bedroom

Bedrooms should have convenient access to bath and toilet rooms. There should be a light switch accessible at the bed, and the telephone should be within easy reach. The bed should be placed with adequate space around it to allow easy wheelchair access and movement. The height of the bed should be level with the wheelchair seat height. Storage next to the bed can be conveniently used for the easy reach of braces, prostheses, or clothing. A pullout storage system under the bed can be an efficient use of wasted space.

Furniture can be placed on casters so that the pieces can be easily moved by the wheelchair user. Drawers should be such that only one hand is needed to open them. Stops should be used so that drawers cannot be pulled all the way out accidentally. Shelving units with narrow shelves for single-row storage can be used. Bottom shelves should be 18 inches from the floor. Bedside tables with drawers can be utilized to provide storage top area for a clock, telephone, and the like.

Doorways and Doors

The minimum clear width for doorways is 32 inches (Figure 19–16). This usually is adequate space for wheelchair passage, but consideration should be taken for the person's arms and hands while turning the wheels. The wheelchair will need more space if a turn is to be made.

To modify a narrow doorway, fold-back hinges can be installed, increasing clear width by 1½ to 2 inches. A 5-foot space inside and outside the doorway should be provided. This space needs to be level to prevent the wheelchair from rolling when the person releases the wheel grips to reach for the door. Doors should not open directly to the top of a staircase. In small rooms, especially bathrooms, doors should open outward, allowing better access and eliminating door blockage should the person fall and require assistance.

Evaluation is needed in choosing suitable doors for individual needs. Side-hung doors may be suitable for people with limited arm and hand usage. Remote controls may be needed by other individuals. Some types of doors to consider are pocket-sliding, sliding, folding, automatic, remote controlled, those equipped with opening and closing devices, pneumatically assisted closers, and pulley-operated openers and closers.

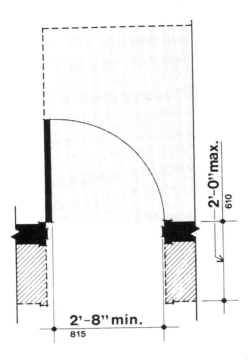

Figure 19–16 Hinged door clearances.

Kick plates may be used to protect the door from wheelchair footrests. Where glass doors are used, the bottom frame should be 7½ inches high. Mat wells should be provided for doormats to provide level surfaces.

Door Hardware

Handles, pulls, latches, locks, and other operating devices on doors should have a shape that is easy to grasp with one hand and does not require tight grasping, pinching, or twisting of the wrist to operate. Lever, push type, and U-shaped handles can be used. There are handles available that slip over existing round doorknobs to convert them to lever handles.

There should be a clearance of 2 inches between the handle and the door. Door handles should be placed between 3 feet and 3 feet 3 inches high for comfortable operation and should not exceed 4 feet. An auxiliary handle or rail may be installed that aligns with the door handle and is used to pull the door. Sliding doors should have an exposed pull handle on each side of a door where ingress and egress are required. Where locks are used, they should be of a type to avoid the need for simultaneous use of both hands.

Thresholds

Raised thresholds should be avoided. If they are installed, they should be no higher than ¾ inch high, and the floor on either side should be at the same level. Wooden thresholds that are beveled on each side act as miniramps. Weather stripping can be obtained by using a flexible threshold with a spring action. In some cases, weather stripping can be attached directly to the door. When sliding doors are used, there should be no upstanding door guides or upward projections.

Floors

Floors should be constructed of hard surfaces such as wood, vinyl, or tile. When carpeting is used, it should be installed tight to the floor (Figure 19–17). When possible, it is better to exclude padding under the carpet. Tightly woven fabric should be used; avoid loose weave or shag.

Hard floors should have a flat, nonskid surface. Bathroom floor surfaces should be such that they do not become slippery when wet. Wax for floors should be used sparingly or not at all. Flooring material that looks slippery but has a nonslip surface should be avoided. Tiles instead of continual flooring can be used because the joints between the tiles provide a measure of friction. Pick a tile with a pattern or color so as to mask marks made by wheelchair tires and other scuffing.

Hallways

Hallways should be 4 feet wide wherever possible to allow easy access to and egress from adjoining rooms. Where narrow hallways must be used, doors should be widened to achieve the same effect. Turning room should be provided at the beginning and end of a hallway where possible (Figures 19–18 and 19–19).

Routes

During the evaluation of a home for modification or in the design of a new home, one should look at routes from a wheelchair point of view. Starting from the street curb, drive, or garage, look at the route to the front door. From the front door, examine the routes around furniture, appliances, and bath and kitchen fixtures. Consider each task to be performed and the time required to accomplish it. Structures that impede free

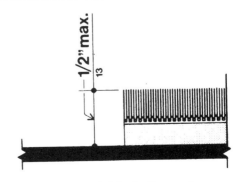

Figure 19–17 Carpeting height for floor surface.

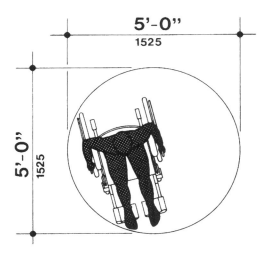

Figure 19–18 Minimum clear space for 180°/360° turn.

wheelchair movement should be removed. There should be 360° turn areas throughout the home.

Walls

Clear plastic corner edging or metal plaster bead can be used to protect corners from damage. Walls should be of a material that is easy to clean and maintain. Clear plastic shields can be used in hard wear areas such as above the sink and where wheelchair footrests touch the walls. Insulation should be used inside the walls to reduce heat and air conditioning expenses.

Windows

Windows should open outward and be easy to operate. Casement windows are the most difficult to operate. When casement windows are used, keep the area in front of them clear so that the wheelchair user has easy access. If radiators are in front of a window, it is advisable to cover the radiator with a solid cover to minimize heat transference and possible burns. In an environment where wall space is minimal for furniture placement, windows may have to be installed at a level that makes them inaccessible. In this case, windows can be power operated. Horizontal sliding windows should be considered when one is designing or planning window treatment.

HOME MECHANICAL

Light Switches

When light switches are adjacent to doors, they should be positioned horizontal to the handle for ease in locating them. At staircases and hallways, there should be two-way switching. A wheelchair person's most comfortable range for forward reach begins 1 foot 3 inches from the floor and generally does not exceed 4 feet (Figure 19–20). Switches should be placed at a height between 3 feet and 3 feet 6 inches.

For persons with limited hand or finger mobility, rocker action switches can be utilized. Light switch extenders, which

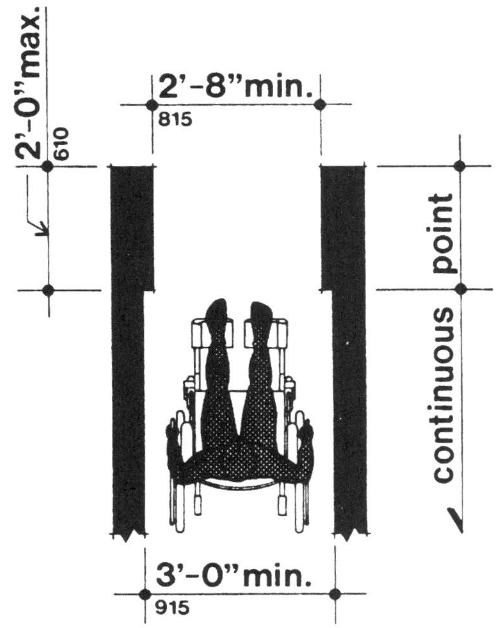

Figure 19–19 Moving wheelchair clearances.

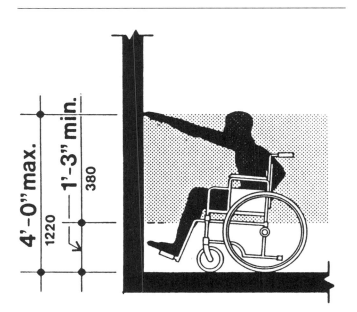

Figure 19–20 Forward reach limitations.

slip over the existing switch, can be used to adapt existing light switches. There should not be more than two switches per plate. Switches should be placed at the point of entry to all rooms, staircases, and hallways. Wireless remote control switches are available from local hardware stores. Cord switches, dimmer switches, timer switches, and pull chains are the most suitable for persons with limited finger function.

Lighting

Wall-bracket lighting that is placed within easy reach is convenient, accessible for light bulb changing, and stable when securely fastened to the walls. Table lamps should have wide bases to allow for maximum stability. Pull chains or pressure-sensitive push switches are useful. Lighting can be used to enhance the beauty inside the home and to be of practical function in the kitchen, bathrooms, and bedrooms. Outside lighting should be considered for access paths at night.

Receptacles

Receptacles should be located where they are most needed. They should be unobstructed and accessible. Most receptacles are placed too low and are difficult to reach. They should be placed at a height between 18 and 24 inches. Fuses and circuit-breaker switches should be within easy reach. An electric tabletop strip console of switches and outlets can be used alongside the bed to control television, stereo, radio, lights, and so forth. One of these strips in the kitchen at a key point can be used to operate and control the kitchen appliances, radio, television, and the like.

Heating and Air Conditioning

The thermostatic controls should be positioned at a level so as to be read and operated easily. There may be a need for space heating, especially in bedrooms and bathrooms, where much time is spent in dressing, washing, and personal grooming. Air conditioning is imperative for those with impaired lung function or breathing problems. Most people with quadriplegia require air conditioning. Ceiling-mounted circulating fans can provide more even heat, circulate air, and reduce heating and air conditioning expenses.

Shelves and Counters

When there needs to be some part of a storage wall suitable for the wheelchair user (Figure 19–21), the ambulatory person with disability, and the able-bodied, all of whom have different minimum and maximum areas of reach, shelves should be full height from floor to ceiling. The usual system of shelves above and below counters does not make use of the space directly above the counter, the most convenient height for disabled people. A full wall of shelves therefore offers storage

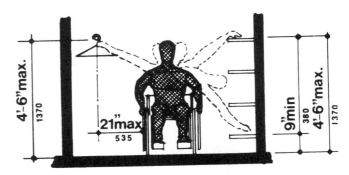

Figure 19–21 Closet and storage area for the wheelchair user.

within reach of the ambulant and wheelchair users. Where a writing surface is required, at least one 30- to 33-inch high counter or tabletop should be provided. Where possible, shelves should be constructed narrowly for single-row storage.

Special Construction

Access to recreation has been one of the major goals of the accessibility movement. Many homes, condominiums, and apartment complexes are equipped with swimming pools, pool tables, and tennis and basketball courts. Horseback riding, archery, hiking, skiing, and boating are some outdoor activities that may require consideration for accessibility.

Swimming pools should be designed with built-in stairs on the shallow end of the pool or in a corner with hand rails for stability. A recessed alcove should be formed into the concrete to provide a rest area. A continuous grab bar installed around the inside perimeter of the pool, just above the water line, should be avoided because it protrudes from the wall and restricts safe entry and exit. Overhead hoists, hydraulic lifts, and ramps can be used for transfer. Changing areas with raised transfer mats should be supplied for dressing at all facilities.

Safety

In the event of fire, an emergency evacuation plan should be designed. The home should have fire detectors, fire extinguishers, and smoke alarms. Preparations should be made for a fireproof area and a shielded balcony or deck for evacuation purposes. Where mechanical lifts are used for primary access, a ramp should be used for secondary access at the opposite end of the home. Emergency phone numbers should be readily available at all phones.

Central Vacuum Cleaning System

To eliminate the problem of using a vacuum cleaner from a wheelchair, a central vacuum system may be useful. The suction hose and attachments are plugged into special outlets built into the walls in each room. Debris is gathered in a storage canister and must be removed periodically.

Mailboxes

A large slot letterplate at the door with a letter basket inside at a 2-foot 4-inch height is a good way to provide accessibility to outside mail delivery. An outdoor shelf for newspapers, milk, and package delivery will eliminate the difficulty of having to lift these items from the ground. Post-mounted drive-up mailboxes should be positioned to allow access from the vehicle window without leaving the vehicle.

HOME ACCESSIBILITY

Individual Lifts and Hoists

Individual lifts and hoists are utilized to allow a person inconvenienced through disability to transfer from bed to wheelchair and to the bath tub, toilet, exercise mat, and back to the

wheelchair. There are several types of these devices available, such as manual hydraulic, electrically powered, or portable. Some require assistance; others can be operated independently. These lifts provide accessibility inside the home for the individual and reduce or eliminate the need for attendant care. When attendant care is utilized, these devices will eliminate back strain and unnecessary exertion for the attendant.

Ramps

Ramps are the most reasonable means of access to and from a home. They can be installed to beautify the home by blending into an altered façade and accenting the grounds with flowers and shrubbery. It is important to go beyond standards of measure and into the imagination. The results will be a home that is accessed more easily by all family members and guests (Table 19–1, Figure 19–22).

The ability of the person to navigate through a ramp as well as the ramp's location, convenience, style, and materials should be considered before a ramp is built or purchased. Ex-

Table 19–1 Slope Chart for Ramps

Suit Ramp to the User	Slope Requirements	If the Step Is This High . . .	. . . Ramp Must Be This Long	Ramp Slope Often Referred to as:
Gentle slope for most wheelchair users	For each inch in height, the ramp must extend 12 inches	1″/25 mm	1′/305 mm	1 in 12
		2″/51 mm	2′/610 mm	1 in 12
		3″/76 mm	3′/914 mm	1:12
		4″/102 mm	4′/1.2 m	1/12
		5″/127 mm	5′/1.5 m	5°
		6″/152 mm	6′/1.8 m	
		7″/179 mm	7′/2.1 m	
For wheelchair users with strong arms; those who must be pushed by able-bodied; motorized chairs	For each inch in height, the ramp must extend 5 inches	1″/25 mm	9″/228 mm	6°
		2″/51 mm	18″/457 mm	
		3″/76 mm	27″/686 mm	
		4″/102 mm	36″/914 mm	
		5″/127 mm	45″/1.1 m	
		6″/152 mm	54″/1.4 m	
		7″/179 mm	63″/1.6 m	
Only for wheelchair users who are unusually strong; when disabled is lightweight and pusher is strong; for extra-powerful motorized chairs	For each inch in height, the ramp must extend 7 inches	1″/25 mm	7″/179 mm	8°
		2″/51 mm	14″/356 mm	
		3″/76 mm	21″/533 mm	
		4″/102 mm	28″/711 mm	
		5″/127 mm	35″/889 mm	
		6″/152 mm	42″/1.0 m	
		7″/179 mm	49″/1.2 m	
Steepest slope only suitable for motorized vehicles or mechanical assists such as incline lifts and power hoists	For each inch in height, the ramp must extend 5 inches	1″/25 mm	5″/127 mm	10°
		2″/51 mm	10″/457 mm	
		3″/76 mm	15″/381 mm	
		4″/102 mm	20″/508 mm	
		5″/127 mm	25″/635 mm	
		6″/152 mm	30″/762 mm	
		7″/179 mm	35″/889 mm	

Note: A step of ⅝″/15.9 mm or less need not be ramped.

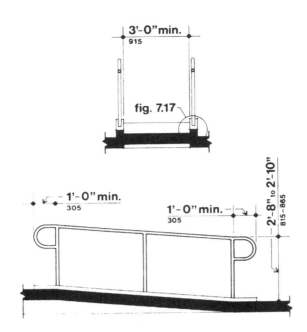

Figure 19–22 Ramp with curb and hand rails.

panded metal provides traction but is a poor choice for some kinds of heeled shoes. Concrete ramps can be constructed with nonskid surfaces. Wood should be treated to resist rotting and should maintain space of no more than ½ inch to allow elements to pass through as well as provide better grip. Carpeting should be avoided because it holds water and is more difficult to push on. People using crutches or canes often prefer stairs.

A manual wheelchair weighs from 25 to 65 pounds, and it can be tiring for some people to push themselves up a ramp, especially at the maximum slope of 1:12. On a long or steep ramp, there is the possibility of loss of control; the downward speed could cause friction burns on the hands. Level rest platforms are therefore necessary at 10-foot intervals for ascent and descent on a long ramp. Level platforms are also necessary to turn a wheelchair on a slope. Continuous hand rails should be installed on each side, extending beyond the slope at the top and bottom of a ramp. Ramps should have curbs on both sides so that a wheelchair cannot accidentally run off the ramp; curbs also are used to help brake a wheelchair in an emergency.

There should be at least 5 feet of straight clearance at the bottom of a ramp. Nonskid surfaces are essential. If possible, ramps should be protected from the elements. In any case, they should be kept free from ice and snow.

Mechanical Lifts

In remodeling homes where several stairs exist and space for ramps is not available, mechanical lifts may be the only solution to access for people with mobility limitations. There

are both vertical and inclined platform lifts for wheelchairs. Vertical lifts are placed at the bottom of stairs, and the upper landing may need to be extended to meet them. Inclined platform lifts are mounted on walls or stairs or are post-mounted on tracks along the stairs. Both lifts can be installed with enclosing walls and electrically interlocked gates for safety. There should be enough space to propel the wheelchair directly onto the lift without the need for turning. Controls should be easy to use and conveniently located. Chair lifts have built-in seats for people with mobility limitations who can walk but cannot climb stairs. This type of lift does not serve wheelchair users well and therefore is of limited use.

Elevators

Elevators often are used to provide access between floors. Some companies will manufacture residential type elevators with special car sizes to accommodate a wheelchair (Figure 19–23). They are constructed in a convenient location inside the home where a corner or closet area common to all floors exists (Figure 19–24). Local coding authorities should be consulted before design begins.

Transportation

When planning the home environment, consider the transportation of the person and his or her family. Transportation is the link to life; in most areas of the country, public transportation is either nonexistent or poor and undependable. An available vehicle to allow a person the dignity to be transported or to transport himself or herself is a necessity, not a luxury. The

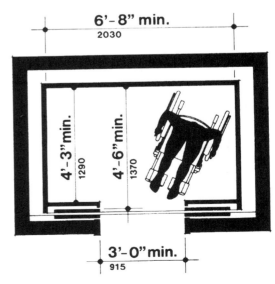

Figure 19–23 Elevator car floor area with side-opening center door.

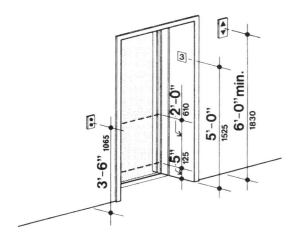

Figure 19–24 Elevator entrance and control positioning.

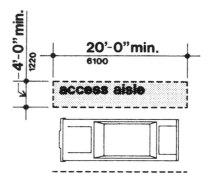

Figure 19–25 Automobile transfer and loading area.

vehicle provides access to employment, recreation, and social functions as well as medical and dental care while stimulating an overall feeling of independence that is primary to the physical and psychological strength of the person. Equally important is the need to provide proper recommendations and choice of equipment. Traditionally, medical facilities and rehabilitation providers have had to rely on vendors to recommend equipment. Unfortunately, this tends to limit knowledge of technology and choices to only those brands distributed by a particular vendor. All too often the individual is unaware of other choices available that might better enhance his or her abilities.

Transportation needs can be divided into three major groups: individuals requiring assistance, those who transport themselves using a power wheelchair or cart, and those who utilize a standard vehicle with hand controls. For individuals requiring assistance or who transport themselves using power wheelchairs, special transportation such as wheelchair vans, taxis, or custom-built private vans are used. Parking should be provided in a garage or covered area with access to the home whenever possible. The overhead door and floor of the garage may require modification to accommodate a tall vehicle, and the door should be automated. An automobile requires a 12-foot wide space, and a van requires a 15-foot wide space. An entry ramp is used to provide access to the single-entry door to the home (Figure 19–25). Careful research should be conducted on daily activities and home environment before a vehicle is purchased.

SAMPLE CONSTRUCTION DESIGN

Attendant Care Environment

Figures 19–26 and 19–27 portray room additions for a person requiring attendant care. The original home (light line areas) provided 600 square feet of usable living space. A room addition (dark line areas) has been added to provide an additional 800 square feet of space to accommodate the person, family, and attendants. The addition features include the following:

- accessible bath with roll-in shower
- exercise and therapy area in bedroom
- storage for disposable and medical supplies and equipment
- wheelchair lift for direct access to garage
- attendant access to laundry
- exterior deck for recreation and emergency fire waiting area
- expanded eating and passage areas to accommodate wheelchair
- front-enclosed sunroom with attached front ramp for emergency evacuation, recreation, and front access to yard
- expanded kitchen area
- access to back yard from garage
- extra-wide sidewalk connecting rear, side, and driveway to street for recreation and outside activities
- oversize garage door to accommodate raised van roof

Quadriplegic Environment

Figure 19–28 portrays a room addition for a young C-5 quadriplegic husband and father of a 2-year-old child. Working closely with the disabled person and the Rehabilitation Institute of Chicago staff, this 800-square-foot home addition was designed to provide an environment to allow the person to begin his retraining for employment through education at a local college. Additions, indicated by heavy black lines, were added to the original structure. These additions also provide

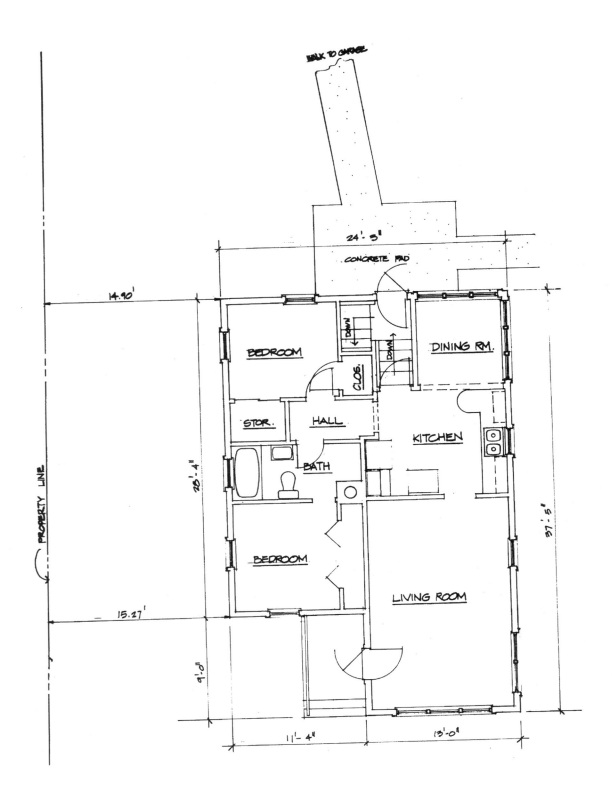

Figure 19–26 Original floor plan of existing house (see area labeled "Existing House" in Figure 19–27).

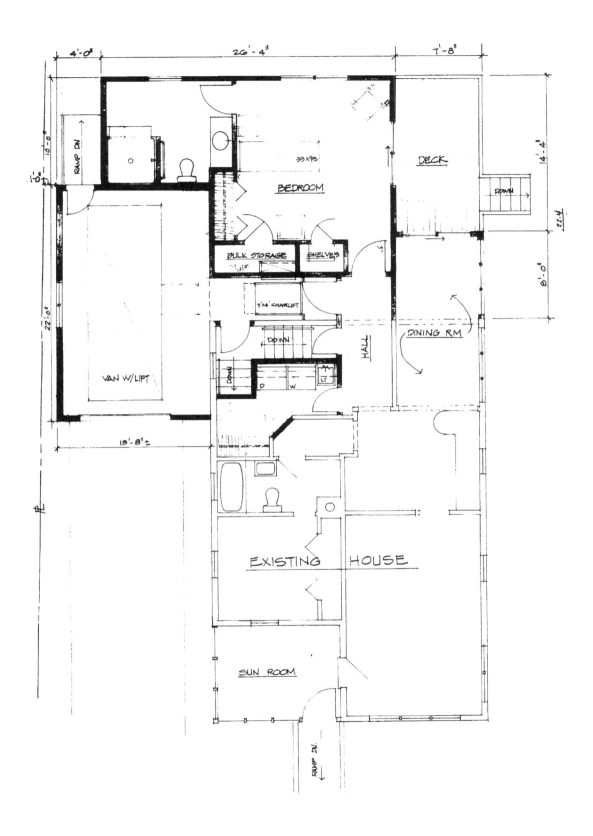

Figure 19–27 Floor plan showing room addition.

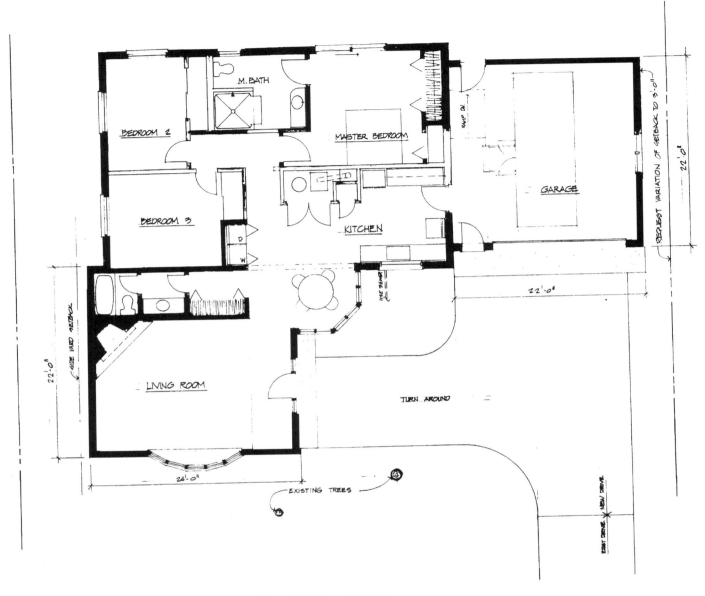

Figure 19–28 Floor plan of home addition for a patient with C-5 quadriplegia.

unrestricted movement for other family members. They feature the following:

- master bedroom converted from living room
- wheelchair bathroom with roll-in shower and accessible toilet and sink areas
- second bedroom converted to a study
- existing master bedroom converted to child's room
- extra-wide doorways for easy movement
- 4-foot-wide hallways
- expanded kitchen and eating areas for wheelchair maneuverability

- central air conditioning easily accessible
- galley type kitchen for wheelchair access
- convenient access to washer and dryer
- gas fireplace in living room to supply emergency heat
- level front access and emergency access
- rear emergency access from master bedroom to patio
- level access to level garage area for van access
- outside turnaround area to park van
- oversize automatic garage door and approach ramp to front and rear of home for recreation and exercise

- additional bathroom to accommodate family members and guests

Paraplegic Environment

Figures 19–29 and 19–30 portray modifications to a two-story home for a T-12 paraplegic husband and father of two. After careful evaluation and review, it was decided to modify the first floor of existing home (Figure 19–29) as a short-term solution to provide transition from the Rehabilitation Institute of Chicago to home. Modifications include the following:

- new entry door from garage to first-floor foyer
- raised platform and ramp for access to garage and patio
- rear-entry ramp from existing deck to patio
- chair lifts from first to second floor
- wheelchair on second floor

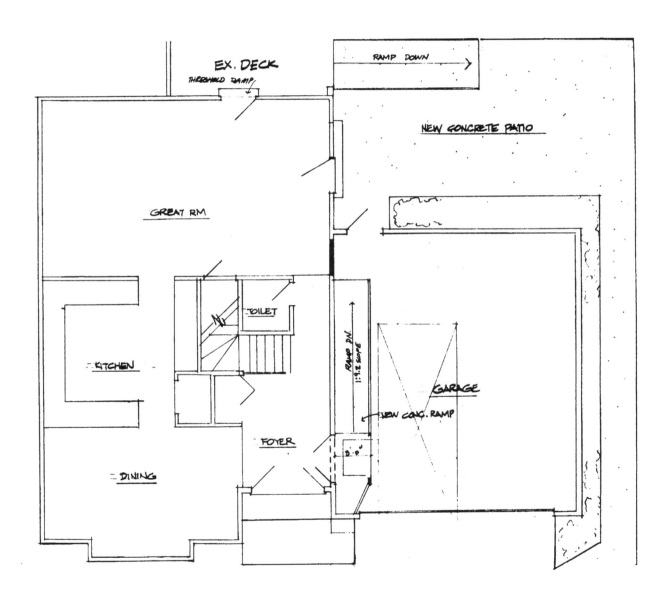

Figure 19–29 First-floor plan with modifications.

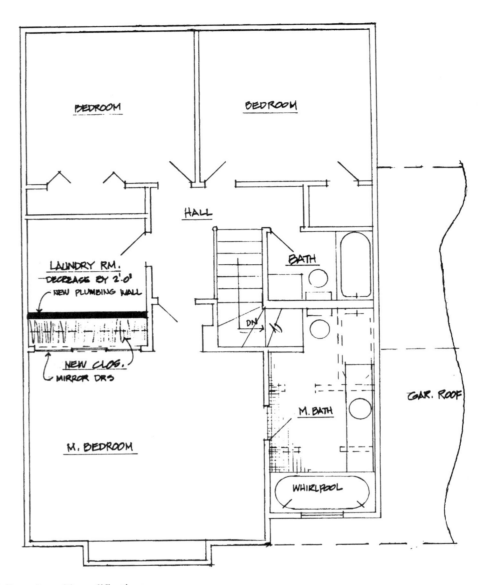

Figure 19–30 Second-floor plan with modifications.

- modified master bath and walk-in closet to provide additional wheelchair space
- relocation of closet for better access

Because this person was to return to work for his company, the two-story style home would restrict his ability to meet time frames and job responsibilities. The sale of the old home would provide funds for a more suitable, new home to be designed and constructed.

CONCLUSION

We are living at a time when society is making major scientific and technological advancements that have created opportunity for people with disabilities to reach their maximum potential. Meaningful employment, recreation, and travel are now a reality. The home environment must provide a comfortable, relaxing, and stimulating atmosphere where a person with a disability can coexist with family and friends. The home must be a place where one can rejuvenate energy and creativity, a place that reflects accomplishment in life and contributions to society, a place in which to feel pride and dignity.

Life must be an adventure where those who are physically challenged go beyond standards and the status quo by continuing to be creative and objective about themselves and the way the world perceives them. Indeed, they must become the teachers of the meaning of life.

* * *

Please note that although the various products described in this chapter are not specifically required, they can solve problems, lower costs, and ensure accessibility more efficiently, especially in rental apartment and condominium living, where major changes are not feasible. The author seeks to present only a range of useful products that can be acquired by contacting manufacturers. Certainly there are good products and manufacturers of which we are not aware; many of these manufacturers have access to products in addition to those mentioned here. Inclusion of a product in this book is in no way an endorsement or guarantee of either the manufacturer's claims or the product's acceptability under any jurisdiction. The graphics for this chapter are taken from: A Guidebook to: The Minimum Federal Guidelines and Requirements for Accessible Design, *United States Architectural and Transportation Barriers Compliance Board, 1331 F Street NW, Suite 1000, Washington, DC 20004-1111.*

Chapter 20

Driver Assessment

Kirsten M. Kohlmeyer and Christi Rom

A driver rehabilitation program can enhance the traditional rehabilitation program because driving is a high-level activity of daily living skill that facilitates independent functioning within the community. An interdisciplinary approach to driving allows most patients with spinal cord injury an opportunity to drive. It may also facilitate getting unsafe drivers off the road, a definite public safety issue.

TEAM APPROACH

The driver rehabilitation team can be quite extensive. It includes the client and family members and a counselor or funding source (e.g., workers' compensation, litigation, department of rehabilitation services, or third party payers). Evaluators may include an occupational therapist, who evaluates physical functioning, cognition, vision, perception, and potential adaptive equipment needs. A rehabilitation engineer usually evaluates with an occupational therapist and helps assess for new technology and equipment needs and recommends, modifies, and/or designs adaptive devices. A driver instructor conducts the on-the-road assessment and training. The vehicle modifier provides current information regarding adaptive controls and vehicle modification, installs devices, modifies vehicles, trains the client on secondary and accessory control operation once installed, and provides vehicle service and maintenance. The physician is a primary referral source who provides the medical history and acts as a liaison with the secretary of state as a reporting mechanism. Clients may be referred back to a physician if the evaluators have questions or concerns regarding medical, cognitive, or visual status. The department of motor vehicles most often performs driver license examinations and basic vehicle safety inspections and imposes restrictions and suspensions. Authority and reporting mechanisms regarding licensing recommendations should be investigated because they often vary from state to state. Last, the client's family provides emotional and financial support as well as a good perspective on the client's day-to-day functioning. Family support is imperative for successful follow-through with training and driving once the license is obtained (Pierce 1987; Shipp 1989; Smith 1987; Strano 1987).

EVALUATION

Referral sources for a driving program often include physicians, rehabilitation professionals, insurance companies, family members, or patients themselves. Reasons for referral may include evaluation for safety issues, equipment needs, training, or recommendations for a passenger vehicle. Once a referral is received, a significant amount of background information is obtained to ensure smooth entry into the program. Upon establishing initial contact and rapport, the therapist gathers client information regarding medical history (e.g., disability type, secondary disability, and current therapies), physician clearance (e.g., any concerns, precautions, or current medication), and current level of functioning (e.g., mobility, cognitive, and physical status). Potential problems with program entry, such as funding and licensure, are identified and rectified. Communication with the secretary of state may be necessary at this time. The therapist then makes the preliminary estimate of needed adaptive equipment (Latson 1987; Shipp 1989; Smith 1987; Strano 1987).

During the patient interview, the therapist obtains a basic medical history regarding seizures, spasticity, heterotopic ossification, past or planned surgery, pressure sores, hospitalizations, medications and side effects, living situation, and current daily activities. A preinjury and postinjury driving history is obtained, including education, violations, and accidents, as well as driving goals and overall general attitude toward driving (Latson 1987; Shipp 1989).

The clinical assessment is based functionally and obtains a gross picture in a number of areas. Physically, the therapist evaluates upper and lower extremity proprioception and range of motion, active arm placement, strength, balance, reflexes, tone, and any orthoses or prostheses. The wheelchair assessment evaluates the type, condition, and dimensions of the chair as well as the patient's positioning, postural stability, and ability to manage parts regardless of whether the patient plans on transferring to a car or captain's seat or will drive from the wheelchair level. The visual/perceptual screening measures visual acuity, stereodepth, lateral and vertical phoria convergence, night vision, contrast sensitivity, glare recovery, saccades, fixation, tracking, and color discrimination. The cognitive screening evaluates attention (divided, alternating, and sustained), sign recognition, driving knowledge, and problem-solving abilities.

A patient often is evaluated in a driving simulator to look at brake reaction time; bilateral coordination; environmental visual scanning; threat recognition; the ability to identify, predict, and execute in a variety of situations; transfer skills; and potential equipment needs for accelerating, braking, and steering. The behind-the-wheel assessment is invaluable in providing information about basic vehicle control (brake, gas, and steering), bilateral upper extremity control, balance and postural stability, vehicle maneuvers (turns, backing up, and parking), and in-traffic performance (Latson 1987; Shipp 1991; Smith 1987; Strano 1987).

VEHICLE RECOMMENDATIONS

After the clinical assessment, the team usually decides among a car (two- or four-door), full-size van, or minivan. Considerations before vehicle purchase include transfer ability, wheelchair type, and mobility status.

To drive independently a two- or four-door car, one needs to be able to transfer quickly in and out of the vehicle as well as load and unload the wheelchair. This is one reason why the selection of manual wheelchair styles is so important. If a client purchases a folding frame wheelchair, then a two-door car is necessary for loading unless one has an automatic car top carrier that carries the wheelchair above the vehicle. If the client purchases a rigid style wheelchair, then either a two- or

four-door car may work, but increased dexterity and mobility are needed for the breakdown and loading of the wheelchair (Sabo & Shipp 1989).

If the client cannot transfer or maneuver the wheelchair into or out of the car easily, then one may consider the option of a minivan or full-size van. By choosing a minivan or full-size van, one has the option of driving from a powerbase captain's chair or the wheelchair, depending on the person's transfer status (Claus 1987; Shipp 1991).

When exploring the feasibility of driving a minivan (Figure 20–1), one must consider the following: Can one safely maneuver a ramp, or is a lift indicated? Is there sufficient turning radius for proper positioning of the wheelchair to transfer or drive? If one does need to drive from a wheelchair, will there be sufficient height in the driver's station to accommodate full visual field and access to primary controls?

If the client is unable to maneuver the wheelchair into the proper position or appears to sit too high in the driver's station, then a full-size van may be indicated. Vendors can modify vans for safe access to primary controls if the client needs to drive from a wheelchair level.

The static behind-the-wheel evaluation follows the clinical evaluation. This is performed in a methodical manner from the outside to the inside of the vehicle. First, can the client open the vehicle? Adaptations to key and door handles can be made to make access into the car easier. When accessing minivans and full-size vans, one may choose from key entry, toggle switches, magnetic switches, or a remote control unit. These can open and close the doors as well as operate the lift or ramp (Shipp 1989).

When entering the minivan or full-size van, the width of the wheelchair is crucial. If a client has a manual wheelchair with oblique pegs and cambered wheels, or if the client may camber the wheels in the future, then the lift may need to be wider than a standard lift. The length of the wheelchair must also be

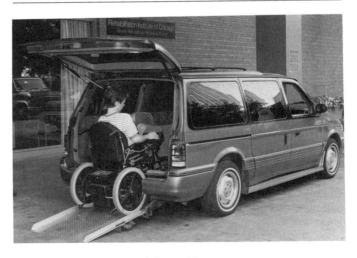

Figure 20–1 Rear entry minivan with a ramp.

addressed, especially for the self-reclining electric wheelchair. If the wheelchair does not easily fit into the lift, then an extra-long lift may be indicated. To accommodate the client's individual needs, one may choose from electric and hydraulic standard platform lifts, swingaway lifts, and split lifts (Figures 20–2 and 20–3). Each type of lift has its own pros and cons and must be individually explored to best meet the client's needs (Beck 1990).

Once a lift is chosen that accommodates the client's life style and wheelchair style, vehicle entrance is addressed. Entrance into the vehicle must be quick and easy. If the client needs to bend over or recline the wheelchair just to have head clearance to enter the van, then a raised roof and/or lowered floor may be indicated. The amount of the raised roof or lowered floor will again depend on the client's individual needs (Shipp 1989, 1991) (see Figure 20–4).

Once the client has accessed the vehicle, transfer into the driver's station is evaluated. In a car, a sliding board is often used to increase ease and safety during the transfer. A power seat is also recommended to increase ease in allowing room for loading and unloading the wheelchair and for final positioning in the driver's station (Shipp 1989, 1991).

If a client requires a minivan or full-size van but can still transfer, then one may need a six- or eight-way powerbase captain's seat (Figure 20–5). This type of seat has a set of switches that move the seat backward, forward, up, and down and swivel the chair. These movements facilitate the transfer process and positioning into the driver's station. Once the client has transferred into the captain's seat, the client locks the wheelchair into an unoccupied wheelchair tie down (Shipp 1989, 1991).

For the client who cannot transfer, an automatic tie-down system can be placed on the floor in the driver's station. The

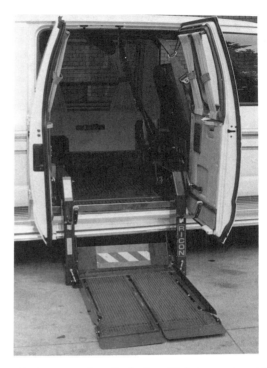

Figure 20–3 Automatic split platform lift in lowered position.

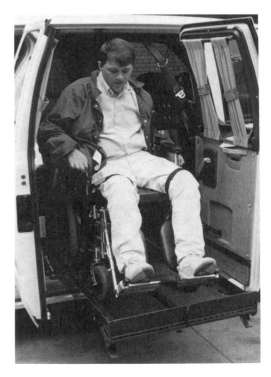

Figure 20–4 Vehicle entrance modified with cargo doors, platform lift, and a 5-inch drop floor.

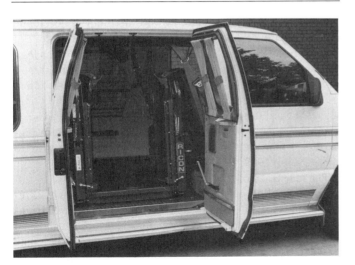

Figure 20–2 Automatic split platform lift in stored position.

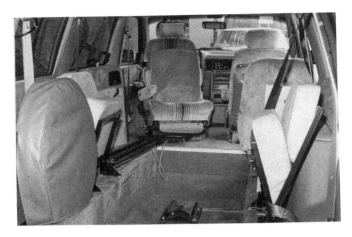

Figure 20–5 Eight-way powerbase captain's chair and a 10-inch dropped floor.

client pushes the wheelchair into the driver's station to lock the wheelchair automatically into the tie-down system. A standard captain's seat can usually be stored in the back of the van if an individual who does not use a wheelchair drives (Shipp 1989, 1991) (Figure 20–6). When the client is utilizing the vehicle solely as a means of transportation, a four-point tie-

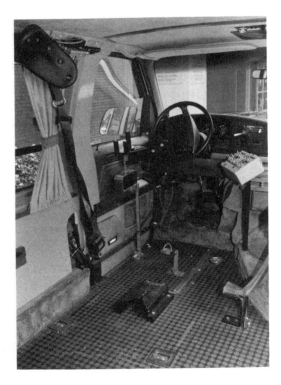

Figure 20–6 View of driver's station. On the floor is an automatic tie-down system.

down system can be positioned on the floor in the center station with the client facing forward. In addition to the four-point tie down, a three-point restraint system should be utilized to assist in keeping the client secure (Shipp 1989, 1991).

Once the client is positioned in the driver's station of the car or van, the type of primary controls needs to be addressed. Primary controls are the basic controls needed to maneuver the vehicle (brake, accelerator, and steering system). When assessing the need for adapted controls, one must look closely at the physical evaluation (especially the manual muscle test). Level of injury, strength, and endurance determine the type of primary control used.

As a general rule, the strongest, most coordinated upper extremity is normally used to operate the steering system. Steering systems can be modified in many ways. Most commonly a device is put on the wheel to assist in steering. Many are prefabricated and increase the client's ability to move the wheel quickly and accurately. Spinner knobs, palm cups, V-grips, and tri-pins are some of these devices. Customized steering devices can also be fabricated if a client presents with contractures or other difficulties (Shipp 1989, 1991).

In addition to actual steering devices, steering wheel resistance can be adjusted. To assess accurately the correct amount of resistance needed, a spring scale method to calculate strength or trial and error can be used. Steering columns can also be modified by placing the wheel off to one side and tilting it in a horizontal plane. This type of modification is done primarily for clients with C5–6 quadriplegia presenting with a weak clavicular portion of the pectoralis major.

Besides steering, the correct type of brake and accelerator must be recommended. There are three general types of hand controls: push–right angle, push–twist, and push–pull. For a client with a diagnosis of paraplegia or a strong individual with C7–8 injury, a push–right angle hand control may be appropriate. To operate this type of control, one must push the control down at a right angle toward the thigh to accelerate and toward the dashboard to brake. Occasionally this control may not be appropriate, as in the case where the client has long legs and they interfere with acceleration. In this situation, a push–twist control may be indicated. To accelerate, the client uses a twisting motion on the control; to brake, the client pushes toward the dash. If a client presents as a strong C-6 or weak C-7, then a push–pull hand control is often used (Figure 20–7). One pulls back to accelerate and pushes forward to brake (Shipp 1989, 1991).

The resistance of the brake and accelerator may also be adjusted depending on the client's muscle strength. Stock, reduced, and zero effort are different types of resistance. High-technology systems are also available and are primarily used by patients with high-level quadriplegia (C5–6). These range from driving systems requiring less than zero effort (pneumatic or electric) to joystick systems. Joystick systems have the client operating the brake/accelerator and steering systems

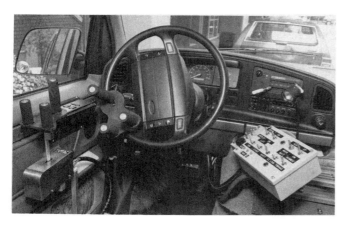

Figure 20–7 Pictured on the left is a pneumatic push–pull hand control adapted with a tri-pin. The steering wheel is also adapted with a tri-pin.

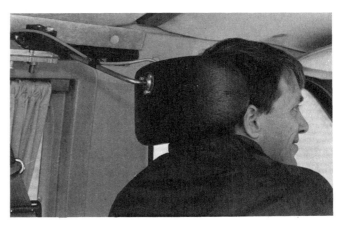

Figure 20–9 Power head rest in position for operation of the secondary controls.

using one joystick (similar in concept to a power wheelchair). Because of the complexity of these systems, cost can be a significant factor. Many times the client needs to assess the need of the driving task and whether it is worth the financial expenditure (Shipp 1989).

Once the correct primary system has been determined, the use of secondary controls must be assessed. Secondary controls are the controls that are needed while the vehicle is in motion, such as the horn, turn signals, windshield wipers, cruise control, and dimmer switch. The controls can be left in the original form or accessed via basic extensions, elbow switches, or head controls (Shipp 1989) (see Figures 20–8 and 20–9). Accessory controls are the controls on a vehicle that are used when the car is stationary, such as the ignition, gear selector, heater, and parking brake. Adaptations may include

toggle extensions, D rings, and touch pads (Shipp 1989) (see Figure 20–10).

Several medical and safety issues for individuals with spinal cord injury may necessitate other vehicle adaptations. A remote ignition switch to heat or cool the vehicle before entering as well as an air conditioning option help reduce problems with temperature regulation (Shipp 1989, 1991).

Curtains or blinds and a back bench seat that folds out into a bed are also recommended for a variety of reasons. First, if the client begins to have symptoms of autonomic dysreflexia, the bed gives room to address the issues and resolve the problem. The bed also allows the client to take an extended pressure relief during long trips. Besides addressing the issues of autonomic dysreflexia and skin care, the bed and curtains provide a private place to deal with incontinency issues. A portable or voice-activated telephone is also recommended in case of ve-

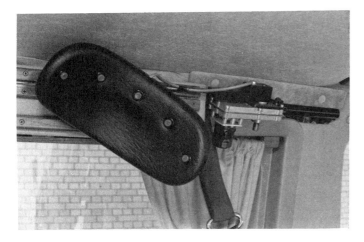

Figure 20–8 Power head rest. Each button performs a secondary function.

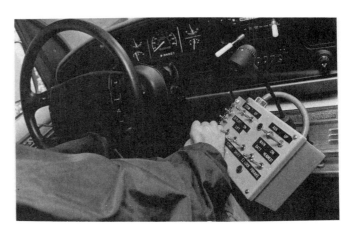

Figure 20–10 Accessory controls.

hicle breakdown, emergency situations, or physical problems (Shipp 1989, 1991).

Upon completion of the static behind-the-wheel evaluation and initial equipment assessment, the client begins the actual behind-the-wheel assessment to assess the equipment functionally. A driver instructor teaches the client how to operate the primary, secondary, and accessory controls before the actual driving experience. Often, especially in more complex cases, the occupational therapist and rehabilitation engineer will accompany the driver instructor on the actual behind-the-wheel evaluation to observe and make equipment recommendations (Smith 1987).

Upon completion of the above assessments the team compiles overall results, which are discussed with all involved parties. Therapists may recommend that the patient is safe to drive, unsafe to drive, able to drive upon completion of a certain number of training hours, or able to drive with a certain type of vehicle or equipment. Equipment options are discussed, determined, and written in a specific, descriptive, and inclusive manner. Failure to do this could result in a costly mistake if there is confusion with the vendor or, worse, injury to the patient or other people on the road. One should also consider the able-bodied driver when making equipment recommendations (e.g., type of lift and vehicle entry). Things to consider when choosing a vendor include inventory, product lines, insurance coverage, turnaround time, and travel distance for repairs. Previous consumers may also provide helpful insight and information (Shipp 1991).

For more complicated cases such as a fully modified van, a bidding conference may be helpful. Participants include evaluators, client, family, funding source, and potential vendors. The purpose is to meet involved parties, review and discuss recommendations, determine client preferences, establish delivery time and inspection locations, and choose the vendor for the job. A vehicle/equipment inspection with the client, evaluators, funding source, and vendor is strongly suggested.

Therapists can compare recommended to installed equipment, check installation against the manufacturer's specifications, and evaluate client positioning, equipment fit, and ability to operate equipment safely and efficiently in a standstill and on-the-road assessment. The client and family should be trained in the use of all equipment, not just adaptive equipment.

The amount of time needed for driver's training depends on the client's physical functioning, endurance, and previous driving experience as well as the complexity of the driving system and the client's skills exhibited with the adaptive equipment. Standards for instructor qualifications, use of the rehabilitation facility's versus the client's vehicle, performance criteria, and when to discontinue training should be established up front (Smith 1987).

DOCUMENTATION

Documentation states the results of the driving evaluation, behind-the-wheel training, and distribution of information. Functional and/or medical needs for equipment such as air conditioning for temperature regulation often facilitate funding. Documentation is also key for liability and reporting purposes. It is important to know state vehicle codes regarding who can report, what can be reported, the mechanism of reporting, and the types and timing of restrictions. Clients should sign an informed consent regarding program risks and potential program outcomes. Insurance needs should be identified for the rehabilitation facility, vendor, and client. Drivers of modified vehicles usually pay higher insurance premiums because of high-cost vehicles and the added value of equipment (Pierce 1993).

Funding for driver's training is often hard to come by because driving is not seen as a medical necessity. Documentation to support increased independence, decreased attendant care needs, and ability to return to work or school may facilitate financing for the driver rehabilitation program.

REFERENCES

Beck, K. (1990, June). Wheelchair lifts for vans: Is there a company that makes a lift to fit your van and you? *Paraplegia News*.

Claus, C. 1987. Van evaluators for the severely disabled. *Physical Disabilities Special Interest Section Newsletter* 10:4.

Kein, C.M., and E. Irwin. 1990. "Driver assessment and training of the disabled client." In *Rehabilitation engineering*, ed. R.V. Smith and J.H. Leslie, Jr. Boca Raton, Fla.: CRC Press, Inc.

Latson, L.F. 1987. Overview of disabled drivers' evaluation process. *Physical Disabilities Special Interest Section Newsletter* 10:4.

Pierce, S. 1987. Formula for developing a driving program for the disabled. *Physical Disabilities Special Interest Section Newsletter* 10:4.

Pierce, S. 1993. Legal consideration for a driver rehabilitation program. *Physical Disabilities* 16:1.

Sabo, S., and Shipp, M. 1989. *Disabilities and their implications for driving.* Ruston, La.: Louisiana Tech University.

Shipp, M. 1989. *Adaptive driving devices and vehicle modification.* Ruston, La.: Louisiana Tech University, Center for Rehabilitation Science and Biomedical Engineering.

Shipp, M. 1991. Adaptive Driving Program Manager, Ruston, La.: Louisiana Tech University, Center for Rehabilitation Science and Biomedical Engineering, personal communication.

Smith, D.L. 1987. Evaluation of disabled drivers: An instructor's perspective. *Physical Disabilities Special Interest Section Newsletter* 10:4.

Strano, C.M. 1987. Driver evaluation and training of the physically disabled driver: Additional comments. *Physical Disabilities Special Interest Section Newsletter* 10:4.

Chapter 21

Therapeutic Recreation after Spinal Cord Injury

Thomas H. McPike

In the rehabilitation of persons with spinal cord injury, therapeutic recreation utilizes recreational experiences as a modality to address the treatment goals of the patient, particularly those obstacles to leisure behavior. Therapeutic recreation activities are not ends in themselves but an enjoyable, individualized educational process to bring about a patient's awareness of and ability to provide for his or her leisure needs and desires. The therapeutic use of recreation requires a well-planned process of assessing the patient's goals of treatment, analyzing and selecting appropriate activities, and intervening in an appropriate interaction style pointed toward a realistic discharge plan.

The philosophy of therapeutic recreation services at the Rehabilitation Institute of Chicago maintains that leisure is a vital part of living and must be taken seriously as an integral factor in the rehabilitation process and social reintegration. Individuals with spinal cord injuries have the right to direct their recreational life style in the pursuit of satisfaction by accessing the esthetic, healthful, and social aspects of recreation. Patients should be supported to achieve their highest potential for personal fulfillment and quality of life in and through recreation.

Therapeutic recreation services at the Rehabilitation Institute of Chicago are divided into three main service components:

1. Rehabilitation/treatment addresses the treatment needs of the patient utilizing recreational activities and services as a method of treatment. The Therapeutic Recreation Department provides specifically designed services to improve one's physical, psychological, social, and emotional well-being (e.g., conducting a volleyball activity to improve balance, eye–hand coordination, and endurance).

2. Leisure education/counseling strives to increase the patient's knowledge and effectiveness in recognizing, identifying, and successfully providing for his or her leisure involvement. Leisure education/counseling provides opportunities for patients to acquire the necessary leisure skills, knowledge, attitudes, and understanding related to their leisure involvement. Whether instructing the person in a specific physical skill, such as a swimming stroke, or educating the individual about the opportunities available for social recreation, this component attempts to expand the patient's knowledge of how personal values, needs, opportunities, and skills affect his or her life choices.

3. Recreation participation provides opportunities of interest to the patient with spinal cord injury for enjoyable recreational experiences. These services recognize the importance of recreational opportunities for a normalized, balanced life style for all people but emphasize their essential role for the hospitalized individual who still experiences free time and is in need of opportunities for self-expression, release, socialization, and enjoyment. These experiences allow learning and practicing of rehabilitation skills in a realistic setting for patient and family. Using transferring techniques in movie theaters or negotiating crowds at a concert to

achieve an enjoyable evening focuses the rehabilitation experience for many patients and positively rewards patients' work in therapy.

Assisting patients with spinal cord injury to achieve a satisfying leisure life style is a cooperative effort at the Rehabilitation Institute of Chicago. Therapeutic recreation is supported by other members of the rehabilitation team. Conversely, therapeutic recreation programs incorporate supportive goals of other disciplines. Therapeutic recreation and other individual therapies foster the philosophy of the institute to promote individuals' functioning at their maximum level based on their abilities and to return individuals to their community enjoying the highest quality of life possible.

The main objectives of therapeutic recreation services are the following:

- to provide recreational opportunities to the patient with spinal cord injury
- to complement and promote carryover of newly learned skills to real-life situations through recreational activities
- to increase client understanding of leisure needs and to develop necessary skills to address them
- to complete discharge plans including referrals to community programs and agencies

ASSESSMENT

An individual assessment initiates involvement in the therapeutic recreation program. The therapeutic recreation assessment helps the therapist determine the patient's strengths, interests, expectations, and the nature and extent of problem areas in recreation participation. The therapeutic recreation assessment analyzes:

- information about the patient's personal leisure values
- significance and pattern of the patient's leisure behavior
- appropriateness for participation in specific programs
- social needs and relationships
- individual strengths and assets
- life-style adjustments necessary for healthy leisure functioning
- available leisure support systems or resources in home and community
- economic factors influencing the patient's leisure
- how the patient views recreation and the impact of his or her disability

From the assessment, the patient and therapeutic recreation clinician together plan a program that builds upon the abilities of the patient and either remediates problem areas or develops coping strategies.

Effective program planning requires the therapeutic recreation specialist to understand the individual needs of the patient and related roles in working with the patient. Therapeutic recreation activity planning incorporates several elements into a continuum of developmental services. Individual treatment, group programs in the hospital and the community, interdisciplinary programs, wheelchair sports, equipped activity areas, and outpatient therapeutic recreation services provide a range of options to individualize a treatment plan.

Individual Treatment

Individual treatment encompasses assessment of the particular needs of the patient, provision of supportive teaching, and problem solving of barriers to participation. It then applies the treatment experience to a long-range discharge plan. As the patient progresses in treatment, the therapist additionally acts as a resource to assist the patient to carry over therapy skills into independent leisure activities alone or with others during free time and home passes.

ACTIVITY ANALYSIS

A major responsibility in individual treatment is analyzing activities for leisure application. Activity analysis is the process of breaking down and examining the components of a particular activity to determine how an activity would contribute to the treatment objectives. The goal of activity analysis is to gain information that allows selection of appropriate activities relevant to patient goals. This information will facilitate sequencing and modification of instructional design. Activity analysis provides the following (Peterson & Gunn 1984):

- better understanding of expected outcomes
- greater understanding of the complexity of activity components, which then can be compared with the functional level of an individual to determine appropriateness of the activity
- information about whether the activity will contribute to the desired behavioral outcome when specific goals or objectives are being used
- direction for the modification or adaptation of an activity for individuals with limitations
- useful information for selecting intervention, instructional, or leadership techniques
- rationale or explanation for the therapeutic benefits of activity involvement

The therapist strives to instruct the patient to independently analyze and problem solve activities of personal interest. This skill will expand the patient's ability to address leisure needs in areas of physical and social function.

ACTIVITY MODIFICATION

An activity analysis indicates the participation requirements for physical, cognitive, and social skills. Activity modification assesses the patient in relation to these standards. When functional abilities are impaired or absent, modification is required for successful participation. This often requires the collaboration of occupational therapy or other disciplines.

Common modification begins with proper body mechanics in terms of the patient's position in relation to the desired activity skill. This can be accomplished by increasing the patient's awareness of his or her body space by utilizing augmentative sensory aids. Similarly, the patient can be provided with added stability through a chest strap or positioning. Additional adaptations include reachers; Velcro to augment grip; Dycem, a nonskid material to augment fine motor control and stability; orthoplast splints to substitute gross movement for fine motor movement; guides or handles; battery-operated switches; and electronic controls.

IN-HOSPITAL GROUP ACTIVITIES

Organized group recreation strives to provide a supportive, realistic environment to learn and apply skills through enjoyable activities. Programs conducted within the hospital duplicate community leisure and social experiences. Activities are scheduled pertinent to needs and interests for a balanced range of leisure options. A comprehensive calendar of activities such as the following will include identified need areas:

* social activities
* hobbies
* art
* entertainment
* special events
* holiday programs
* arts and crafts
* music
* drama
* physical activities
* games
* intellectual activities

COMMUNITY TRIPS

Trips into the community challenge the patient's ability to plan, problem solve, generalize therapy skills, and deal effectively in variable real-life situations. This will be critical to the patient's view of the promise (or anxiety) of returning home and embarking on an independent life style. It is intended that the skills learned from successfully enjoying a community recreation experience will generalize to independent recreation participation in the patient's home community. When the patient voluntarily chooses a community out trip of interest and experiences the problems and accomplishments of participation, the patient often is remotivated to take a more active role in the design of his or her rehabilitation program and discharge plan. A balanced schedule of community out trips includes the following range of experiences (sports are omitted because they are included in the wheelchair sports program):

* spectator sports
* shopping
* clubs
* restaurants
* concerts
* outdoor nature experiences
* theater
* holidays
* special events
* sightseeing/tours
* museum exhibitions
* movies
* educational tours/presentations

INTERDISCIPLINARY GROUPS

The purpose of interdisciplinary groups is to facilitate problem-solving skills in the areas of physical, social, and leisure functioning by an interdisciplinary treatment approach. Recreation therapists, occupational therapists, physical therapists, and nurses conjointly staff the group, addressing the joint discipline goals for successful reintegration of the patient with spinal cord injury into the community. Group experiences of interpersonal dynamics with subsequent supervised group processing are utilized. The content of the group includes three areas:

1. *Planning*: Patients are responsible for appropriately planning for the leisure and educational experiences (finances, schedules, and admissions) decided upon by the group. Factors to be considered include medical issues, personal needs, wheelchair maintenance, architectural barriers, transportation options, and potential social interactions.
2. *Participation*: After making the necessary arrangements, participants will conduct the activity with emphasis on acquiring the necessary analytical and coping skills to increase independence in a community setting.
3. *Processing*: Patients are involved in individual and group processing with facilitators to identify problem

areas and successes. Together, strategies are shared to improve each individual's problem-solving behavior.

RECREATION AREAS

A recreation area equipped with stereo, television, quiet area, reading material, table games, and recreation equipment such as pool tables, ping-pong tables, and videos is maintained in the hospital for independent, spontaneous free-time recreation. It is an area for patients to pursue an unstructured recreational activity with family and friends or alone. The area provides a diversion from the therapy areas and nursing floor. It is important to allow for a normalized leisure environment, which will promote socialization and self-directed activity. Patients can practice skills necessary for favorite activities such as billiards, cards, or reading, or they can utilize the area with a therapist to assess and investigate necessary adaptations for independent participation.

WHEELCHAIR SPORTS

Athletics for persons with spinal cord injury trace their origins to the efforts of World War II veterans, who were determined to make the most of their abilities despite their war injuries. Wheelchair basketball and bowling were the first activities, and since 1957 men and women have been competing in track and field, swimming, archery, table tennis, softball, football, rugby, road racing, marathoning, and other sports.

The wheelchair sports program of the Rehabilitation Institute of Chicago Therapeutic Recreation Department offers a range of opportunities in recreational and competitive sports and educational programs. The program strives to:

- provide coaching, training, and organization of a range of sports programs
- educate persons with disability about physical fitness and well-being
- advocate and promote community-integrated facilities and sports programs for all persons
- educate the community about the potential of athletes with disabilities

In addition to the recreative value of wheelchair sports, Sir Ludwig Guttmann, medical authority in spinal cord injury rehabilitation and leader in the development of wheelchair sports, concluded that "from a physical point of view, sports prove of immense therapeutic value in restoring the disabled person's strength, coordination, and endurance," (Guttmann, 1976, p. 617).

Vigorous physical activity in the form of sport stimulates circulation, helping prevent skin breakdown. It increases fluid intake, contributing to decreased kidney and bladder infections. Conditioning, which is essential to sports participation,

enables the body to cope better with minor diseases and infections. Another positive outcome is increased wheelchair mobility in day-to-day activities from the refinement of techniques and development of upper extremity strength.

OUTPATIENT SERVICES

For patients who require ongoing therapeutic recreation services to reach their goal of independent social/leisure functioning, outpatient services focus on assisting the patient in eliminating barriers that presently prevent him or her from participating in community recreation programs and self-satisfying use of leisure time. Individual counseling assists the patient in acquiring the skills, knowledge, and attitudes to enhance leisure functioning, and group programs are designed to facilitate the development of social/leisure skills within a group structure. The patient is able to develop new peer relationships, share information, and continue to improve self-confidence and rehabilitation skills.

DISCHARGE PLANNING

After an assessment of strengths, deficits, and teaching intervention, the emphasis is directed toward raising the patient's awareness about the positive need for constructive leisure experiences. The patient is exposed to leisure options, and strategies are developed to return the patient to past meaningful activities. At this time, it is necessary to incorporate the discharge plan into the treatment plan. Discharge leisure planning identifies agencies and services needed for continued support of the patient's leisure goals upon conclusion of hospitalization. Common referrals include the following:

- special recreation associations
- wheelchair sports organizations
- specialists in adaptive recreation equipment
- outdoor programs and accessible outdoor facilities
- continuing education programs
- public parks and recreation departments
- YMCAs, YWCAs, and health clubs
- state and federal departments of parks
- accessibility guides to cities
- travel agencies and books
- special interest clubs
- volunteer opportunities and bureaus
- independent living centers
- national organizations concerned with spinal cord injuries
- therapeutic recreation departments in other hospitals

CONCLUSION

Leisure has become a dominant part of American life. Most Americans value their leisure for self-expression, release, social interaction, recognition, and stimulation; there are as many individual values as there are people. An individual's self-expression through leisure is one of the most personal, although often least acknowledged, aspects of human needs. Persons with spinal cord injury historically have been faced with limited opportunities and services in relation to their leisure options. Not enough effort has been exerted in assisting this group to achieve the socioleisure skills essential to other members of society. The patient with spinal cord injury shares the common need, and may have a greater need, for self-development and expression of enjoyable self-directed recreation that refreshes and "re-creates."

The goal of therapeutic recreation for the patient with spinal cord injury is to assist the individual to make informed, self-directed, and personally satisfying leisure choices. The processes involved in developing the patient to the point of being able to choose and effectively participate in meaningful options can be intricate and complex.

The recreation therapist must be capable of identifying clients' needs and helping them develop basic functional skills. By coping with individuals and their problem areas through thoughtful manipulation of the clients' abilities along with various activity tools and facilitation techniques, the professional therapeutic recreation specialist promotes adaptation to or the amelioration of problematic behaviors and conditions. The therapeutic recreation specialist then seeks, through leisure education, to promote growth toward meaningful, self-directed leisure choices (Peterson & Gunn 1984).

Comprehensive therapeutic recreation services address patient needs through educational goals, prescriptive programming, and facilitation of community integration. By this process, therapeutic recreation promotes the goal of rehabilitation: adequate training and understanding to use available resources to optimize independence through life.

BIBLIOGRAPHY

Adams, R., et al. 1982. *Game, sports and exercises for the physically handicapped.* 3rd ed. Philadelphia: Lea and Febiger.

Austin, D. 1991. *Therapeutic recreation: Process and techniques,* 2nd ed. Champaign, Ill.: Sagamore.

Auxter, D., et al. 1993. *Principles and methods of adapted physical education and recreation,* 7th ed. St. Louis, Mo.: Mosby.

Carter, M., et al. 1990. *Therapeutic recreation: A practical approach.* Prospect Heights, Ill.: Waveland.

Cotton, M. 1983. *Outdoor adventure for handicapped people.* London, England: Souvenir Press.

Haun, P. 1973. *Recreation: A medical viewpoint.* New York: Teachers College.

Hill, J.P. 1986. *Spinal cord injury: A guide to functional outcomes in occupational therapy,* Gaithersburg, Md.: Aspen Publishers.

Kennedy, D.W., et al. 1986. *Special recreation.* Philadelphia: Saunders.

Nixon, V. 1985. *Spinal cord injury: A guide to functional outcomes in physical therapy management.* Gaithersburg, Md.: Aspen Publishers.

Paciorek, M., and J. Jones. 1989. *Sports and recreation for the disabled: A resource manual.* Indianapolis, Ind.: Benchmark.

Peterson, C., and S. Gunn. 1984. *Therapeutic recreation program design: Principles and procedures,* 2nd ed. Englewood Cliffs, N.J.: Prentice Hall.

Schlein, S., et al. 1993. *Integrated outdoor education and adventure programs.* Champaign, Ill.: Sagamore.

Winnick, J., ed. 1990. *Adapted physical education and sport.* Champaign, Ill.: Human Kinetics.

Winslow, R., and K. Halberg, eds. 1992. *The management of therapeutic recreation services,* Arlington, Va., NRPA Publications.

Chapter 22

Vocational Rehabilitation and Spinal Cord Injury

Brian C. Walker and Susan S. Holstein

Although there are a myriad of individuals concerned with the physical restoration and medical maintenance of a patient with spinal cord injury, it is the vocational rehabilitation specialist who has the primary concern of returning the individual to some degree of vocational productivity, which often enhances self-esteem. After a spinal cord injury, the patient often feels hopeless in regard to future vocational goals. The sense of self, once defined by work or school, may be lost, and with this the individual's own sense of worth or purpose. The patient looks to the vocational rehabilitation specialist for hope, especially early on in the adjustment phase. Encouragement about residual abilities and moving on with one's life is critical. During this adjustment period, the role of the vocational rehabilitation specialist is to provide supportive vocational counseling and guidance. The belief that options still exist after injury is often beyond the purview of the person with spinal cord injury. It is also the role of the vocational rehabilitation specialist to instill hope by assisting the patient in identifying realistic vocational options. There is no other individual within the hospital setting that is more sensitive to the vocational needs of the patient, and none more qualified or skilled in vocational planning. Factors relating to leading a successful life have been identified (Trieschmann 1980):

- prevention of medical complications (activities of daily living and mobility skills)
- maintenance of a stable living environment (all the social skills necessary to cope with family, friends, and attendants)

- productivity (vocation, educational, volunteer, and hobby)

Rehabilitation has been defined as a facilitative process that enables a person with a disability to live as satisfactory and fulfilling a life as possible (Wright 1980). This chapter discusses what traditionally has been the emphasis of vocational rehabilitation efforts: securing gainful employment. This emphasis appears to be based in part on the assumption that those with spinal cord injuries expect some recovery and desire a resumption of their premorbid work role.

Work means different things to different people, but common to all definitions of work is some kind of goal-directed activity. It is not sufficient to do something; something must be done for a purpose. The extent of satisfaction one derives from work depends upon the kind of work and the personal value placed in it.

Employment may not be an appropriate goal for everyone, and there are obstacles within the system that prevent everyone who desires a job from becoming employed. Therefore, it seems reasonable to consider productivity one goal, which includes education and avocational activities, group membership, and family and community participation in addition to employment (Trieschmann 1978).

Young and Northrup (1979) have pointed out that reports regarding postinjury employment of those with spinal cord injury produce discrepancies resulting from the lack of standardized definition regarding the term *working*. They suggest that working be defined as employment in the competitive labor market and that a broader category be adopted that would include worker, homemaker, and student. Hallin (1968) similarly classified these patients into a single group of those engaged in self-directed activities.

The onset of spinal cord injury may have profound effects on existing roles and personal relationships. It is the role of the vocational rehabilitation specialist to examine the extent to which individuals with spinal cord injury will experience a vocational handicap.

WORK: A HEALTH MAINTENANCE ACTIVITY

The role of work is an integral part of the way in which we structure our time. Work imposes a needed structure; it provides one with a reference point from which to organize other aspects of one's life. In this respect, work has been referred to as a health maintenance activity. That is, work provides the sense of purpose and consequently the motivation to keep oneself healthy and active.

While hospitalized, the person with spinal cord injury finds that his or her day is structured through prescribed therapy programs; upon discharge, however, the individual often is faced with a loss of this structure, especially if a return to school or work is not immediately forthcoming. For some patients, it is true that discharge is the first time that they fully begin to consider how they will utilize their free time.

The individual whose main daily activity is sitting at home and watching television may feel bored and depressed. Further medical complications are common; pressure reliefs are ignored, and basic health maintenance activities become unimportant. Consequently, life adjustment issues must be addressed before gainful employment is a feasible option. Once these concerns have been addressed, purposeful activity, self-care, and medical maintenance are of primary concern, and each promotes the others.

REHABILITATION PHILOSOPHY AND PRACTICE

It is counterproductive to involve someone in a vocational rehabilitation program aimed at full-time employment until he or she has had a chance to master the skills necessary for survival in the community. Oftentimes, inpatient rehabilitation programs do not teach the person these skills or offer the opportunity to practice social and survival skills in the community before discharge.

Jellnik and Harvey (1982) compared patients who participated in an inpatient program before the addition of on-site vocational/educational staff with those who participated after professional staff were added. Availability of professional vocational/educational staff in the hospital phase of rehabilitation was found to enhance an individual's likelihood of becoming interested in returning to school or seeking employment. Also, vocational/educational placement rates increased from 19% or lower to as high as 78% in cases where vocational/educational services were appropriate.

The Rehabilitation Institute of Chicago (RIC) provides vocational services early on in the rehabilitation of the person with spinal cord injury. An initial contact is made with the patient shortly after admission to alert him or her to the available services. Vocational planning is often not a priority to the newly injured patient, but this initial contact with the vocational rehabilitation specialist is critical in the process of instilling hope that future possibilities exist for work. Furthermore, a skilled professional is available to assist the patient in exploring vocational potential and thereby reestablishing his or her sense of self as it is defined by work or school.

VOCATIONAL REHABILITATION

Rehabilitation candidates in the population with spinal cord injury have been categorized in the research as follows:

- 20% are young with a strong family background, without significant psychological problems, and with a history of educational/vocational planning; these individuals are believed to succeed with or without rehabilitation
- 20% are poor candidates because of poor history of coping and an environment full of obstacles
- 60% have average potential; their spinal cord injury has significantly challenged their ability to cope, and they have no outstanding talents or environmental supports

GOALS AND MOTIVATION

The goals selected by clients have been seen as extremely important by practitioners (Trieschmann 1978), and the number of discreet goals stated by persons with spinal cord injury have been positively related to postrehabilitation productivity (Kemp & Vash 1971). Practitioners often cite low motivation as a reason for rehabilitation failure (Zadney & James 1979). Goal-directed behavior is often used as a synonym for motivated behavior (Madsen 1973), and motivation has been regarded as the most important factor of the rehabilitation process. Cook (1981) found that, of 110 patients with spinal cord injury receiving services with the explicit treatment goal of vocational rehabilitation, only 23% chose a vocational goal. It could be assumed from these results that at least some clients would be labeled as unmotivated because of staff–patient goal incongruence. Yet Cook found that in grouping patients on the basis of five motivational variables the clearest discriminator was the type of goal chosen and the perceived importance of that goal.

PREDICTORS OF PRODUCTIVITY AFTER SPINAL CORD INJURY

Trieschmann (1978) reviewed the variables associated with productivity after spinal cord injury. Findings indicated that previous education and employment may be predictive of re-employment after disability but may not correlate with overall productivity. The investigator stated that productivity encompasses more than employment; it involves creativity and the ability to set goals related to productive living. Productivity is defined as vocational endeavors, education pursuit, volunteer activities, and avocational pursuits.

Dvonch et al. (1965), however, found that predisability employment is an effective predictor only when combined with an educational level of high school or better. Siegel (1971) found that patients with quadriplegia who were college students had a better chance of employment than those who were not college students. Overall, the data suggest that persons with paraplegia are somewhat more likely to obtain employment than persons with quadriplegia (Brown & Chanin 1974; Goldberg & Freed 1976; Seybold 1976); definitions of what constitutes work are not always clear, however, and consequently it is difficult to compare these studies.

POSTHOSPITAL ADJUSTMENT

It appears that education and training after onset of spinal cord injury are important because they:

- provide the physically disabled individual with a meaningful and constructive way to spend time
- contribute to feelings of self-worth
- increase the probability of social interaction because the individual is in contact with others with similar interests
- increase the likelihood of obtaining productive employment

Interests, work values, and rehabilitation outlook of 29 patients with spinal cord injury due to trauma were explored within the context of the rehabilitation hospital (Goldberg & Freed 1973). Education and vocational plans made before injury contributed significantly to postinjury adjustment. Persons who had formulated concrete plans to accomplish a vocational objective tended to be employed full time or involved in school full time.

Investigators also have found that motivation to work and rehabilitation are related negatively to the level of neurological impairment; persons with a lower level of impairment are more optimistic in their outlook toward their disability and have a greater motivation to work. The best predictors 4 years after discharge are vocational plans, work interests, work values, remotivation, and rehabilitation outlook. In some studies, educational grade best predicted rehabilitation status after discharge. Other predictors were the number of children (the

more children, the more persons were employed) and educational status (training correlated positively with employment). Marital status was not associated with employment. The follow-up study by Goldberg and Freed (1982) 8 years after discharge revealed that employment levels did not change significantly after another 4 years in the community.

El Ghatit and Hanson (1982) surveyed 745 male veterans with spinal cord injury. Their findings similarly indicated that those with a higher educational status and those who improved their education after injury had better vocational outcomes. Contrary to Goldberg and Freed, they found that postinjury education was not related to the level of injury.

Webb et al. (1982) found that employment decreased 1 year after injury but increased with changes in the types of employment, showing a general upgrading of job levels. Although fewer people were employed 2 to 6 years after injury than at the time of injury, the number increased over that at 12 to 18 months after injury. Of those individuals reportedly employed, three fourths worked full time (40 hours per week), and 13% had more than one job.

Onset of traumatic spinal cord injury often necessitates that these plans be postponed completely, somewhat modified, or completely altered, and it is the vocational rehabilitation specialist who must work with the patient to assess these options realistically. When this is not the case and return to former vocational plans is possible, the vocational rehabilitation specialist can assist the individual with adjustment issues related to reintegrating into the school or work community.

EVALUATION TECHNIQUES

The foundation of a comprehensive vocational evaluation for the disabled individual relies on a complete assessment of the person's basic skills, both academic and applied.

The process of vocational evaluation measures a variety of traits. Some specific traits can be negated immediately when one is investigating the employability of individuals with spinal cord injury according to the corresponding level of injury (e.g., finger dexterity, manual dexterity, and gross motor coordination). The vocational evaluation unit at RIC is equipped with a variety of work samples and simulated work activities. Over the years, it has been found that the lack of certain residual functional capabilities negates the utilization of these activities with the population with spinal cord injury; that is not to say, however, that an individual with paraplegia cannot benefit from a work sample. It is necessary to keep in mind the actual physical limitations of the individual in comparison with the physical capabilities necessary to perform the work sample activities. These work samples may not be measuring specific physical capabilities. For example, the Valpar numeric sorting work sample is one that purports to measure an individual's capability of working within an organizational format to perform sorting and data-gathering activities. The actual physical make-up of the work samples requires an individual to pick up a small, numbered plastic chip and move it approximately 3 feet to place it into a slot slightly larger than the chip itself. The physical requirements of locating, picking up, and moving these small chips are, at times, beyond the capabilities of a patient with spinal cord injury, but failure is not indicative of the patient's ability to work within a data-gathering and organizational format.

The remaining categories and traits reflect the individual's cognitive capabilities and therefore can be measured. Difficulties arise, however, when we attempt to use a paper and pencil test under a standardized time format with an individual who has severe problems with finger and manual dexterity because the time necessary for a patient with quadriplegia to place answers on a standardized answer sheet negates the ability to present his or her true cognitive capabilities. It has therefore been our practice to provide a writer or to utilize a specialized computer program developed at RIC to allow an individual independent power and control during the evaluation process.

The computer program that we currently use is *Answer Sheet*. This program allows the individual with spinal cord injury, with the use of assistive devices such as balanced forearm orthosis (mobile arm support) and a writing or typing splint, to access a video display terminal through a computer keyboard. For each answer, two keys must be pressed, which then activate the recording device and generate a screen to accept the next answer. This program has been designed to accept any style of answer (number, letter, or word) to allow the flexibility needed for the great diversity of paper and pencil measures available for use with the population with spinal cord injury.

It is important to note that, even with the use of an adaptive computer program, the time necessary to perform these activities is outside the standardization procedures of test development. It is therefore generally our practice that the test will be given in a timed format according to the standardized procedures.

After the allotted amount of time per the test guidelines, the individual will be allowed to finish the activity. The test is scored for both time periods. It is important to note that administering a standardized, time-loaded test in an untimed manner requires careful consideration of the results. The vocational rehabilitation department of RIC refers to this as power test. Reporting and analyzing require careful interpretation, keeping in mind that the power score obtained is an inflated indicator of an individual's maximum potential.

As the field of vocational rehabilitation has understood for many years, interest development is a lengthy, time-consuming process. There are times during the vocational rehabilitation of an individual when interests will change. These times generally appear at or about the same time that an individual's self-perceptions or the acceptance of the disability emerges in an integrated body image. It is extremely important for the vocational evaluator and/or rehabilitation specialist working with a newly injured individual to understand that, just as the patient's physical body is in a fluctuating state, so too is his or her emotional component of viewing himself or herself as he or she fits into the working world.

DISINCENTIVES TO WORK

Financial Disincentives

Intrinsic factors within the system often do not enable those persons with spinal cord injury who desire to return to work to do so. Monthly benefits received from Social Security insurance and/or Social Security disability insurance often far exceed what the individual with disability could earn upon returning to work. Deyoe (1972) found that veterans with a service-related disability often could not afford to work because their monthly benefits exceeded what they could earn if employed. Although a desire to work may exist, the patient must then face the insecurity of maintaining a job for less pay and the loss of the security of consistent disability payments.

Employer Attitudes

Employment rates of the disabled are distressing. Only about 10% of the vocationally rehabilitated population that is working are in normal, competitive employment settings (Rhyne 1984). There has been a slow but gradual change in the negative attitudes of employers toward hiring the disabled. Although strong efforts to educate employers as well as the public have been made, employer attitudes are frequently a barrier to placing the individual with disability back into the workforce.

Bressler and Lacey (1980) designed a study to test the hypothesis that, given a vocational environment and sociologic climate in which the perceptibly physically disabled have the same opportunities for career progression and self-actualization as nonimpaired employees, there would be few differences between the two groups in career progression and contribution. For the orthopedically impaired (66% of the sample), a significant difference was found in the mean salary between workers with and without disabilities ($1,765). These investigators speculated that this may have occurred for the following reasons: lower educational level of the group with disabilities compared with the nondisabled group; some degree of discrimination or prejudice exercised by nonimpaired supervisors in the selection for promotion process; a large amount of travel involved in some of the higher positions (it has been speculated that a great deal of the required travel may have offered a basis for rationalizing prejudices); the possibility that some orthopedically impaired individuals did not pursue positions that required extensive travel; and perceptibility of the orthopedic impairment, which also may have influenced decisions regarding promotions.

AMERICANS WITH DISABILITIES ACT OF 1990

In July of 1990, the 101st Congress passed the Americans with Disabilities Act (ADA). This Act makes it unlawful to discriminate against a qualified individual with a disability in state and local government services, public accommodations, transportation, telecommunications, and employment. The portion of the ADA that outlaws job discrimination is effective for all employers with 25 or more employees after July 26, 1992, and for all employers with 15 or more employees after July 26, 1994.

The ADA defines a disability as a physical or mental impairment that substantially limits one or more of the major life activities. It is readily apparent that an individual with a permanent spinal cord injury falls within this definition. The ADA makes it unlawful to discriminate in all employment practices including but not limited to recruitment, hiring, job assignments, pay, layoff, firing, training, promotions, benefits, and leave.

The Act specifically provides that an employer may not discriminate against a qualified disabled person applying for a job if the individual satisfies the employer's requirements for the job, such as education, skills, or license, and the individual can perform the essential functions of the job with or without reasonable accommodation.

The essential functions of a job will be defined in each specific instance. Factors that must be considered include whether the reason the position exists is to perform that function; the number of employees available to perform the function or among whom the performance of the function can be distributed; and the degree of expertise or skill required to perform the function, hopefully documented by a job analysis or job description.

A disabled individual may request a reasonable accommodation in order to be capable of performing the essential functions of a job. The ADA does not define all reasonable accommodations but it appears that making the workplace accessible, adjusting or modifying examinations or training materials, restructuring a job, modifying equipment, or acquiring new devices would all be reasonable accommodations. If, however, an accommodation would require significant difficulty or expense, an employer may claim an undue hardship and decline the provision of an accommodation.

The ADA will be enforced by the United States Equal Employment Opportunity Commission (EEOC). Both individuals with disabilities and employers can consult with the EEOC for assistance in defining their specific accommodations.

The enactment of the ADA is a significant step in eliminating many of the rationales used by employers for not employing disabled individuals. The Act also provides for money damages to an individual who is discriminated against. Much of the specific information necessary for each individual case and each individual job is not spelled out in the ADA or in the regulations promulgated by the EEOC. Only time and case-specific rulings by the EEOC and courts of law will provide the answers to the many specific questions surrounding essential functions and reasonable accommodations.

The ADA provides substantial incentive to both employers and individuals with disabilities to work together in increasing the distressingly low employment rate among Americans with disabilities.

COMMUNITY RESOURCES

A community advisory group called the TEAM committee has been assisting the Vocational Rehabilitation Department at RIC. TEAM stands for training, employment, advisory, and marketing. Each subcommittee focuses its activities within a specific area to facilitate the employment of the disabled.

- *Training:* The training subcommittee of the TEAM committee works with RIC patients and staff. For the patient population, this subcommittee provides job-seeking skills training and mock interview activities and presently is contemplating organizing an alumni group of former patients who currently are employed.
- *Employment:* The employment subcommittee focuses its activities on assisting the RIC patient population in attaining employment. The most significant activity of this subcommittee is an annual job fair, which is involved with other community rehabilitation agencies, including the Chicago Lighthouse for the Blind, Jewish Vocational Services, Projects with Industry, and Schwab Rehabilitation Hospital.
- *Advisory:* This subcommittee is composed of the chairpersons of all the subcommittees. It functions as a governing board of the TEAM committee.
- *Marketing:* This subcommittee is responsible for publicizing the actions of the TEAM committee. It publishes a newsletter and hosts quarterly luncheons and an annual awards banquet, at which awards are presented to the Chicago business community for excellence and tenacity in the hiring and employment of the disabled.

In addition to assisting RIC patients and staff, the TEAM committee provides the business community with an arena where it can network with regard to successes and difficulties in the employment of the disabled. A significant motivation for company involvement in the TEAM committee is a combination of personal altruism and a necessity to document affirmative action. This large group of approximately 30 companies in Chicago is a definite asset to RIC's link with the realistic practices of the business community.

ADDITIONAL VOCATIONAL REHABILITATION SERVICES

A unique aspect of the Vocational Rehabilitation Department at RIC is that placement specialists were hired with no rehabilitation background. Their background is sales or business oriented so that they can interact appropriately with the business community.

TOTAL REHABILITATION

It is clear that rehabilitation, whether vocational or medical, must address disability acceptance in terms of life-adjustment issues. It is not enough to assume that the patient's adjustment while in the hospital is predictive of adjustment once he or she is discharged from the hospital. The goal must be acceptance of the disability into one's overall life style.

BIBLIOGRAPHY

Americans with Disabilities Act. 1990. 42 U.S.C. 12101, *et seq.*

Alfred, W.G., et al. 1987. Vocational development following severe spinal cord injury: A longitudinal study. *Arch. Phys. Med. Rehabil.* 68(12):854–857.

Bressler, R., and A. Lacey. 1980. An analysis of the relative job progression of the perceptibly physically handicapped. *Acad. Manage. J.* 23:132–143.

Brown, B., and I. Chanin. 1974. *Patterns of education and employment: Rehabilitation from severe spinal cord injury, FY 1972–73* (Rehabilitation Research Reports). Sacramento, Calif.: Department of Rehabilitation.

Cook, D. 1981. A multivariate analysis of motivational attributes among spinal cord injured rehabilitation clients. *Int. J. Rehabil. Res.* 4:5–15.

Crewe, N.M., and J.S. Krause. 1990. An eleven year follow-up of adjustment to spinal cord injury. *Rehabil. Psych.* 35(4):205–210.

Crisp, R. 1990. Return to work after spinal cord injury. *J. Rehabil.* (January/February/March): 28–35.

Devivo, M.J., et al. 1987. Employment after spinal cord injury. *Arch. Phys. Med. Rehabil.* 68:494–498.

Deyoe, F. 1972. Spinal cord injury: Long-term follow-up of veterans. *Arch. Phys. Med. Rehabil.* 53:523–529.

Dvonch, P., et al. 1965. Vocational findings in post-disability employment of patients with spinal cord dysfunction. *Arch. Phys. Med. Rehabil.* 46:761–766.

El Ghatit, A., and R. Hanson. 1982. Vocational development of spinal cord injury patients: An eight-year follow-up. *Arch. Phys. Med. Rehabil.* 63:207–210.

Goldberg, R.T., and M.M. Freed. 1973. Vocational adjustment, interests, work values and career plans of persons with spinal cord injuries. *Scand. J. Rehabil. Med.* 5:3–11.

Goldberg, R.T., and M.M. Freed. 1976. The vocational development, interests, values, adjustment and rehabilitation outlook of spinal cord patients: A four-year follow-up. *Arch. Phys. Med. Rehabil.* 57:532.

Goldberg, R.T., and M.M. Freed. 1982. Vocational development of spinal cord injury patients: An 8 year follow-up. *Arch. Phys. Med. Rehabil.* 63:207–210.

Hallin, R. 1968. Follow-up of paraplegics and tetraplegics after comprehensive rehabilitation. *Int. J. Paraplegia* 6:128–134.

Jellnik, H., and R. Harvey. 1982. Vocational/educational services in a medical rehabilitation facility: Outcomes in spinal cord and brain-injured patients. *Arch. Phys. Med. Rehabil.* 63:87–88.

Kemp, B., and C. Vash. 1971. Productivity after injury in a sample of spinal cord injured persons: A pilot study. *J. Chronic Dis.* 24:259–275.

Krause, J.S. 1990. The relationship between productivity and adjustment following spinal cord injury. *Rehabil. Couns. Bull.* 33(3):188–199.

Madsen, K.B. 1973. "Theories of motivation." In *Handbook of general psychology,* ed. B.B. Wolman. Englewood Cliffs, N.J.: Prentice-Hall.

Rhyne, D. 1984. IE's can play vital role in bringing the disabled into economic mainstream. *Ind. Eng. Soc. Issues* 60:66.

Rohe, D.E., and G.T. Athelstan. 1985. Change in vocational interests after spinal cord injury. *Rehabil. Psych.* 30(3):131–143.

Seybold, J. 1976. Rehabilitation and employment status report. *Paraplegia News* 29:34–36.

Siegel, M. 1971. "Improving employment horizons for the severely disabled." In *Research utilization in rehabilitation facilities,* ed. R. Pacinelli. International Association of Rehabilitation Facilities.

Trieschmann, R. 1978. The psychological, social, and vocational adjustment to spinal cord injury: A strategy for future research (Final report and executive summary of Rehabilitation Services Administration, grant 13-P-59011/9-01, Easter Seal Society of Los Angeles County).

Trieschmann, R. 1980. *Spinal cord injuries: Psychological, social and vocational adjustment.* New York, N.Y.: Pergamon.

Webb, S., et al. 1982. Marital, educational, employment, income and general financial status prior to and one to six years post-spinal cord injury. *Paraplegia* 20:108–109.

Wright, G. 1980. *Total rehabilitation.* Boston, Mass.: Little, Brown.

Young, J., and N. Northrup. 1979. Statistical information pertaining to some of the most commonly asked questions about s.c.i. *Spinal Cord Inj. Digest* 1:11–27.

Zadney, J., and L. James. 1979. The problem with placement. *Rehabil. Couns. Bull.* 22:439–442.

Chapter 23

Spinal Injury and Psychotherapy: A Treatment Philosophy

Jeri Morris

The following chapter is intended not as a theoretical discussion or research review but rather as a description of the philosophy and resulting strategies that are used in the psychological treatment of patients with spinal injury at the Rehabilitation Institute of Chicago. The philosophy was developed and adapted by the author through her clinical experience with these patients and reflects her biases.

THE MENTAL HEALTH VS. THE CONSULTATION (MENTAL ILLNESS) MODEL

The cornerstone of this treatment philosophy (which I call the mental health model) is the fundamental assumption that spinal injury is a catastrophic event that influences almost every sphere of a patient's life, the adjustment to which presents a major challenge for even the most mature, emotionally stable individual. The enormity of this challenge cannot be overstated. Awareness of its magnitude can be dulled as we work with patients over time and as dealing with this traumatic event becomes part of the experience of our everyday life.

After the injury, patients are faced with an endless series of questions about their lives, ranging from specific, pragmatic issues to broad and basic concerns about self-concept and world view: "Will I ever work again, and if so, at what kind of job?" "Will my spouse/parents still love me?" "Will anyone ever find me attractive again?" "How can I like myself with my changed body?" "How will I relate to my friends? To new people I meet?" "How will I get to there from here?" "Will I be able to drive a car?" "Will I spend the rest of my life in the house?" "Who will help me with my care?" "Is there sex after spinal injury?" "How does this affect my masculinity/femininity?" "How will I be able to afford to take care of my family? To make alterations in my house/apartment?" "What will my children think of me?" "Why did this happen to me?" "How could my life be so different than I believed it would be?"

Patient uncertainty about the future is generally so extensive that patients feel themselves to be virtually without a life style. The concept of mental health model implies that, given the magnitude and extent to which spinal injury affects the life of any patient, it is valuable to make available the services of a trained psychologist to all such patients so that they are afforded the opportunity to begin to explore feelings, thoughts, and questions engendered by the injury and its consequences. The model presumes that neither the willingness of patients to avail themselves of these services nor the need for such services as seen by the psychologist implies poor adaptation to the injury or emotional or personality maladjustment on the patient's part.

This approach can be contrasted with the mental illness or consultation model currently employed in many rehabilitation facilities, where patients are not routinely seen by the psychologist but rather are referred for psychological treatment only after they have been identified as problem patients on the nursing unit or in their therapies and have exhibited behavior seen as pathological by the treatment team. Using this model tends to encourage staff (including psychologists) to see intense reactions on the part of patients as crazy behavior. It also does little to foster a therapeutic relationship between patients and the psychologist, who quickly becomes identified as someone who works with emotionally ill patients. In addition, it does not give well-behaved patients the opportunity to begin to work through the normal but nevertheless extensive reactions to the catastrophe that has occurred.

The use of a mental health model suggests strategies that can be employed in treatment. The first hurdle that generally must be leaped for the psychologist is being useful to patients in establishing a therapeutic alliance. When patients appear for their first appointment, scheduled by the psychologist, they cannot be expected to be willing participants in the therapeutic process. Patients often begin such treatment with negative ideas about psychotherapy, and many would never have sought anyone to discuss thoughts and feelings, much less have chosen an individual who might be able to read their minds, analyze their personalities, or make judgments about their emotional health or adjustment. Because it is the psychologist who has requested the session (a rather unusual arrangement under most circumstances outside the hospital/rehabilitation setting), the burden falls upon the psychologist at the outset to help patients understand why they are being seen and, in general, what use can be made of psychological services within the rehabilitation setting. One way to approach this would be to initiate the first session with some variant of the following "I am Dr. Smith, and I am in the psychology department. Before you tell me about yourself, let me tell you a little about me and my job. Every patient in the hospital sees someone from the psychology department because it is assumed that anything that is serious enough to land you in this place will have some impact on various parts of your life."

There are several ideas communicated by this message. First, there is the suggestion that patients will, in fact, talk about themselves. Second, patients are being told that their visit is routine and a customary part of the course of treatment within the setting. Furthermore, the remarks are made in the form of understatement. It is difficult to argue with the thoughts set forth in the last sentence, and most patients nod in agreement. Finally, the remarks lay a foundation for acknowledging that it is normal to have a reaction to spinal injury which is of a magnitude that makes the extraordinary experience of talking to a psychologist a natural event.

The use of a mental health model also tends to shape the attitudes and behaviors of the psychologist throughout the period of treatment. It is a reminder to the psychologist as well as to patients that intense emotional reactions, confusion, and the use of psychological defenses are normal responses to an abnormal situation. It is imperative that the experience with the psychologist not be an assault upon the dignity of individuals who may already be feeling quite vulnerable and uncertain about their self-worth. This model may lead psychologists to adopt a somewhat more active stance than they might in other, more traditional settings and to avoid behaviors that might be perceived as stereotypic of psychologists as depicted in the media (e.g., psychologists as the blank screen). This does not imply relinquishing the boundaries of the therapeutic relationship (e.g., becoming a friend to patients); rather, it underscores the need for sensitivity to the perspective of patients who may not previously have valued what psychologists have chosen as their work. Patients may even have thought that only crazy people see psychologists.

A LONG-TERM GOAL OF REHABILITATION

One premise of this treatment philosophy is that a major goal of rehabilitation is for patients to reach the point where the disability is no longer the focus of their lives. It is quite apparent that if this goal is ever to be accomplished it will not be during the acute rehabilitation stay. Nevertheless, while in the rehabilitation setting, patients can begin a path that leads toward this goal. A necessary requirement for achieving this goal involves exploring and discovering ways in which patients can lead satisfying lives. They must sort through what they will need to give up, what they will have to do differently, and what can be enjoyed as before their injuries; the psychologist can help them with this process while they are in the rehabilitation facility. One task of treatment, therefore, is to help patients expand their world view into one that includes the possibility of finding satisfying lives after spinal injury. We want to help them live as full a life as possible without giving up anything they do not have to.

Such an exploration, however, requires that patients contemplate life as individuals with spinal injury. Given the number of concerns that patients typically have immediately after spinal injury, it is not at all unusual for them to believe that they have lost everything, that life has nothing more to offer, and that acceptance of the reality and permanence of the consequences of the injury is equivalent to acceptance of a permanent state of unhappiness and loss. These beliefs lead to a variety of responses on the part of patients, which often involve some form of denial of permanence or effects of the injury. The following examples are only a few of the more typical responses:

- Patients do not recall receiving information about their prognosis.
- Patients recall being given information but do not agree with the physician about their prognosis and say that they expect to recover fully.
- Patients report that they know that a miracle will occur that will heal them.
- Patients state that they know their injury is permanent but that it will not change their lives in any way.

These reactions are commonly believed to be normal, adaptive defenses (Power & Del Orto 1980). Thus the patient may not be anxious to cooperate with the explorative process described above. To ask patients who believe they have lost everything to consider what life will be like as individuals with spinal injury is often to invite patients to abandon their defenses in favor of despair, something most patients are understandably reluctant to do. It follows, then, that it is the task of the psychologist to encourage patients to expand their world view without undermining their defenses. In the meantime, patients who are using these defenses present, at the very least, a challenge and frequently a problem to the treatment team.

THE PROBLEM OF ACCEPTANCE OF DISABILITY

Patients who maintain a position of denial or minimalization of the effects of their injury are using an adaptive coping mechanism because it serves to maintain psychological equilibrium by preventing them from becoming overwhelmed emotionally. Treatment staff must recognize, however, that if this position is maintained indefinitely little adjustment and adaptation to the injury will be possible. Moreover, this position is troubling and frustrating to staff, who face dealing with the ramifications of these defenses. It is not simply that staff are miffed because patients' versions of reality do not match their own. The patients' ideation generally is reflected in a variety of behaviors encountered by the team, and many of these cannot be ignored.

One of the more common behavioral reactions of patients under these circumstances is the expression of anger. Often nursing personnel receive the biggest share of patient anger, but other therapists and family members certainly are frequently on the receiving end of temper outbursts and expressions of hostility. Understandably, staff often feel that patients' angry outbursts are personally insulting or demeaning. They may feel that their competency is in question or that their caring is being rejected (Gans 1983). Consequently, they may respond angrily or may come to view patients as having a bad personality or a poor adjustment to their disability.

Let us consider what may be prompting patients to misbehave. Whether or not patients are contemplating the long-term consequences of their disability, they usually are faced with some terrifying prospects: being confronted with their own vulnerability, perhaps for the first time in their lives; being in a position where they are forced to accept caregiving from others; being expected to behave casually about invasive procedures or those that they may feel are humiliating (e.g., catheter care or bowel program); having to follow the rules of the institution, whether or not they understand or approve of them; having to face the fact that life is not fair; not having much control over their lives; not being able to scratch their noses; being trapped in bed at night. There is no end to the immediate problems, frustrations, indignities, and differences faced by patients during their acute rehabilitation stay.

It is not difficult to understand why staff tend to get out of touch with these issues, seal over, and develop defenses themselves in dealing with patients. We cannot afford to be empathic to the point where we become immobilized. Furthermore, the angry, complaining patients tend to make us feel incompetent, and we tend to take patient anger personally. At times, we can get so far away from the patients' reality that we become angry or avoid the patients in return. Staff members become alarmed, concerned, angry, and/or surprised at the intensity or inappropriateness of patient anger; if staff would ask, "What do patients have to be angry about?" however, the answer would seem obvious: Almost everything.

In addition to anger, there are numerous other behavioral responses exhibited by patients who have not accepted the permanence of their disability. Patients may resist treatment by reporting late to therapies, find excuses for staying in bed, or exhibit a lack of compliance with the requests of the staff. They may refuse equipment or adaptive devices; they may be unwilling to make realistic discharge plans. They may refuse to leave the hospital for recreational trips because they do not want to be seen in a wheelchair; they may avoid associating with other patients because they are disabled. Or they may simply insist, "The doctors are wrong; I'm going to walk out of here," leaving staff feeling compelled to convince them otherwise. Staff correctly see adjustment as a significant part of the rehabilitation process and become alarmed when patients appear to set up barriers that impede progress and prevent them from taking advantage of all that the setting has to offer. Responding with anger or avoidance to the patients' bad behavior (or, as happens with the consultation model, labeling the patients as behavior problems and referring to the shrink) is an understandable and common reaction on the part of staff but is likely to increase the patients' anger and resistance.

It is probably less obvious, and therefore important to emphasize, that intensifying efforts to persuade patients to accept the permanence of their disability is another common reaction on the part of staff; this, too, is likely to have negative consequences. If this were effective, it would be a fine idea. Unfortunately, all these responses, including the last, tend to create an adversarial relationship between staff and patients. They provoke a power struggle, which increases patient resentment and distrust of the staff and is antitherapeutic because it motivates patients to entrench further into their position of resistance.

OVERCOMING THE RESISTANCE

It follows, then, that the immediate goal of the psychologist is to encourage a willingness by patients to think about the long-term effects of spinal injury. This is important for their psychological adjustment if they are to make any progress toward the goal, set forth above, of getting to where the disability is no longer the focus of their lives. It is also important to minimize problematic responses and resistance on the part of the patients so that they may make optimal use of the resources of the rehabilitation facility. To accomplish this, it is critical that the psychologist first develop an alliance with patients. The psychologist must get on the side of patients rather than make himself or herself their adversary. Let us consider what is involved in this therapeutic process.

Asking patients to expand their world views means asking them to alter their belief systems. Thus the process dictates that the psychologist must begin by coming to an understanding of their current belief system. One approach is to begin by asking patients what their physicians have told them with regard to the long-term effects of their injury. Then inquiry can be made as to the patients' own beliefs, guesses, or gut feelings about what they can expect. Often these questions yield two different responses. If patients say that they have been told by physicians that their disability is permanent, failure to ask the second question can lead the psychologist to an erroneous conclusion about the patients' current beliefs about their futures.

If the patients indicate that they have been told by their physicians that their disability is permanent but they do not believe it will be, reflecting reality to them by confronting them with the facts may seem to be the responsibility of the psychologist. Actually, this is the time when psychologists must ally themselves with patients but without colluding with the patients' denial.

The psychologist might begin with the following comments: "I understand that the physician has told you that your injury is permanent, and, naturally, you hope that this is not true." This is an empathic comment that acknowledges that you are aware of the patient's thoughts and feelings. "It's natural that you hope. In fact, it's really impossible not to hope. The fact is, I hope that you will fully recover, although I know that the physician has said it will be permanent." This is a direct statement giving the patients permission to have hope, which is virtually impossible to give up. The impossibility of giving up hope is underscored in the next statement, an acknowledgment on the part of the psychologist that he or she cannot help but hope as well. This acknowledgment is also an empathic statement that places the patient and psychologist on the same side, able to work together to contemplate the problem out there. The last sentence is crucial because it reiterates what the physicians have said is the prognosis and emphasizes the expectations for outcome, given the best medical opinion. It is critical to include because without emphasizing this point psychologists risk colluding with the patient's denial system. Also, if omitted, there is a risk that patients and psychologists will become allied with the physicians on the other side. In fact, it may be helpful to acknowledge that physicians also hope that patients will recover fully, although it is not the outcome they expect. The psychologists would love to be wrong even though they are entirely confident that they are not.

THE DIFFERENCE BETWEEN HOPES AND EXPECTATIONS

With this approach, the psychologist can give patients permission to do what they cannot help but do: hope for full recovery while knowing that the best medical opinion is that they should not expect to do so. In this way, the psychologist can help the patients begin to see the differences between their hopes and their expectations. They can also appreciate that what the physicians expect may be different from their own expectations. The distinction between hoping and expecting is often not obvious to patients and frequently is blurred by professionals as well. A lack of sensitivity to this issue on the part of staff can leave patients with the impressions that the physician said that there is no hope for recovery. If one shares the opinion that there is a difference between hope and expectation and believes that it is virtually impossible not to have hope, the physician's statement either makes no sense or asks the patients to do the impossible.

Once having allied themselves with the patients and having made the distinction between hopes and expectations, psychologists are in a position to explain to patients that they can consider the permanence of this disability on a "what if" or hypothetical basis. For example, the psychologist may explain to the patient, "If your hopes come to pass and you are able to run out of here, you already know how to behave. What's going to happen while you're in this place is that everyone will try to help you learn ways you can handle yourself given the level you're at right now. If you learn what they are trying to teach you, you can be prepared for any outcome."

Thus the psychologists can suggest that patients do not have to stop hoping in order to consider life as a person with spinal injury. The patients can be encouraged to feel that they can contemplate the effects of permanent injury without necessarily expecting this outcome and with the understanding that it is what the physicians expect. They can begin to explore what life with permanent spinal injury might mean for them without giving up hope. They can have these thoughts without relinquishing their defenses and giving in to despair.

THE PROCESS OF DEVELOPING REALISTIC EXPECTATIONS

Developing realistic expectations is generally a process rather than an event, and most patients will vacillate between the expectation of recovery and the expectation that the injury is permanent. It is as though for a time the patients have two selves (i.e., self-images, egos, or self-concepts) from which they perceive the world and their places in it and that they alternate between these two perspectives. Typically for a time, the patient's thoughts are primarily dominated by the old self that expects recovery and return to a life relatively unchanged by the trauma. From this perspective, the patients' self images are quite clear: They have a reasonable degree of certainty about how they view themselves and others, and they have more confidence about what decisions they will make about vocational and social pursuits. At this point, the new selves usually are only vaguely formed, and the patients operate from this perspective less frequently. As patients gradually develop a greater sense of confidence and hopefulness about the possibility of leading a satisfying life despite the permanent effects of their disability, the new selves are envisioned more clearly and completely by the patients, and they are able to spend more time operating from this perspective. The patient usually shows no awareness of having two selves and may often express mutually exclusive or contradictory statements without feeling or expressing any sense of conflict. For instance, it is not unusual for patients to state that they know they will be fully recovered by the time they leave the hospital and, in the next statement, to report happily that they have just discovered that they will be able to return to their former workplaces because they have learned that it is wheelchair accessible. This model suggests that it is the role of the psychologists and the treatment team to create an environment in which the patients' new selves can become more fully formed. The vacillation should not be viewed with concern by the staff but should be seen as normal within the context of adjustment to the effects of the injury. The shifts represent the patients' current ability to tolerate the reality of their situations. During the course of their stay in the rehabilitation facility, it is hoped that patients will operate more and more frequently from the perspective of these new selves and that they will be able to work through feelings about this new self-concept as well as begin to plan realistically about their futures.

THE COURSE OF PSYCHOTHERAPY: DIRECTIONS AND APPROACHES

Once having established the rudiments of a therapeutic alliance, dealt with the patients' initial resistance to treatment, and encouraged the patients to separate their hopes from their expectations, it would follow within the context of this model that the psychologists would then work with patients to develop their new selves. This includes helping patients in their exploration of life so that they can begin to determine which aspects of their lives will remain the same, which will need to be modified, and which are actual losses to be acknowledged and mourned. The psychologists also must help patients deal with their confusion and fears about themselves and their places in the world.

A fundamental assumption of this model is that, at this point, development of a treatment plan depends upon the individual personality of the patient. The patients' concerns are a direct reflection of their own personalities, their ways of acting upon and reacting to the world, their history, their intellectual and emotional resources, and their character structures

and life circumstances (e.g., socioeconomic status and degree of family and social support). Those who work with patients with spinal injury see a wide range of adjustments in the long term with regard to issues relating to social and vocational spheres, personal satisfaction, and self-acceptance. It is not the injury itself that determines the adjustment of patients. We have all seen patients with quadriplegia who return to work or college, resume or initiate satisfying relationships, raise families, and achieve the long-term goal of getting to the place where the disability is no longer the focus of their lives. Other patients have more difficult adjustments. They may be virtually inactive, spending years (or a lifetime) waiting for physical recovery; they may withdraw from friends and live in relative isolation; or they may persist in thinking that they have little worth socially or vocationally. This model posits that it is not the injury itself that determines adjustment; long-range adjustment is largely dependent upon pretrauma personality.

The health care team, the institution, third party payers, and the families of the injured must accept the fact that there is no template or canned treatment when one is going from the theoretical to the specifics of individual patients. Therefore, it follows that there is no substitute for devoting time to assessing the patient's personality in formulating the case. Despite the fact that, once stated, this may seem obvious, the most common mistake made by psychologists working with these patients is finding solutions without giving adequate consideration to personality assessments. This error is more likely to be made either by psychologists who do not ascribe to any theoretical orientation or synthesis of orientations to personality theory or by those who adhere to treatment models that deemphasize personality theory and emphasize focus on symptoms. A common example is psychologists who tend to categorize and describe patients by their symptoms (e.g., depressed or anxious) rather than by their personality descriptors. Such psychologists tend to look for ways in which to delimit the problem and for techniques that can be applied to deal with the specific problem. An example, which is extreme but unfortunately not unusual, is the psychologist who determines that the patient is depressed (in this case, as a consequence of injury) and goes to a five-step approach to treat depression using techniques such as increasing the patient's awareness of negative thoughts. If the real problem the psychologist faces is how to help the patient develop his or her new self, attempting to delimit the problem to make it more manageable (for the psychologist) is likely to subvert the process. Defining the problem through classification of the patient by symptoms may help bind the anxiety of the psychologist, who can then go to his or her bag of treatments for a method of action. Indeed, working with patients can be difficult and anxiety producing, and it would be lovely if such a short-cut method were productive; no reasonable treatment can take place, however, if personality is not assessed, if the psychologist does not first ask, in some form or another, "Who is this person? How does this injury affect this person's life?" It appears obvious that having some orientation in terms of personality theory is advisable.

The use of this rather traditional method of case formulation that I am suggesting, however, does not imply that we cannot have an active intervention strategy. Our patients are in crisis, and we do not have the time, nor is it necessary, to employ only patient-initiated strategies. Early interpretations, suggestions, and even outright teaching can be a part of treatment from the beginning. Cognitive/behavioral techniques can be employed. Active strategies and techniques can be effective if the case has been adequately formulated with current functioning seen in the context of the individual's lifelong functioning.

CASE EXAMPLES

For purposes of illustration, consider the psychologist's role in helping patients deal with feelings of "Why me? Why did this happen to me?" This is certainly a commonly asked question. It is the meaning of the question in the context of the personality of the individual that will determine what approach the psychologist should take.

Case 1

Let us take the case where the psychologist after evaluation reached the working hypothesis that the patient had considerable strengths in terms of psychological functioning before injury. The psychologist may have determined the following about the patient: Before the injury, the patient had a relatively well-integrated sense of self; the patient has a history that shows a capacity to establish and maintain mature relationships with others; the patient has the capacity to see himself or herself in a relatively realistic way; the patient has had enough impulse control and judgment to have a history of success experiences; and the patient uses defense mechanisms and coping strategies that are not destructive to self or others and that show flexibility in functioning.

To this individual, the psychologist's role in helping the patient answer "Why me?" may involve helping the patient articulate, in relation to this event, something that the patient already believes: There are things in the world over which we have control (e.g., our actions, decisions, and thoughts), others over which we have only some influence (e.g., other people), and a great many over which we have little or no control (e.g., the drunk driver in the car next to us). Such patients may find it a relief to hear stated openly that which they already believe: that a percentage of events occur that affect us adversely because we simply cannot control everything. Working with these patients might then involve helping them make use of their strengths by assisting them in examining, given their new circumstances, what they do control in their lives, how they can take charge of these parts of their lives, and how they can maximize their ability to be productive and lead satisfying

lives. For these individuals, the answer to the question "Why me?" may simply be, "Why not? Sometimes cornices fall off buildings. Some things are not in my control." For other patients, this answer may be excruciatingly difficult to accept.

Case 2

In the second case, let us think of individuals who ask "Why me?" because they have had a lifelong belief that if you behave in a kind, fair, and ethical manner good things will happen to you. These individuals may believe that, if events occur that adversely affect them, it is because they have done something bad to deserve them. Let us assume that before their injuries these individuals, like the patient described in case 1, had a relatively well-integrated sense of self and good impulse control and judgment as well as a history of success experiences. Let us assume, however, that they have less flexibility in functioning as a consequence of having less capacity to see themselves and others in their complexity and a tendency to be somewhat more polarized in their views, seeing themselves and others in terms approaching good versus bad and other such dichotomies.

To these individuals, admitting that there are things in the world over which we have no control may be contrary to their lifelong world views. They may have believed that they could, in fact, control their lives by acting in a manner (e.g., kind, fair, and ethical) that would ensure that reasonably good things would happen to them. This view is often associated with religious beliefs but also is common to individuals who profess no religious ideology whatsoever. When these individuals have a spinal injury, asking them to accept that there are things over which they have no control is asking them not only to change their belief systems but also to deal with an idea that may be frightening to them because it shakes their sense of security about the predictability of their lives. Thus such individuals may initially prefer to blame themselves for their injuries even when this is not logical (i.e., they did not contribute to the accident, and they were not particularly bad people). Having feelings of guilt about their injuries may be preferable to living with the ambiguity of having less control over their lives and living in a world that is less predictable than they once believed. In contrast to the situation in case 1, therapists may need to begin by helping these individuals accept this ambiguity and manage the feelings this engenders before attempting to work on other issues.

Case 3

Now let us take a different but not atypical case, wherein the psychologist has formulated a working hypothesis that a particular patient has a significant character pathology. In this example, let us assume that this patient has a rather poorly integrated sense of self. Such patients have a history of loss; for example, the mother abandoned the family when they were toddlers, a compensatory environment did not exist in which they were able to establish close relationships with others on whom they could rely when they were young, and they have responded to this difficult childhood by becoming counterdependent (i.e., becoming almost phobic of being dependent on others). These patients have decided that they do not need to rely on others and that they can control their lives and avoid being injured by the world. In contrast to the individual described in case 1, such individuals have a considerably poorer ability to view themselves realistically, are limited in their ability to establish and maintain mature relationships with others, and have had fewer success experiences. Furthermore, they have a lifelong pattern of responding rather impulsively with little consideration of the consequences of their actions, and they regularly use defenses (e.g., denial and splitting) that support their pathology at the expense of functioning. They tend to respond to their frequently felt negative feelings (e.g., rage and depression) or to adverse events (e.g., being left by a girlfriend or boyfriend) with alcohol and/or drugs, by fleeing a situation (leaving home for days at a time), and/or by engaging in a dangerous activity (e.g., getting drunk and jumping from the garage roof into the swimming pool). Often the activities are selected as a means of proving, primarily to themselves but also to the rest of the world, that they do in fact have control over their lives, that they are different and less vulnerable than others. This patient asks "Why me?" and concludes that the injury will not be permanent and that he or she will not have to answer the question.

Naturally this is an individual who has significantly greater difficulties in adjusting to injury than the individual described in case 1 because this type of personality includes significant character pathology. Nevertheless, after spinal cord injury even problems that are characterologic can be addressed. One common view of character disorders is that they are defined as personality constellations that include symptomatology that is syntonic to the individuals who possess the pathology and is thus a problem for those around the individuals but not a problem for the persons themselves. Consequently, such pathology is often not amenable to treatment not only because it is significant, deeply ingrained, and complicated but also because the individuals are not motivated to change. After spinal injury, however, what was once ego syntonic for the patients may no longer be. What was only a problem for others around the patients may, in fact, now be a problem for the patients as well (e.g., not planning ahead or drinking to excess as a means of escape). For many patients with such characteristics, the period after their spinal injury may be the first time in their lives that they are able to profit from treatment. The patients are then in a situation where their customary defense coping skills (e.g., running away or taking physical action) are not typically available. It is a time when patients may well be motivated to make rather significant changes and when they may benefit from hearing interpretations that on other occasions probably would not have been heard, much less considered.

Therefore, it is a mistake to assume that character pathology in patients is an indicator that treatment will not be effective. In fact, it may be an indicator that the timing of treatment for these individuals is optimal. The treatment would be quite different for these patients than for those described in the first two cases. A more confrontive technique in making interpretations might be needed; special attention would need to be given to being certain that the patients understand that these interpretations are made from a position of benevolence on the part of the therapist.

THE THERAPIST WAS NOT PROMISED A ROSE GARDEN

The desire to control one's situation is not limited to patients with spinal injury. In fact, it is basic to the human condition. Consider humanity's attempts from prehistoric times to the present, from cave drawings to meteorologic charts, to understand and gain mastery over the environment. Neither can the psychologist walk between the raindrops. There is no simple recipe for treating patients with spinal injury; each must be evaluated individually. Given the catastrophic nature of their trauma and the consequent devastation of their previous lives, complete adjustment by patients is unlikely to occur during their rehabilitation stay. Therefore, one of the more difficult problems for therapists is that they may not see conclusive results of their work in the near term. At times our efforts fail, we cannot help everyone. Some patients derive minimal benefit from working with us, whereas others may not incorporate what occurred during treatment until long after their discharge from the rehabilitation facility.

This model assumes that the enormity of the challenge of adjustment on the part of patients with spinal injury cannot be overstated. Similarly, the magnitude of the challenge to psychologists in working with these patients is great as well. Therapists therefore must develop realistic expectations of themselves so that they do not become overwhelmed by feelings of being inadequate to the task.

REFERENCES

Gans, J.S. 1983. Hate in the rehabilitation setting. *Arch. Phys. Med. Rehabil.* 64:176–179.

Power, P.W., and A.E. Del Orto. 1980. "Impact of disability/illness on the adult." In *Role of the family in the rehabilitation of the physically disabled,* ed. P.W. Power and A.E. Del Orto. Baltimore, Md.: University Park Press.